Pocket Guide to
Basic Skills and Procedures

Pocket Guide to
Basic Skills and
Procedures

Anne Griffin Perry, RN, MSN, EdD

Associate Professor
Saint Louis University School of Nursing
Coordinator, Critical Care Education
Saint Louis University Hospital
St. Louis, Missouri

Patricia A. Potter, RN, MSN

Director of Nursing Practice
Barnes Hospital
St. Louis, Missouri

THIRD EDITION

illustrated

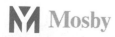 Mosby

St. Louis Baltimore Boston Chicago London Philadelphia Sydney Toronto

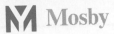
Mosby

Dedicated to Publishing Excellence

Editor: Susan R. Epstein
Developmental Editor: Beverly J. Copland
Project Manager: Gayle May Morris
Production Editor: Donna L. Walls
Manufacturing Supervisor: John Babrick
Designer: Susan Lane
Cover Photograph: © Bill Leslie Photography, Inc.

THIRD EDITION

Copyright © 1994 Mosby–Year Book, Inc.

Previous editions copyrighted 1986, 1990

Printed in the United States of America
Composition by Clarinda
Printing/binding by R.R. Donnelley Press

Mosby–Year Book, Inc.
11830 Westline Industrial Drive
St. Louis, Missouri 63146

Library of Congress Cataloging in Publication Data
Perry, Anne Griffin.
    Pocket guide to basic skills and procedures / Anne Griffin Perry,
Patricia A. Potter. — 3rd ed.
        p.   cm.
    Includes bibliographical references and index.
    ISBN 0-8016-6879-4
    1. Nursing—Handbooks, manuals, etc. I. Potter, Patricia Ann.
II. Title
    [DNLM: 1. Nursing—handbooks. WY 39 P462p 1994]
RT51.P37   1994
610.73—dc20
DNLM/DLC   93-40805
for Library of Congress   CIP

96 97 98 / 9 8 7 6 5 4 3 2

Reviewers

Patricia A. Castaldi, MSN, RN

Assistant Dean
School of Nursing
Elizabeth General Medical Center
Elizabeth, New Jersey

Dorothy Thomas, RN, MSN

Assistant Professor
St. Louis Community College at Florissant Valley
St. Louis, Missouri

Preface

The *Pocket Guide to Basic Skills and Procedures,* third edition, is a practical, portable reference for students and practitioners in the clinical setting. Grouped according to specialty area, nearly 100 commonly performed skills are presented in a clear, step-by-step format that includes:

the purpose for performing each skill

a list of actual or potential nursing diagnoses

a list of equipment needed

rationales for each step

Skills conclude with helpful clinical aids including Nurse Alerts, client teaching, and special considerations for pediatric and geriatric clients.

To address realities of practice, current universal precautions and BSI (body substance isolation) guidelines are incorporated throughout. Photographs and drawings provide realistic visual reinforcement of the steps. Appendix A is a current list of NANDA-approved nursing diagnoses to facilitate planning client care.

New features include five new skills to prepare nurses for current practice: assessing pulse oximetry, assessing central venous pressure, teaching self-catheterization, using a hypothermia blanket, and measuring peak expiratory flow rate (PEFR). Appendix B, Normal Reference Lab Values, provides assessment criteria for quick reference in the clinical setting. An index has been added for quick location of specific content.

For a more complete discussion of information presented here, refer to Perry/Potter: *Clinical Skills and Techniques,* third edition.

Anne G. Perry
Patricia A. Potter

Contents

Unit VII   HYGIENE

Unit VIII   ELIMINATION

Unit IX   CARE OF THE SURGICAL CLIENT

Unit X   NUTRITION

Pocket Guide to
Basic Skills and Procedures

PRELIMINARY
SKILLS

Admission into the Health Care System

A client can access the health care system in various ways (e.g., at a hospital, emergent care center, clinic, or physician's office). Whether a client is entering a hospital, a nursing home, or a rehabilitation center, the admission process can be stressful. It is essential that as much information as possible be collected during the admission process so that the client ultimately receives individualized health care. Including friends or family members in the admission process increases their ability to support the client during the experience in the health care setting.

Although each institution follows a different set of admission practices, the purposes of admission remain the same. The admission process initiates data collection for nursing care and discharge planning, reduces anxiety and fear, provides an opportunity to present information to the client and family, ensures client comfort and safety, and maintains the client's legal rights as a health care recipient.

Potential Nursing Diagnoses

Client data derived during the assessment process reveal defining characteristics to support the following nursing diagnoses for clients requiring this skill:

Anxiety
Fear

Equipment

Admission Office

Necessary admitting forms
Identification band
General consent form

Nursing Unit

Room preparation: *Obtain personal care items:* Bed pan and urinal, wash basin, bath towel and washcloth, toiletries, tissue paper, water pitcher and glass, and emesis basin. *Bed:* Arrange room for easy access to bed and adjust the bed to lowest adjustable height to facilitate the client's safety and ease in getting into and out of bed. *Special equipment:* Verify that necessary items such as suction equipment, oxygen supplies, and intravenous (IV) equipment are readily available and in working order.

Assessment forms

Equipment to perform physical assessment: Scale, watch with a second hand, thermometer, sphygmomanometer, urine collection cup, and additional equipment as needed by type of assessment.

Steps	Rationale
Admitting Area	
1. Welcome client and family, introduce yourself by name and title and escort to interviewing area.	Reduces anxiety about first encounter with agency personnel. Interviewing area provides privacy for client.
2. Acquire pertinent identifying information, including client's: Full legal name Age Birthdate Address Next of kin Physician Religion Previous admissions Allergies	Ensures correct legal identification on client's medical records.
3. On client's wrist place identification band containing the following information: Client's full legal name Hospital or agency number	Serves as means to officially identify client when therapies or procedures are performed (e.g., medication administration, surgical procedures, x-ray examinations).

Steps	Rationale
Physician's name Client's birthdate Be sure that band is secure.	
4. Instruct client (or legal guardian) to read general consent form for treatment. Assess client's understanding of consent form. ■ Request client (or family member) to sign form if he agrees to be admitted for treatment.	Gives agency right to perform routine procedures and therapies, select room placement, and provide required nursing care.
5. Provide any brochures that describe purpose and organization of agency as well as policies or rules that affect client's conduct.	American Hospital Association's "Patient's Bill of Rights" states that the client must have access to this information.
6. Assign a room on basis of client's condition, health care needs, and personal preferences.	Clients requiring frequent observation and therapy should be close to central nursing station. Consideration of client's personal preferences during room selection minimizes anxiety and prevents conflict with other clients. Room environment can provide sensory stimulation.
7. Direct client to area where technicians in admitting office will collect routine blood specimens and perform chest x-ray and electrocardiographic (ECG) examinations. ■ Instruct client on method for collecting urine specimen.	Routine diagnostic testing serves to screen clients for presence of common physical alterations. Specimen may be collected in admitting area or on nursing division.

Steps	Rationale
8. Notify nursing division of client's admission. ■ Report client's name, assigned room and bed, admitting physician's name, diagnosis, and pertinent information relating to client's condition (e.g., IV line infusing, need for oxygen).	Allows nursing personnel to prepare room and obtain necessary equipment for client's arrival. Client may be admitted directly from emergency room.
9. Transport client and family members to nursing division, using an escort.	Promotes timely and safe arrival of patient to nursing division.
10. In nursing division, introduce client and his family to nurse who is assuming client's care.	Provides client a sense of personalization during admission process.
11. Share with nursing staff pertinent observations about client's behaviors or level of knowledge regarding need for health care.	Promotes continuity of care so nursing staff can assist client in coping with new environment and procedures of care.

Nursing Division

1. Wash hands.	Prevents spread of microorganisms.
2. Prepare assigned room with necessary equipment and personal care items.	Availability of equipment for personal care promotes client comfort by preventing unnecessary delays during care delivery.
3. Prepare client's bed by adjusting it to lowest horizontal position. Turn down top sheet and spread.	Makes it easier and safer for client to get into and out of bed.

Steps	Rationale
4. Greet client and his family cordially. Introduce yourself by name and job title, telling client you are responsible for his care.	Reduces anxiety client may feel regarding admission. Being aware of which nurse is responsible for his care expedites resolution of requests of client.
5. Escort client and family members to assigned room. Introduce them to roommate if semiprivate room is assigned.	Orientation begins with introduction to roommate.
6. Assess client's general appearance, noting signs or symptoms of physical distress.	If client is experiencing any acute physical problems, routine admission procedures should be postponed until problems are resolved.
7. Check physician's orders for any treatment measures that should be initiated immediately.	Delay in initiation of therapies can cause worsening of client's condition.
8. Assess client's and family members' psychologic status by noting nonverbal behaviors and verbal responses to greetings and explanations.	Client's level of anxiety influences his ability to adapt to health care environment.
9. Orient client to nursing division: ■ Introduce staff members who enter room. Always introduce client by surname. ■ Tell client name of head nurse or charge nurse of division and that person's role in solving problems. ■ Explain visiting hours and their purpose. ■ Discuss smoking policy.	Promotes understanding of agency policies and procedures. Family members' willingness to follow visiting-hour policy ensures that client will receive adequate rest.

Steps	Rationale
■ Demonstrate how to use equipment in room (e.g., bed, over-bed table, lighting).	Client safety depends on understanding of policies and of how to use equipment correctly.
■ Show client how to use nurse call light.	
■ Escort client to bathroom (if able to ambulate).	
■ Explain hours for meal time and nourishment.	
■ Describe services available (e.g., chaplain visitation, gift shop, activity therapy).	
■ Explain areas where client and family might visit (e.g., cafeteria, lounge, recreation room).	
■ Warn client against keeping large sums of money or valuables in own room in agency.	Because clients are often required to leave their rooms during day, there is risk of money or valuables being stolen.
■ Inform client about procedure for acquiring television or radio.	
10. Collect any valuables client wishes to have placed in agency safe. Place articles in specially labeled and sealed envelope. Instruct client to sign statement releasing agency of responsibility for valuables.	Protects client from theft.
11. Explain to client that admitting process will include a nursing history and physical examination. Request client to change into appropriate gown. Provide privacy.	Keeping client informed of procedures and their purpose minimizes anxiety. Hospital gown or pajamas makes exposure of body parts during examination easier.

Steps	Rationale
12. Assist client with hanging or storing clothing in closet or locker.	Basic to most people's self-image is keeping personal items neat and properly stored.
13. If client prefers, family members may stay in room during history taking; otherwise, escort family to waiting area.	Client may be embarrassed to share personal information about his health with family members.
14. Wash hands.	Reduces transmission of microorganisms.
15. Prepare equipment for nursing history and assessment.	Prevents delays that might increase client's anxiety or fatigue.
16. Weigh client and record his height.	Determines baseline values and any recent change in weight.
17. Assist client to assume comfortable position in bed or in bedside chair.	Relieves anxiety and thereby increases accuracy of findings.
18. Assess client's vital signs.	Provides baseline measurement to compare with future findings and discloses any alterations from normal expected range.
19. Obtain nursing history: Client's perceptions of illness Past medical history Presenting signs and symptoms Risk factors for illness	Provides data necessary to develop individualized plan of care based on client's identified health problems.
History of allergies. (Nurse provides client with an allergy band, similar in size to an identification band, that lists all foods, drugs, or substances to which client is allergic.)	Alerts nurses to substances to which client is allergic. Prevents accidental administration of substances if client is confused or nonresponsive.

Steps	Rationale
Medication history. (If client brings medications to agency, the nurse sends them home with family or friends; otherwise, medications are stored on division for safekeeping.)	Therapeutic drug administration depends on correct dosages and proper timing as well as avoidance of drug incompatibilities.
Alterations in activities of daily living	Identifying client and family needs early helps in planning for eventual discharge from agency.
Family resources and support	
Potential risk factors affecting discharge planning	
Client's knowledge of health problems and implications for long-term care	Allows nurse to plan for necessary instruction to prepare client for eventual discharge.
20. Conduct physical assessment of appropriate body systems.	Provides objective data for identifying client's health problems.
21. Instruct client on proper technique to provide urine specimen (if not obtained in admitting). ■ While wearing gloves, label specimen and attach requisition form.	Urinalysis is a basic test to screen for renal and metabolic problems, fluid and electrolyte alterations, and lower urinary tract alterations.
22. Explain to client that technicians will be obtaining blood specimens and performing chest x-ray and ECG examinations (if not performed in admitting office).	Complete blood count (CBC) is a routine test used to screen for anemias. Blood typing and cross-match are necessary for clients undergoing surgery or who are expected to receive blood transfusions. Chest x-ray screens for preexisting lung disease. ECG screens for conduction defects of heart.

Steps	Rationale
23. Inform client about any planned procedures or treatments scheduled for next shift or day (e.g., visit by physician, additional x-rays, dietary restrictions).	Client has a right to be informed of any procedures or treatments that he will undergo. Being able to anticipate planned therapies minimizes anxiety.
24. Provide client opportunity to ask questions about any procedure or therapies.	Helps clarify any misconceptions.
25. Allow client and family time together alone.	Admission procedure can be stressful and fatiguing. Client and family often have decisions to make or concerns to share before visitation ends.
26. Be sure call light is within reach, bed is in low position, and side rails are raised, when appropriate for client safety.	Provides for client safety.
27. Wash hands.	Reduces transmission of micro-organisms.
28. Record history and assessment findings on appropriate forms.	Prompt and thorough documentation prevents deletion of data.
29. Notify physician of client's admission and report any unusual findings.	Client's condition may require immediate medical intervention.
30. Begin to develop nursing care plan.	Provides for continuity of individualized care.

Nurse Alert

The nurse should always wear gloves when the risk of contacting moist body substances (e.g., draining wounds, secretions, vomitus) during the admitting process is high. When a critically ill client reaches a hospital's nursing division, extensive examination, diagnostic procedures, and treatment procedures become necessary almost immediately. Time constraints may force the nurse to delay certain steps in the admission process.

Client Teaching

Teaching can occur during the admission process. A nurse can provide information regarding physical assessment findings, planned diagnostic procedures, or hospital routines. A formal teaching plan is designed and implemented after a nursing assessment and care plan are completed.

Pediatric Considerations

Thorough explanation of the hospital experience and related procedures will reduce a child's fear of the unknown. Ideally, children should be prepared for hospitalization *before* admission, either by parents or by the nursing staff. A tour of hospital facilities and the use of dolls, puppet shows, or specially produced children's films to demonstrate procedures will help the child understand hospitalization.

Geriatric Considerations

An elderly person who is to be admitted into a long-term care facility or nursing home often undergoes extensive screening. When such a person enters the hospital, it is very important to orient him to his new surroundings. Gradual loss of sensory perception places the elderly client at risk of sensory overload, resulting in confusion or feelings of isolation.

Making a Referral

for Health Care

Services

Often clients require the services of various departments within an agency or the services of a different facility altogether. The nurse frequently recognizes the need for additional resources and initiates the referral process. Whatever type of referral is needed, it is important that the nurse collaborate with members of other disciplines so that clients' individual needs are met.

The purposes of the referral process are to provide clients with expert services that the nurse or the physician cannot provide, to improve the continuity of care throughout the client discharge and return to home, and to prepare the client adequately for discharge.

Potential Nursing Diagnoses

Client data derived during the assessment process reveal defining characteristics to support the following nursing diagnoses for clients requiring this skill:

Knowledge deficit

Anxiety

Self-care deficit

Steps	Rationale
1. Assess client's need for services from other hospital departments. Consider client's current and posthospital needs.	Other health professionals specialize in skills and knowledge that afford clients services that the nurse often cannot offer.

Steps	Rationale
a. Dietary—recognize factors such as client's repeated intolerance of diet, weight loss, or verbalized discontent with food choices. Client may express poor understanding of newly prescribed diet or diet restrictions.	Registered dietitian can determine nutrients and food sources client requires, based on client's physical condition. Dietitian has educational aides available to teach about diets.
b. Social work—assess client's need for counseling for major crises (e.g., terminal illness, loss of body part, family problems, need for relocation after discharge to nursing home or extended-care facilities; financial resources to cover medical costs; equipment for home health care; transport home following discharge).	Social worker is qualified to conduct regular counseling sessions with client who needs assistance to cope with life crises. Social workers are also knowledgeable about many community resources to help client with health care problems.
c. Physical therapy—assess client's need for regular exercise and mobility training following injury, surgery, or as result of chronic illness. Consider length of client's potential rehabilitation period.	Physical therapist is licensed to assist in examination and treatment of physically disabled or handicapped person. Therapist assists in rehabilitating client and restoring normal function.
d. Occupational therapy—assess client's need to learn new vocational skills or techniques to perform activities of daily living following a disability resulting from injury or illness.	Occupational therapists train client to adapt to physical handicaps by learning new vocational skills or activities of daily living.

Steps	Rationale
e. Speech therapy—assess client's ability to communicate, which has been altered as result of surgery, injury, or illness.	Speech therapist is trained to assist client with disorders affecting normal oral communication.
f. Clinical nurse specialist—assesses client's needs related to a specialized nursing care problem. Consults with nursing staff on appropriate interventions.	Clinical nurse specialist (CNS) is a nurse with a Master's degree in nursing and expertise in a specialized area of practice. The CNS functions as a clinician, educator, manager, consultant, and researcher within the specialty to plan or improve the quality of care for client and family.
g. Home health services— assess client's need for intermittent skilled nursing care or physical/ speech therapy following discharge.	Home health nurses can provide a follow-up visit as well as regular and frequent nursing services (e.g., administration of injections, wound care, ostomy care). This can help to shorten length of client's stay in a hospital.
2. Obtain necessary order for referral and communicate with appropriate department the client's specific health care needs that will influence therapies. (When order is not needed, nurse may confer directly with health care provider.)	Department accepting referral will require basic information about client before visits begin. Information related to nursing care needs may influence type of therapy referral service provides.
3. Explain to client that therapist from another department will visit.	Client has right to know of proposed treatment measures.
4. Consult with referral service about nursing implications related to prescribed treatments (e.g., exercises, diet restrictions, communication techniques).	Therapies initiated by referral service may pose implications for type and extent of care nurse delivers.

Steps	Rationale
5. Determine extent to which client's needs are met by referral service, for example, has client's dietary intake improved or has weight gain occurred? Is client's range of motion or motor strength improving? Is client learning alternative communication techniques?	Nurse is in best position to judge efficacy of care and to coordinate all available resources. Continuing problems may indicate need for different referral or adjustment in nursing care plan.
6. Record information regarding type of referral and frequency of visits in Kardex and care plan.	Provides continuity of care.

Nurse Alert

Availability of services varies according to size and type of health care agency. In many agencies, multidisciplinary team conferences provide excellent opportunity for discussing client's needs and making referrals.

Client Teaching

The client needs to be taught the specifics about the role of each new therapist who is introduced into the care activities. Likewise, if the client is going to receive these services in the home environment, the nurse needs to educate the client about the anticipated services and about how to contact the service provider directly.

Pediatric Considerations

Referrals for pediatric clients may include the siblings as well as the child's parents. In addition, the child's developmental, physiologic, and psychosocial needs are considered when referrals are initiated.

Geriatric Considerations

The needs of the older adult vary according to cognitive and physical impairments. Some services available for the older adult include day care activities and other social services in the areas of nutritional support, transportation, and safety.

Discharge from a Health Care Agency

Successful discharge planning is a coordinated interdisciplinary process that ensures that all clients have a plan for continuing care after they leave the hospital (AHA, 1983).

At discharge, clients must have the necessary knowledge, skills, and resources to meet their self-care needs. Most clients are able to return home. The nurse and health care team determine the resources needed to assist the client in returning to the home environment. Clients requiring more intensive skills may enter a skilled nursing facility or rehabilitation program or may become residents of a nursing home. When clients' needs for discharge planning are identified early during a hospital stay there is a greater likelihood that mutual goal setting with the client and family will occur and that a realistic discharge plan will be developed.

Potential Nursing Diagnoses

Client data derived during the assessment process reveal defining characteristics to support the following nursing diagnoses for clients requiring this skill:

    Bathing/hygiene self-care deficit
    Knowledge deficit
    High risk for injury
    Anxiety

Equipment

Necessary instructional materials
Any ordered prescriptions
Discharge summary form
Utility cart
Wheelchair

Steps	Rationale
Discharge planning	
1. From the time of admission, assess client's health care needs for discharge. Use nursing history, care plan, and ongoing assessments.	The plan for discharge begins at admission and continues throughout course of client's stay in the agency. It facilitates client's eventual adjustment to home setting.
2. Assess client's and family members' needs for health teaching related to home therapies, restrictions resulting from health alterations, and potential complications.	Client's and family's understanding of health care needs will improve likelihood of client successfully achieving self-care at home. Inclusion of family members in teaching sessions provides client with an accessible resource when at home.
3. Assess client and family environmental factors in home setting that might interfere with self-care activities.	Environmental barriers may pose risks to client's safety as result of limitation created by client's illness or need for certain therapies.
4. Collaborate with physician in assessing need for referral to skilled home health agencies.	Clients eligible for home health care are those who are confined to home as a result of illness, are under a physician's supervision, or require skilled nursing care on an intermittent basis.
5. Assess client's acceptance of health problems and related restrictions.	Client's acceptance of health status can affect his willingness to adhere to therapies and/or restrictions after discharge.
6. Consult with other health team members (e.g., dietitian, social worker) regarding client's needs on discharge.	Members of all health care disciplines should collaborate to determine client's needs and functional abilities.

Steps	Rationale
7. Ask client or family members for suggestions on ways to prepare for discharge.	Client should become part of discharge planning team. He may be able to identify additional needs for support or resources that your assessment did not reveal.
8. Suggest methods for altering physical arrangement of home environment to meet client's needs.	Client's level of independence can be maintained within an environment conducive to his safety and ability to retain function. Advanced preparation may be needed before client actually returns home.
9. Provide client and family with information about community health care resources.	Community resources often include services that client or family cannot provide for themselves.
10. Conduct teaching sessions with client and family as soon as possible during hospitalization on topics such as signs and symptoms of complications; injections, wound care, transfer techniques, colostomy care; medications, diet, exercise; and restrictions imposed by illness or surgery.	Gives client and family opportunities to practice new skills, ask questions about therapies, and obtain necessary feedback from you to ensure that learning has occurred.
11. Complete any referral forms indicating client's health care needs as well as existing functional abilities.	Continuity of health care is ensured through communication of individualized plan to all health team members.

Day of Discharge

12. Provide client and family an opportunity to ask questions or discuss issues related to health care needs at home.	Allows for final clarification of information previously discussed. Helps relieve client's anxiety.

Steps	Rationale
13. Check physician's discharge orders for prescriptions, change in treatments, or need for special appliances.	Discharge is authorized only by physician. Checking orders early ensures that any last-minute treatments or procedures can be attended to before client is actually discharged.
14. Determine if client or family member has arranged for transport home.	Client's condition at discharge will determine method for transport home.
15. Offer assistance as client dresses into own clothes and packs all personal belongings. Provide privacy as needed.	Promotes client comfort.
16. Check all closets and drawers to be sure that all client's belongings have been removed.	Prevents loss of client's personal items.
17. Obtain copy of valuables' list signed by client at admission and have security personnel or appropriate administrator deliver valuables to client. Account for all valuables.	Client's signature on list will verify receipt of items. Relieves agency of liability for any losses.
18. Provide client with all prescriptions or medications ordered by physician. Review previous instruction.	Review of drug information provides feedback to determine client's success in learning about medications.
19. Contact agency's business office to determine if client needs to finalize arrangements for payment of bill. Arrange for client or family to visit office.	A source of concern for many clients is whether agency has accepted insurance or other payment forms.

Steps	Rationale
20. Acquire utility cart to move client's belongings. Obtain wheelchair for clients unable to ambulate. Clients leaving by ambulance will be transported on ambulance stretchers.	Provides for safe transport.
21. Use proper body mechanics and transfer techniques in assisting client to wheelchair or stretcher. Escort client to entrance of agency where transportation is waiting (check agency policy).	Prevents injury to you and to client. Agency policy requires escort to ensure client's safe exit.
22. Lock wheelchair wheels. Assist client in transferring to automobile or transport vehicle. Help family member place personal belongings inside vehicle.	Agency's liability ends once client is safely in vehicle.
23. Return to division and notify admitting or appropriate department of time client was discharged.	Allows agency to prepare for admission of next client.
24. Complete discharge summary in client's medical record.	Essential for documenting client's status at time of departure from agency.
25. Document status of health problems at discharge.	Allows final evaluation of plan of care.

Nurse Alert

Do not ignore clients who fail to pose an obvious need for discharge planning. Too often, clients with short stays in a health care agency do not receive teaching or necessary referrals until the day of discharge.

Client Teaching

Individualize any discussions or demonstrations so the client can easily apply what he learns to the home setting.

Pediatric Considerations

A child's developmental age must be considered before attempting to prepare him for any home-care skills. Parents are most commonly involved in any preparation for the child's discharge.

Geriatric Considerations

Elderly clients with mobility restrictions or sensory limitations will benefit from installation of safety and/or assistive devices (e.g., as grab bars around toilets, adequate lighting in bathrooms, or chair height adjustments to make bending easier).

Writing a Nursing
Diagnosis

A nursing diagnosis is a statement that describes the client's actual or potential response to a health problem that the nurse is licensed and competent to treat. The client's actual and potential responses are obtained from the assessment data base and a review of literature, client's past medical records, and consultation with other professionals. The client's actual or potential responses require interventions from the domain of nursing (Carlson et al, 1991).

The diagnostic process includes three major elements: analysis and interpretation of data, identification of client problems, and formulation of nursing diagnoses (Fig. 1).

1. Analysis and interpretation of data require data validation and data clustering. Validation involves determining the relationship between assessment data and health needs and determining the data's accuracy. Data clustering is the process that the nurse uses to group related data.

2. Identification of client problems involves determining what the general health problems are and whether they are actual or potential problems. When identifying client needs, the nurse must consider all aspects of the nursing assessment.

3. Formulation of actual nursing diagnoses identifies the specific nursing care needs of each client. Individualization of such needs allows the nurse to develop a specific nursing care plan for each client.

Clients entering a health care agency may have more than one nursing diagnosis based on their individual health care problem. The appendix at the end of this text includes the nursing diagnoses currently accepted by the North American Nursing Diagnosis Association (NANDA; see appendix beginning on page 533).

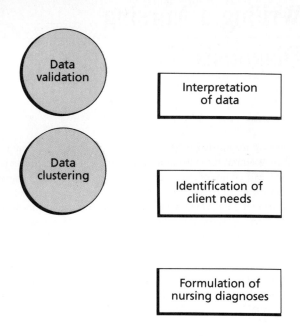

Fig. 1
Nursing diagnostic process.

Steps	Rationale
1. Validate pertinent data identified during history taking and physical assessment. Validation can be achieved from secondary sources of information such as reexamination or results of laboratory tests.	Determines whether data gathered during assessment are complete and accurate. The nurse uses knowledge and experience and analyzes and interprets or draws conclusions from data (Benner, 1984; Carlson et al, 1991; Carnevali et al, 1991).

Steps	Rationale

EXAMPLE
Client states he gets short of
breath climbing stairs. *Data
validation:* Client is re-
quested to climb stairs. After
climbing six stairs, respiratory rate increases from 18
to 32 breaths/min. Nasal
flaring and diaphoresis are
present and pulse rate increases from 82 to 126. BP
is stable at 130/82.

2. Group related data, which
   are generally signs and
   symptoms indicating general
   health problem. Related data
   arc clustered as regards client's mental or emotional
   status, individual body systems, risk factors, family
   data, and community factors.

Clustering of data encourages
the nurse to identify patterns for
health care. Data clustering
groups defining characteristics
from the client's nursing health
history and ultimately leads to
formation of nursing diagnoses.
Defining characteristics are the
clinical criteria that support
(validate) the diagnosis. Clinical
criteria are subjective symptoms
and objective signs, clusters of
signs and symptoms, or risk
factors (Carpenito, 1993).

EXAMPLE
Client states that he has shortness of breath with exertion.
Data clustering: Respiratory
rate is increased from 18 to 32
breaths/min. Pulse rate is increased from 82 to 126 with
exertion. Nasal flaring and diaphoresis are present with exertion.

Steps	Rationale
3. Identify client needs (problems). The nurse first determines what the client's health problems are and whether they are actual or potential problems.	Problem identification step brings the nurse closer to forming a nursing diagnosis and making general analyses of the clustered data, thus assisting the nurse in developing the diagnostic statement.
a. Actual health care problem: one that is perceived or experienced by client.	
b. Potential health care problem: one that client is at risk of developing.	

EXAMPLE
- *Actual* health care problem—shortness of breath with exertion
- *Potential* health care problem—reduced activity level

Steps	Rationale
4. Formulate the nursing diagnosis in two parts.	
a. Problem: actual or potential client need that can be resolved by nursing interventions.	Nursing diagnostic label (NANDA).
b. Cause: direct or contributing factor (condition or situation) that can be affected by nursing interventions.	Helps to individualize nursing diagnosis and subsequent plan of care.

EXAMPLE
- *Problem*—ineffective breathing pattern related to *cause* (exertion)
- *Problem*—high risk for activity intolerance related to *cause* (shortness of breath)

Steps	Rationale
5. Reevaluate list of individualized nursing diagnoses developed for each client contact.	As client's needs (problems) resolve and change, nursing diagnoses are modified. Some may no longer be relevant, while new ones may need to be developed.

Writing a
Nursing Care Plan

The nursing care plan is a written guideline for client care. It documents the client's health care needs, which are determined by assessment and the nursing diagnoses (Table 1). During planning, priorities are set, goals are determined, expected outcomes are developed, and a nursing care plan is formulated. This nursing care plan then coordinates nursing care, promotes continuity of care, and lists expected outcomes (outcome criteria) that are used in evaluating nursing care. In addition, the written care plan communicates to other nurses and health professionals specific individualized nursing therapies.

Steps	Rationale
1. Establish priorities of care. Rank nursing diagnoses and goals in order of importance. Priorities are classified as high, intermediate, or low.	High-priority nursing diagnoses reflect emergency or immediate needs of client that could result in harm to the client or others if left untreated (Gordon, 1987). High priorities occur in psychologic as well as physiologic dimensions. Intermediate-priority nursing diagnoses reflect non-emergency non–life-threatening needs of client. Low-priority nursing diagnoses reflect client needs that may not be directly related to a specific illness or prognosis.

Table 1   Sample nursing care plan

Nursing diagnosis: *High risk for impaired skin integrity* related to immobility resulting from coma
Definition: High risk for impaired skin integrity is the state in which an individual's skin is at risk of being adversely altered.

Assessment	Goals	Implementation	Expected Outcomes
Fever: higher than 102° F for 72 hours Diaphoresis Incontinence of urine	Absence of break in skin Absence of redness Absence of decreased muscle mass over bony prominences	Turn client every 2 hours in following sequence: 8 AM— supine 10 AM— left side Noon— prone Repeat, beginning with supine position.	No skin breakdown is noted. Skin color, temperature, and capillary return are normal. Client is afebrile.
Decreased skin turgor No skin breakdown noted		Keep client's skin dry at all times.	Skin turgor is improved. Skin remains dry and intact.

Steps	Rationale
EXAMPLE	
Nursing diagnoses *High Priority*	*Rationale for priority setting*
Ineffective coping related to an unknown medical diagnosis	Dealing with this early will help client prepare for surgery and his postoperative restorative care.
Ineffective airway clearance postoperatively, related to abdominal incisional pain	Institute preventive client education preoperatively.
Intermediate Priority	
High risk for altered nutrition: less than body requirements, related to decreased nutritional intake	Does not affect client's immediate physiologic or emotional status.
Low Priority	
High risk for infection, related to 20-year smoking history	Reflects long-term needs of client.
2. Develop client-centered goals of nursing care for each nursing diagnosis. A client-centered goal is a specific and measurable objective designed to reflect the client's highest level of wellness and independence in function.	Goals serve as guideposts to the selection of nursing interventions and criteria in the evaluation of care. Setting goals is an activity that includes family and significant others, as well as the client. The goal determines the expected outcomes of the nursing intervention.
EXAMPLE	
Nursing diagnoses Ineffective coping related to unknown medical diagnosis	*Goals* Client assumes responsibility for seeking support resources.
Ineffective airway clearance postoperatively related to abdominal incisional pain	Client's lungs to remain clear postoperatively.

Steps	Rationale
3. For each goal, write expected outcomes anticipated from nursing action. An expected outcome is the step-by-step client response that leads to the attainment of the goal and the resolution of the etiology for the nursing diagnosis. It is the measurable change in the client's status in response to nursing care. Outcomes should reflect goals established in Step 2.	Expected outcomes provide a direction for nursing care (Gordon, 1987), include measurable changes in client status, project a time span for goal attainment, and provide objective criteria to evaluate the effectiveness of nursing interventions.

EXAMPLE

Nursing diagnosis
Ineffective airway clearance postoperatively related to abdominal incisional pain

Goal	*Expected outcome*
Client's lungs to remain clear through postoperative care.	Lungs remain clear to auscultation
	Client able to clear airways
	Client's body temperature remains within normal limits
	Client achieves preestablished incentive spirometry

| 4. Develop and write specific implementation measures directed toward achieving client-centered goals and expected outcomes. Should include when, how much, where, etc. | Choosing nursing interventions is a decision-making process that requires critical thinking. Interventions are based on assessment data, priority setting, knowledge, and experience to select interventions that will successfully meet the goals and expected outcomes (Prescott, Dennis, and Jacox, 1987). They must be specific so that there is continuity of care from one nurse to another. |

Steps	Rationale
5. Modify nursing care plan based on evaluation of the attainment of client-centered goals and expected outcomes as well as changes in the client's status or needs.	Modification requires the nurse to identify factors that interfered with achievement of goals and expected outcomes. Continually individualizes and focuses the nursing care on outcomes of nursing care.

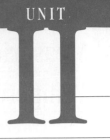

VITAL
SIGNS

Measuring Oral
Temperature

Normally a person's body temperature fluctuates within a relatively narrow range. Under control of the hypothalamus, the core body temperature stays within 0.6° (1°) of the average normal body temperature 37° C (98.6° F). Alterations may result from disease, infection, prolonged exposure to heat or cold, exercise, and hormonal disturbances. The body adapts to temperature changes by conserving or losing heat, depending on the nature of the temperature alteration.

The oral method is the easiest way to obtain an accurate temperature reading. The nurse should delay measurement for 20 to 30 minutes if the client has ingested hot or cold liquids or food or has smoked. Each of these can cause false changes in temperature levels.

The nurse should consider the client's risks of temperature alterations during assessment of body temperature. Conditions or therapies that can cause temperature alterations include expected or diagnosed infections, open wounds or burns, an abnormal white cell count, use of immunosuppressive drugs, injury to the hypothalamus, lengthy exposure to temperature extremes, and reaction to blood products.

Potential Nursing Diagnoses

Hypothermia
Hyperthermia
Ineffective thermoregulation
High risk for altered body temperature

Equipment

Oral or stubby mercury-in-glass thermometer or electronic thermometer with blue probe and plastic probe cover

Tissue paper
Disposable gloves
Pen, pencil, and flowsheet or record form

Steps	Rationale
1. Wash hands and apply disposable gloves.	Reduces transmission of microorganisms.
2. Explain procedure to client.	Certain clients may be unfamiliar with measuring device. Explanation will relieve client anxiety.
3. Obtain oral temperature.	

Glass Thermometer

a. Hold color-coded end of glass thermometer in your fingertips.	Prevents contamination of bulb to be inserted into client's mouth.
b. Read mercury level while gently rotating thermometer at eye level (Fig. 2).	Mercury is to be below 35.5° C (96° F). Thermometer reading must be below client's actual temperature before use. Brisk shaking lowers mercury level in glass tube.

Fig. 2

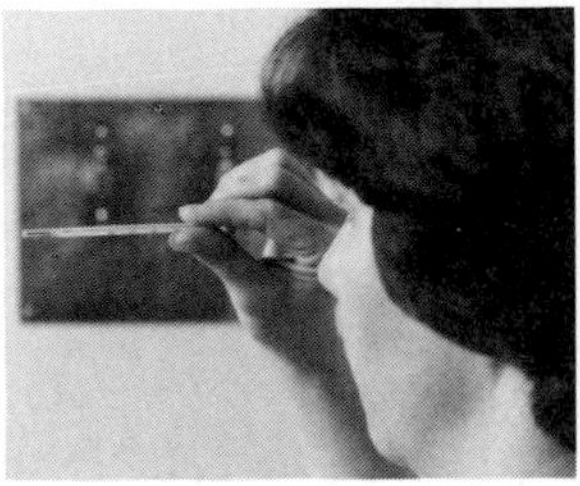

c. If mercury is above desired level, grasp tip of thermometer securely. Sharply flick wrist downward. Continue until reading is at appropriate level.

Steps	Rationale
d. Ask client to open his mouth and gently place thermometer in sublingual pocket (under tongue) lateral to center of lower jaw.	Heat from superficial blood vessels under the tongue produces temperature reading.
e. Ask client to hold thermometer with lips closed.	Maintains proper position of thermometer. Breakage of thermometer may injure oral mucosa and cause mercury poisoning.
f. Leave thermometer in place for 2 minutes or according to agency policy.	Studies disagree as to proper length of time for recording. Graves and Markarian (1980) found that glass thermometers kept in place for 8 minutes recorded values on average only 0.07° F higher than those kept in for 3 minutes. Baker et al (1984) found that 2-minute insertions did not cause clinically significant variations.
g. Carefully remove thermometer and read at eye level. Inform client of temperature reading.	Gentle handling prevents client discomfort and ensures accurate reading.
h. Wipe off any secretions with a soft tissue. Wipe in rotating fashion from tip to bulb. Dispose of tissue.	Prevents contact of microorganisms with your hands. Tip is area of least contamination, bulb area of greatest contamination.
i. Wash thermometer in lukewarm soapy water. Rinse in cool water and dry.	Mechanically removes organic material that can hinder action of disinfectant.

Electronic Thermometer

a. Attach oral probe (blue tip) to electronic display unit. Grasp top of stem, being careful not to apply pressure to eject button (Fig. 3).	Ejection button releases plastic cover from probe.

Steps	Rationale

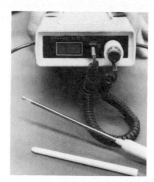

Fig. 3

b. Slide clean disposable plastic cover over temperature probe until it locks in place.

Soft plastic cover will not break in client's mouth and prevents transmission of microorganisms between clients.

c. Ask client to open mouth and gently place probe under tongue, lateral to center of lower jaw.

Ensures accurate readings. Correct techniques prevent injury to client.

d. Ask client to keep probe in place until alarm on electronic unit sounds and temperature reading appears on digital display.

Electronic units are capable of registering client's body temperature in seconds.

e. Remove probe from under client's tongue. Inform client of temperature reading.

f. Push eject button on thermometer probe to discard plastic probe cover into proper receptacle.

Reduces spread of infection.

g. Replace probe in electronic unit.

Battery unit is rechargeable.

4. Wash your hands and dispose of gloves.

Reduces transmission of microorganisms.

5. Record client's temperature in proper chart or flow sheet.

Should be done immediately before it is forgotten.

Nurse Alert

Oral temperature measurement is contraindicated when the thermometer can injure the client or if the client is unable to hold the thermometer properly. Examples of contraindications include infants and small children, clients undergoing oral surgery or with pain in or trauma to the mouth, confused or unconscious clients, mouth breathers, clients with a history of convulsions, and clients with shaking chills.

Client Teaching

Clients susceptible to temperature alterations should know how to measure their temperatures correctly so they can seek medical attention early when alterations occur. Parents of young children should learn how to measure body temperature because children can develop seriously high fevers quickly.

Pediatric Considerations

Oral temperature measurement is not used in infants or small children. Most institutions recommend an age after which taking an oral temperature is permitted (e.g., after 5 or 6 years). The immaturity of a child's temperature regulation mechanisms can cause sudden changes in body temperature. A newborn's body temperature normally ranges from 35.5° to 37.5° C (96° to 99.5° F).

Geriatric Considerations

Disturbances in temperature regulation that normally occur with aging can cause the elderly client to have a lower-than-normal body temperature.

Measuring Rectal
Temperature

The nurse measures a client's body temperature rectally when use of an oral thermometer is contraindicated. The rectal site provides a reliable measure of body temperature. However, a client can easily become embarrassed when rectal temperature must be measured. Thus the nurse should take care to consider the client's privacy and comfort.

Temperature should *not* be measured rectally in the following: infants, clients with rectal surgery or disorders, clients in pelvic or lower-extremity traction or casts, and occasionally, clients with acute myocardial infarction. Rectal temperature measurement is most reliable in young children.

Potential Nursing Diagnoses

Hypothermia
Hyperthermia
Ineffective thermoregulation
High risk for altered body temperature

Equipment

Glass rectal tip thermometer or electronic thermometer with rectal (red tip) probe
Lubricant
Tissue paper
Disposable gloves

Steps	Rationale
1. Wash hands and don gloves.	Reduces transmission of micro-organisms.
2. Explain procedure to client.	Certain clients may be unfamiliar with measuring device. Explanation will relieve client anxiety.
3. Draw curtains around client's bed or close room door. Keep client's upper body and lower extremities covered.	Maintains client privacy and minimizes embarrassment.
4. Assist client in assuming Sims' position, with upper leg flexed. Move aside bed linen to expose only anal area. Children may lie prone.	Provides optimal exposure of anal area for correct thermometer placement.
5. Obtain temperature.	

Glass Rectal Thermometer

a. Hold tip of thermometer in your fingertips.	This prevents contamination of the bulb to be inserted into client's rectum.
b. Read mercury level.	Mercury should be below 35.5° C (96° F) and below client's actual temperature before use.
c. If mercury is above desired level, shake thermometer down. Grasp upper end of thermometer securely and stand away from any solid objects. Sharply flick wrist downward. Continue until reading is at appropriate level.	Brisk shaking lowers mercury level in glass tube. Standing in an open spot away from objects prevents breakage of thermometer.

Steps	Rationale
d. Squeeze liberal amount of water-soluble lubricant onto a tissue. Dip thermometer bulb into lubricant, covering 2.5 to 3.5 cm (1 to 1½ inches) for adult or 1.2 to 2.5 cm (½ to 1 inch) for infant or child.	Inserting thermometer into lubricant container would contaminate all unused lubricant. Lubrication minimizes trauma to rectal mucosa during insertion.
e. With nondominant hand raise client's upper buttock to expose anus.	Retracting buttocks fully exposes anus.
f. Gently insert thermometer into anus in direction of umbilicus. Insert 3.5 cm (1½ inches) for adult. Do not force thermometer. Ask client to take deep breath and blow out. Insert thermometer as client breathes deeply. If you feel resistance, withdraw thermometer immediately.	Proper insertion ensures adequate exposure to blood vessels in rectal wall. Gentle insertion prevents trauma to mucosa or breakage of thermometer. Taking deep breath helps to relax anal sphincter.
g. Hold thermometer in place for 2 minutes or according to agency policy. You may have to hold an infant's legs.	Holding thermometer prevents injury to client. Nichols and Kucha (1972) identified optimal placement time as 2 minutes.

Electronic Thermometer

a. Attach rectal probe (red tip) to electronic display unit. Grasp top of stem, being careful not to apply pressure to eject button.	Ejection button releases plastic cover from probe.

Steps	Rationale
b. Slide clean disposable plastic cover over temperature probe until it locks in place.	Prevents transmission of microorganisms.
c. With nondominant hand raise client's upper buttock to expose anus.	Retracting buttocks fully exposes anus.
d. Gently insert thermometer into anus in direction of umbilicus. Insert 3.5 cm (1½ inches) for adult. Do not force thermometer. Ask client to take deep breath and blow out. Insert thermometer as client breathes deeply. If you feel resistance, withdraw thermometer immediately.	Proper insertion ensures adequate exposure to blood vessels in rectal wall. Gentle insertion prevents trauma to mucosa or breakage of thermometer. Taking deep breath helps to relax anal sphincter.
e. Hold electronic probe in place until electronic unit's alarm sounds and temperature reading appears on digital display.	Electronic units are capable of registering client's body temperature in seconds.
f. Carefully remove probe from client's rectum. Inform client of temperature reading.	
g. Push eject button on thermometer probe and discard plastic probe cover into proper receptacle.	Reduces spread of infection.
h. Replace probe in electronic unit.	Battery unit is rechargeable.
6. Wipe client's anal area to remove lubricant or feces.	Provides for client's comfort.
7. Help client return to a more comfortable position.	Restores client's comfort.

Steps	Rationale
8. Remove gloves and wash hands.	Reduces transmission of micro-organisms.
9. Record client's temperature in proper chart or flow sheet. Signify rectal reading by capital *R*.	Vital signs should be recorded immediately after measurement. *R* prevents later confusion with oral or axillary measurements.

Nurse Alert

Always hold a rectal thermometer while it is in place. Sudden movement by the client could cause the thermometer to break in the rectum.

Client Teaching

Instruct mothers of young children on how to position infant or small child. Infant or small child should be prone on the mother's lap or on a bed. The mother should gently retract both buttocks to expose the anus. The lubricated rectal thermometer is inserted 1.2 cm (½ inch) in an infant or small child.

Pediatric Considerations

Rectal temperature recording is contraindicated in newborns. Do not allow infants or young children to kick their legs or roll to the side while the thermometer is in place. The immaturity of a child's temperature regulation mechanisms can cause sudden changes in body temperature. A newborn's body temperature normally ranges between 35.5° and 37.5° C (96° and 99.5° F).

Geriatric Considerations

Disturbances in temperature regulation that normally occur with aging can cause elderly clients to have a lower-than-normal body temperature. An elderly person may have difficulty flexing his knee or hip to assume the Sims' position. In that case, allow him to lie on his side with legs straight.

Measuring Axillary
Temperature

Axillary temperature measurement is the safest way to assess body temperature in a newborn. However, an axillary temperature is the least accurate of the three temperature measurement techniques because the thermometer must be placed against an external body site instead of an internal site. Whenever an oral or rectal thermometer can be safely used, the nurse should avoid using the axillary thermometer.

Potential Nursing Diagnoses

Hypothermia
Hyperthermia
Ineffective thermoregulation
High risk for altered body temperature

Equipment

Oral or stubby mercury-in-glass thermometer or electronic thermometer with a rectal (red tip) probe, plastic probe cover
Tissue paper

Steps	Rationale
1. Wash hands.	Reduces transmission of micro-organisms.
2. Explain procedure to client.	Reduces anxiety and promotes cooperation.
3. Draw curtains around bed and/or close room door.	Provides privacy and minimizes client embarrassment.

Steps	Rationale
4. Assist client to a sitting or supine position. Move clothing or gown away from client's shoulder and arm.	Provides optimal exposure of axilla.
5. Obtain temperature.	

Glass Thermometer

a. Hold upper end of thermometer in your fingertips.	Prevents contamination of the bulb.
b. Read mercury level. If mercury is above desired level, shake thermometer down. Grasp upper end securely and stand away from any solid objects. Sharply flick wrist downward. Continue until reading is at appropriate level.	Mercury should be below 35.5° C (96° F) and below client's actual temperature before use. Brisk shaking lowers mercury level in glass tube. Standing in open spot prevents breakage of thermometer.
c. Insert thermometer into center of client's axilla, lower arm over thermometer, and place forearm across his chest (Fig. 4).	Maintains proper position of thermometer against blood vessels in axilla.

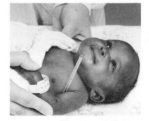

Fig. 4

d. Hold thermometer in place for 5 to 10 minutes or according to agency policy.	Eoff and Joyce (1981) recommend 5 minutes for children. Recommended time varies among agencies.

Steps	Rationale
e. Remove thermometer and wipe off any secretions with tissue. Wipe in rotating fashion from fingers toward bulb. Dispose of tissue.	Avoids contact with microorganisms. Wipe from area of least contamination to area of most contamination.

Electronic Thermometer

Steps	Rationale
a. Attach rectal probe (red tip) to electronic display unit. Grasp top of stem, being careful not to apply pressure to eject button.	Ejection button releases plastic cover from probe.
b. Slide clean disposable plastic cover over temperature probe until it locks in place.	Prevents transmission of microorganisms.
c. Insert probe into center of axilla, lower client's arm over thermometer, and place arm across client's chest.	Maintains proper position of thermometer against blood vessels in axilla.
d. Hold electronic probe in place until electronic unit alarm sounds and temperature reading appears on digital display.	Electronic units are capable of registering client's body temperature in seconds.
e. Carefully remove probe from client's axilla.	
f. Read thermometer and inform client of temperature.	Promotes understanding of health status.
g. Push eject button on thermometer probe to discard plastic probe cover into proper receptacle.	Reduces spread of infection.
h. Replace probe in electronic unit.	Battery unit is rechargeable.
6. Assist client in replacing clothing or gown.	Restores client's sense of well-being.

Steps	Rationale
7. Wash hands.	Reduces transmission of micro-organisms.
8. Record temperature in proper chart or flow sheet. Signify axillary reading by capital *A*.	Vital signs should be recorded immediately after measurement. *A* prevents later confusion with oral or rectal measurements.

Nurse Alert

It may be necessary to hold the child's arm gently against his side.

Client Teaching

Instruct mothers of young children on how to position and restrain the child properly. Also explain the importance of keeping the thermometer in place at least 5 minutes (Eoff and Joyce, 1981).

Pediatric Considerations

Stay with the child throughout the procedure. The immaturity of a child's temperature regulation mechanisms can cause sudden changes in body temperature. A newborn's body temperature normally ranges between 35.5° and 37.5° C (96° and 99.5° F).

Geriatric Considerations

Disturbances in temperature regulation that normally occur with aging may cause the client to have a lower-than-normal body temperature.

Measuring Tympanic Temperature

A newer form of temperature measurement involves use of the tympanic membrane thermometer, which consists of a temperature-sensitive probe inserted into the opening of the external ear canal. Within seconds the probe registers the temperature of the blood flowing near the tympanic membrane. Tympanic membrane temperature matches core-rectal temperature reliably (Shinozaki, Deane, and Perkins; 1988). This thermometer looks similar to an otoscope, is battery powered, and is kept in its own rechargeable case (Fig. 5).

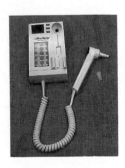

Fig. 5

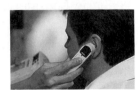

Potential Nursing Diagnoses

Hypothermia
Hyperthermia
Ineffective thermoregulation
High risk for altered body temperature

Equipment

Tympanic thermometer with ear probe cover
Disposable gloves

Steps	Rationale
1. Wash hands. Don gloves if appropriate.	Reduces transmission of micro-organisms.
2. Explain procedure to client.	Reduces anxiety and promotes cooperation.
3. Expose client's external ear canal. Client may be more comfortable in a sitting, side-lying, or supine position.	Provides optimal exposure to tympanic membrane.
4. Attach tympanic probe cover to thermometer unit.	Probe cover prevents transmission of microorganisms between clients.
5. Insert probe into ear canal, applying a gentle but firm pressure.	Gentle pressure seals ear canal from ambient air and improves accuracy.
6. Maintain probe in ear canal until a reading is displayed on digital unit, approximately 2 seconds later. Remove thermometer and inform client of temperature reading.	Tympanic core temperature readings are rapid (less than 2 seconds) and extremely accurate (Shinozaki, 1988; Erickson et al, 1991).
7. Dispose of probe cover in proper receptacle.	Reduces transmission of micro-organisms.
8. Return thermometer to storage unit.	Most units are battery powered and recharge while in storage.
9. Remove gloves and wash hands.	Reduces transmission of micro-organisms.
10. Record temperature in proper chart or flow sheet. Signify tympanic reading by capital T.	Vital signs should be recorded immediately after measurement. T prevents later confusion with other temperature measurements.

Nurse Alert

Use whatever precautions are necessary to restrain the client or to hold the probe in place without injuring the client. Do not use tympanic membrane thermometer when blood or fluid is present within ear canal.

Client Teaching

Tympanic thermometers are rarely used in the home setting. Thus explanation of the procedure is all that is necessary.

Pediatric Considerations

Tympanic membrane thermometers quickly obtain a child's temperature. Children may be less threatened if they are allowed to play with the equipment before temperature is measured.

Geriatric Considerations

An elderly person's body temperature can normally be lower than that of a younger adult.

Assessing Radial Pulse

The character of a client's pulse provides valuable data regarding the integrity of his cardiovascular system.

The nurse commonly assesses the radial artery pulse during routine measurement of a client's vital signs or when a change is expected in his condition. The radial pulse is usually the most accessible. When it is inaccessible because of a dressing, cast, or other encumbrance, the apical pulse can be assessed instead. This involves auscultating heart sounds with a stethoscope placed medially below the left nipple (see Skill 2-6).

Before assessing a client's pulse, the nurse attempts to control four factors—exercise, anxiety, pain, and postural change—that might cause false elevations or decreases in heart rate. The nurse should also be able to anticipate how certain medications or disease processes will affect the client's heart rate.

Potential Nursing Diagnoses

Altered tissue perfusion
Decreased cardiac output

Equipment

Wristwatch with second hand or digital display
Pen, pencil, and flow sheet

Steps	Rationale
1. Wash hands.	Reduces chances of transmitting microorganisms.
2. Explain purpose and method of procedure to client.	Relieves client anxiety and facilitates his cooperation during procedure.

Steps	Rationale
3. Have client assume a supine or sitting position. If supine, place his arm across his lower chest with wrist extended and palm down. If sitting, bend his elbow 90 degrees and support his lower arm on chair or on your arm. Extend his wrist with palm down.	Proper positioning fully exposes radial artery for palpation.
4. Place tips of first two or middle three fingers of your hand over groove along radial or thumb side of client's inner wrist (Fig. 6).	Fingertips are most sensitive parts of hand to palpate arterial pulsations. Nurse's thumb has pulsation that may interfere with accuracy.

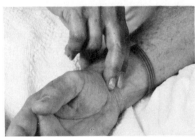

Fig. 6

5. Lightly compress against radius, obliterate pulse initially, and then relax pressure so pulse becomes easily palpable.	Pulse is more accurately assessed with moderate pressure. Too much pressure occludes pulse and impairs blood flow.
6. When pulse can be felt regularly, use watch's second hand and begin to count rate, starting with 0, and then 1, etc.	Rate is determined accurately only after assessor is certain that pulse can be palpated. Timing should begin with 0. Count of 1 is first beat felt after timing begins.

Steps	Rationale
7. If pulse is regular, count for 30 seconds and multiply total by 2.	Research indicates that 30-second pulse check is most accurate for rapid pulse rates, and that a 15-second check is often inaccurate for resting and rapid heart rates (Hollerbach et al, 1990).
8. If pulse is irregular, count for full minute.	Ensures accurate count.
9. Assess regularity and frequency of any existing dysrhythmia.	Inefficient contraction of heart fails to transmit pulse wave and can interfere with cardiac output.
10. Determine strength of pulse. Note whether thrust of pulse against fingertips is bounding, strong, weak, or thready.	Strength reflects volume of blood ejected against arterial wall with each heart contraction.
11. Assist client to comfortable position.	Promotes sense of well-being.
12. Record characteristics of pulse in medical record or flow sheet. Report abnormalities to nurse in charge or physician.	Provides data for monitoring changes in client's condition. Abnormalities may necessitate medical therapy.
13. Discuss findings with client.	Promotes client's participation in care and understanding of health status.
14. Wash hands.	Reduces transmission of microorganisms.

Nurse Alert

If the nurse detects an irregular rhythm, it is important to assess for a pulse deficit. Compare the pulses at the radial artery and the apex of the heart. A difference between rates indicates a deficit.

Client Teaching

Certain clients should learn how to assess their own pulse. Those receiving medications that affect heart function should assess their pulse as well as any undesirable effects of medications. Clients undergoing cardiovascular and pulmonary rehabilitation should also assess their pulse to determine exercise tolerance.

Pediatric Considerations

A 1-week-old to 3-month-old infant's resting heart rate ranges from 120 to 140 beats per minute (Whaley and Wong, 1993). By the age of 2 years, a child's resting heart rate ranges from 80 to 150 beats per minute. From the ages of 2 to 10 years, the rate ranges from 70 to 110. By the time the child is 10 years of age, the resting heart rate ranges from 55 to 90 beats per minute. The apical rate is most accurate in children (Whaley and Wong, 1993).

Geriatric Considerations

The resting heart rate should range between 60 to 100 beats per minute in the healthy older adult. Older adults with cardiovascular, pulmonary, or other chronic illnesses are at risk for rapid, slow, or irregular heart rate and rhythms.

Assessing Apical
Pulse

The apical pulse is assessed with a stethoscope. The stethoscope is placed over the apex of the client's heart. The stethoscope enables the sounds originating from the valves of the heart to be transmitted via the rubber tubing to the nurse's ears for pulse assessment.

The apical pulse is the best site for assessing an infant's or young child's pulse. When a client takes medication that affects heart rate, the apical pulse may provide a more accurate assessment of cardiac rate and rhythm.

Potential Nursing Diagnoses

Decreased cardiac output
Altered tissue perfusion

Equipment

Stethoscope
Wristwatch with second hand or digital display
Pen, pencil, and flow sheet

Steps	Rationale
1. Clean earpieces and diaphragm of stethoscope with alcohol swab as needed.	Controls transmission of microorganisms when nurses share stethoscope.
2. Wash hands.	Reduces transmission of microorganisms.
3. Close door or draw curtains around client's bed.	Maintains client's privacy.

Steps	Rationale
4. With client in supine or sitting position, turn down bed linen and raise gown, or remove client's upper garments to expose sternum and left side of chest.	Exposes portion of chest wall for selection of auscultatory site.
5. Palpate angle of Louis, located just below suprasternal notch at point where horizontal ridge is felt along body of sternum. Place index finger just to the left of client's sternum and palpate second intercostal space below and proceed downward until fifth intercostal space is palpated. Move index finger horizontally along fifth intercostal space to left midclavicular line (Fig. 7). Palpate point of maximal impulse (PMI), also called Erb's point.	Use of anatomic landmarks allows correct placement of stethoscope over apex of heart. This position enhances ability to hear heart sounds clearly. The PMI is over the apex of the heart.

Fig. 7

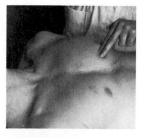

| 6. Place diaphragm of stethoscope in palm of your hand for 5 to 10 seconds. | Warms diaphragm and reduces risk of client being startled. |

Steps	Rationale
7. Place diaphragm over PMI and auscultate for normal S_1 and S_2 (lub, dub) heart sounds (Fig. 8).	Heart sounds are the result of blood moving through cardiac valves.

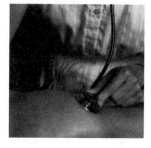

Fig. 8

Steps	Rationale
8. When S_1 and S_2 sounds are heard with regularity, observe watch's second hand and count for 30 seconds and multiply by 2.	Rate is determined accurately only after nurse is able to auscultate sounds clearly.
9. If heart rate is irregular or client is on cardiovascular medications, count for 60 seconds.	Rate determined is more accurate when assessed over a longer interval.
10. Note regularity of any dysrhythmias, (i.e., every third or fourth beat is skipped).	Regularly occurring dysrhythmias with 1 minute may indicate inadequate cardiac dysfunction and require further testing.
11. Replace client's garments and bed linen.	Maintains client comfort and privacy.
12. Discuss findings with client.	Promotes client's understanding of health status.
13. Wash hands.	Reduces transmission of microorganisms.

Steps	Rationale
14. Record characteristics of pulse on flow sheet. Report any abnormalities to nurse in charge or client's physician.	Provides data for monitoring changes in client's condition. Abnormalities may require medical therapy.

Nurse Alert

The nurse should note the presence of any irregularity. If this irregularity is new to the client, it should be reported to the nurse in charge or the client's physician. In addition, irregularities can be associated with adverse effects of cardiac medications, (e.g., digoxin).

Client Teaching

Family members may need to learn to take the client's apical pulse in the home setting. The nurse needs to teach the caregiver how to use the stethoscope correctly as well as how to obtain an apical pulse correctly.

Pediatric Considerations

The most accurate site for pulse assessment in infants and small children is the apical site.

Geriatric Considerations

The healthy older adult has a normal cardiac rate and rhythm. However, in the presence of chronic illnesses or if the client is on cardiac medications the nurse should assess the pulse apically.

Assessing

Respirations

When the nurse assesses a client's respirations, the procedure involves observing the rate, depth, and rhythm of his ventilatory movements. The nurse must be able to recognize normal passive breathing compared with ventilations that require muscular effort. Minimal effort is required to inhale and even less to exhale. If a client is having respiratory difficulties, the intercostal and accessory muscles will work more actively and the nurse will be able to see pronounced movement of his shoulder, neck, and chest muscles.

The nurse should be familiar with factors that normally affect respirations as well as conditions that place a client at risk of respiratory alterations.

Potential Nursing Diagnoses

Ineffective airway clearance
Ineffective breathing pattern
Activity intolerance

Equipment

Wristwatch with second hand or digital display
Pen, pencil, and flow sheet

Steps	Rationale
1. Be sure that client is in comfortable position, preferably sitting.	Discomfort can cause client to breathe more rapidly.

Steps	Rationale
2. Place client's arm in relaxed position across his abdomen or lower chest, or place your hand directly over client's upper abdomen.	This position is used during assessment of pulse. Both your own and the client's hands rise and fall during respiratory cycle. Measuring respirations immediately after pulse assessment makes measurement inconspicuous.
3. Observe complete respiratory cycle (one inspiration and one expiration).	Ensures that count will begin with normal respiratory cycle.
4. Once a cycle is observed, look at watch's second hand and begin to count rate: when second hand reaches a number on dial, count "one" to begin first full cycle.	Timing begins with count of one. Respirations occur more slowly than pulse; thus count begins with one.
5. For an adult, count number of respirations in 30 seconds and multiply by 2. For infant or young child, count respirations for full minute.	Respiratory rate is equivalent to number of respirations per minute. Young infants and children breathe in an irregular rhythm.
6. If an adult's respirations have irregular rhythm or are abnormally slow or fast, count for full minute.	Accurate interpretation requires assessment for at least 1 minute.
7. While counting, note whether depth is shallow, normal, or deep and whether rhythm is normal or contains altered patterns.	The character of ventilatory movements may reveal specific alterations or disease states.
8. Record results in chart or flow sheet. Report any signs of respiratory alterations.	Provides data for monitoring change in client's condition. Abnormalities may indicate need for therapy.

Nurse Alert

Clients' respiratory patterns can change for a variety of reasons. Some reasons, such as an asthmatic attack or the presence of foreign body airway obstruction, are more critical than others and require rapid interventions. In addition, pain and anxiety can also alter respiratory patterns. The nurse should not dismiss changes in respiration without further assessment.

Client Teaching

Clients with chronic lung disease can benefit from diaphragmatic breathing exercises (see Skill 12-1).

Pediatric Considerations

The nurse should plan on respirations being the first vital sign assessed in an infant or child. Startling or arousing an infant for other preliminary measurements can falsely increase respirations. Usually the nurse can simply observe respirations as the infant or young child lies in bed with his chest and abdomen uncovered.

A newborn breathes at a rate of 30 to 60 respirations per minute. A 2-year-old breathes 20 to 30 respirations per minute. A 6-year-old has a rate of 18 to 26 breaths per minute.

Geriatric Considerations

An adult normally breathes 12 to 20 respirations per minute at rest. The average respiratory rate increases with advancing age, and chest expansion tends to decline because of increased rigidity of the chest wall.

Assessing Blood Pressure by Auscultation

Blood flows throughout the circulatory system because the heart pumps it into the arteries under high pressure. Pressure within the aorta at the time of left ventricular contraction (systole) is approximately 120 mm Hg in a healthy adult who is upright but not exercising. Once the aorta distends, a pressure wave traveling through the arterial system sends blood to the peripheral tissues. As the ventricles relax, pressure in the arterial system falls. The diastolic pressure (normally about 80 mm Hg) is the minimal pressure exerted against the arterial walls. The nurse records blood pressure with the systolic before the diastolic reading (e.g., 120/80).

The nurse's assessment of blood pressure helps determine the balance of several hemodynamic factors: cardiac output, peripheral vascular resistance, blood volume and viscosity, and elasticity of the arteries. A client's blood pressure should be carefully compared with pulse rate and character in addition to other cardiovascular assessment findings so that an intelligent conclusion can be drawn regarding the client's circulatory status.

Potential Nursing Diagnoses

Decreased cardiac output
Altered peripheral tissue perfusion

Equipment

Stethoscope
Sphygmomanometer with cuff
Pen, pencil, and flow sheet

Steps	Rationale
1. Determine proper cuff size. Width of inflatable bladder within cuff should be 40% of circumference at mid-point of limb on which cuff is to be used (or 20% wider than diameter). Length of bladder should be about twice recommended width.	Proper cuff size is necessary so correct amount of pressure is applied over artery. Cuffs that are too narrow, too wide, or improperly applied cause false-high or false-low readings, respectively.
2. Determine best site for cuff placement. Avoid extremity with an IV line, arteriovenous shunt, presence of trauma, side of mastectomy, or side of paralysis or paresis after a cerebrovascular accident (CVA).	Application of pressure from an inflated cuff can temporarily impair blood flow and compromise circulation.
3. Explain to client purpose of procedure.	Reassures client.
4. Wash hands.	Reduces transmission of microorganisms.
5. Assist client to comfortable sitting position, with upper arm slightly flexed, forearm supported at heart level, and palm turned up.	Having arm above level of heart produces false-low readings. This position facilitates cuff application.
6. Expose client's upper arm fully.	Ensures proper cuff application.
7. Palpate brachial artery (on lower medial side of biceps muscle). Position cuff 2.5 cm (1 inch) above site of pulsations (antecubital fossa).	Stethoscope will be placed over artery without touching cuff.
8. Center arrows marked on cuff along brachial artery.	Inflating bladder directly over brachial artery ensures that proper pressure is applied during inflation.

Steps	Rationale
9. With cuff fully deflated, wrap cuff evenly and snugly around upper arm.	Loose-fitting cuff causes false elevations in blood pressure readings.
10. Be sure that manometer is positioned at eye level. Observer should be no more than 1 meter (approximately 1 yard) away.	Ensures accurate reading of mercury level.
11. Palpate brachial artery while inflating cuff rapidly to pressure 30 mm Hg above point at which pulse disappears. Slowly deflate cuff and note point when pulse reappears.	Identifies approximate systolic pressure and determines maximal inflation point for accurate reading. Prevents auscultatory gap.
12. Place stethoscope earpieces in your ears and be sure sounds are clear, not muffled.	Each earpiece should follow angle of your ear canal to facilitate hearing.
13. Deflate cuff and wait 30 seconds.	Prevents venous congestion and false elevated readings.
14. Relocate brachial artery and place diaphragm (or bell) of stethoscope over it (Fig. 9).	Ensures optimal sound reception. American Heart Association (AHA) recommends use of bell for detecting low-pitched Korotkoff sounds.

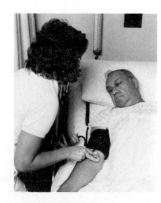

Fig. 9

Steps	Rationale
15. Close valve of pressure bulb clockwise until tight.	Prevents air leak during inflation.
16. Inflate cuff to 30 mm Hg above client's palpated systolic level.	Ensures accurate pressure measurement.
17. Slowly release valve, allowing mercury to fall at rate of 2 to 3 mm Hg per second.	Too rapid or too slow decline in mercury level may lead to inaccurate reading.
18. Note point on manometer at which first clear sound is heard.	First Korotkoff sound indicates systolic pressure.
19. Continue to deflate cuff gradually, noting point at which muffled or dampened sound appears, and point on manometer at which sound disappears in adults. (Note pressure to nearest 2 mm Hg).	Fourth Korotkoff sound may be detected as diastolic pressure in adults with hypertension. AHA recommends it as indication of diastolic pressure in children. AHA recommends recording fifth Korotokoff sound as diastolic pressure in adults.
20. Deflate cuff rapidly and remove it from client's arm unless you need to repeat measurement.	Continuous inflation causes arterial occlusion, resulting in numbness and tingling (paresthesia) of client's arm.
21. If repeating procedure, wait 30 seconds.	Prevents venous congestion and falsely high readings.
22. Fold cuff and store it properly.	Proper maintenance of supplies contributes to instrument accuracy.
23. Assist client to position he prefers and cover his upper arm.	Maintains client's comfort.
24. Record findings on medical record or flow sheet.	Document procedure and client status.
25. Wash hands.	Reduces transmission of microorganisms.

Nurse Alert

Although hypertension may be asymptomatic, be aware of possible signs and symptoms of high blood pressure (hypertension): headache (usually occipital), flushing of the face, nosebleed, fatigue in elderly clients. Be aware also of the signs and symptoms of low blood pressure (hypotension): dizziness, mental confusion, restlessness, pale or cyanotic (dusky) skin and mucous membranes, cool mottled skin over the extremities.

Client Teaching

Clients should understand the risk factors for high blood pressure: obesity, increased sodium intake, increased cholesterol intake, smoking, lack of exercise. When clients are taking antihypertensive medications, review their medication schedules and assess their understanding of the purpose and importance of the medication.

Pediatric Considerations

A newborn (3000 g or 6.6 lb) has an average systolic pressure of 50 to 52, diastolic of 25 to 30, and mean of 35 to 40 mm Hg. At 4 years the average blood pressure is 85/60; at 6 years it averages 95/62; and at 12 years, 108/67.

Geriatric Considerations

With aging there is a reduction in blood vessel compliance and an increase in peripheral resistance to blood flow. Arteriosclerosis is a common disorder with advancing age, although it can begin in early adulthood. Because of vascular changes, elderly clients are at risk of significantly increased systolic and slightly increased diastolic pressures.

Assessing Pulse Oximetry

Pulse oximetry is the noninvasive measurement of arterial oxygen saturation (Sao_2). The pulse oximeter uses fiberoptics to measure the amount of oxygenated hemoglobin in arterial blood. The oximeter probe can be applied to the earlobe, finger, toe, or bridge of the nose in adults, and the foot, wrist, or hand in infants. Noninvasive measurement of oxygenation has few of the risks associated with arterial blood gas samples or in-dwelling arterial catheters. The oximeter is accurate and precise for saturation in the 50% to 100% range but may not be reliable at lower saturations (Spyr and Preach, 1990). Pulse oximetry is clinically indicated in clients who have an unstable oxygen status and in those who are at risk for alterations in oxygenation.

Potential Nursing Diagnoses

Client data derived during the assessment process reveal defining characteristics to support the following nursing diagnoses for client's requiring this skill:

Impaired gas exchange
Inability to sustain spontaneous ventilation
Ineffective airway clearance
Ineffective breathing pattern
Potential activity intolerance

Equipment

Pulse oximeter
Sensor probe
Continuous printout (optional)
Pen, pencil, and flow sheet

Steps	Rationale
1. Wash hands.	Reduces transmission of micro-organisms.
2. Position client comfortably and support dependent extremity to be used for monitoring.	Ensures probe positioning and decreases motion interference with signal.
3. Instruct client to breath normally.	Prevents large fluctuations in minute ventilation and possible changes in Sao_2.
4. Remove finger nail polish (if finger is to be used).	Polish can falsely alter saturation.
5. Attach sensor probe to finger, earlobe, or bridge of nose.	Select sensor site based on peripheral circulation and extremity temperature. Peripheral vasoconstriction can alter Sao_2
6. Watch pulse bar for pulse sensing.	Amplitude of pulse bar sensor indicates how well oximeter monitors pulse.
7. Determine that client's radial pulse correlates with the pulse on the oximeter and read saturation level.	Ensures accuracy of oximeter, double-checks pulse against machine.
8. Record Sao_2 in client's record or flow sheet.	Documents procedure and client's status.

Nurse Alert

Clients who smoke cigarettes or who use nicotine gum may have reduced peripheral circulation, which can make monitoring difficult and reduce accuracy of arterial saturation monitor.

Clients who have peripheral vascular disease or Raynaud's syndrome or who simply have cold hands may be difficult to monitor if using their hands, thus another site should be used.

Decreased pH, increased temperature, and increased $Paco_2$ cause oxyhemoglobin curve to shift to right, resulting in lower saturation for the same Pao_2. Conversely, elevated pH, low temperature, decreased 2,3-diphosphoglycerate (DPG), and decreased

Paco$_2$ shift curve to left, resulting in higher saturation at lower Pao$_2$ (Schnapp and Cohen, 1990).

Pulse oximetry is used in home care to noninvasively monitor oxygen therapy or changes in oxygen therapy.

Client Teaching

Teach significance of monitoring arterial saturation.

Teach signs and symptoms of hypoxemia: headache, somnolence, confusion, dusky color, shortness of breath.

Measuring Central Venous Pressure

Central venous pressure (CVP) measurement is a useful tool in the care of acutely ill patients. The CVP measurement reflects the pressure in the great veins (superior vena cava and the inferior vena cava). It is used to monitor circulating blood volume, right ventricular function, and the central venous return, though it does not directly measure the right atrial pressure (Peterson, 1985).

The central venous catheter is placed by a physician into one of the large veins that empty into the vena cava, such as the internal jugular or the subclavian vein. A manometer and stopcock are then attached to the IV tubing to determine the pressure measurement. Care must be taken by the nurse to prevent contamination of the stopcock and CVP tip, to avoid the entrance of air into the vascular bed, and to take the CVP measurement at the same place on the patient at each time.

Potential Nursing Diagnoses

Client data derived during the assessment reveal defining characteristics to support the following nursing diagnoses for clients requiring this skill:

Fluid volume deficit
Fluid volume excess
Altered peripheral perfusion

Equipment

CVP manometer with vented top and cm H_2O gradations
Three-way stopcock with Luer adaptors
Sterile dead-end caps
Pen, pencil, and flow sheet
IV fluids with tubing

Steps	Rationale
1. Identify client whose potential for fluid imbalance or hypotension may require CVP measurement.	Clients at risk for hypotension or fluid imbalance include those with cardiac decompensation (including cardiomyopathy), overwhelming infection leading to sepsis, hemorrhage, postoperative recovery, any form of shock, and other conditions where rapid fluid shifts occur.
2. Observe for signs and symptoms indicating need for CVP measurement: a. Blood pressure low or labile b. Intake and output widely diverse c. Fluid administration at a rapid rate	CVP measurement helps determine the cause of hypotension and thus the appropriate treatment.
3. Review client's medical record for physician's order to measure CVP and the frequency that was ordered.	CVP measurement must be ordered by a physician.
4. Wash hands.	Reduces transmission of microorganisms.
5. Explain the procedure to the client.	Promotes understanding and reduces anxiety.
6. Position the client supine.	Lateral positions produce significantly higher CVP readings (Banasik and Broderson, 1991). Maintaining the same position for each reading provides for more consistent, comparable results.
7. Mark an "X" with the indelible pen at the level of the right atrium (midaxillary line in the fourth intercostal space).	The zero mark on the CVP manometer should always be placed on this "X" (zero point) to minimize variations in measurement.

Steps	Rationale
8. Connect the IV fluids to the three-way stopcock and flush the other two ports with the fluids.	Flushing IV fluids forces air out of the stopcock.
9. Connect the CVP manometer to the upper port of the stopcock.	Avoid touching the tips of the manometer or the stopcock.
10. Connect the CVP tubing from the patient to the second side port of the stopcock.	Establishes IV line from fluids to CVP catheter.
11. Allow IV fluid to drip rapidly into patient for several seconds, with stopcock closed to manometer.	This ensures patency of the CVP line. If fluids do not flow freely, CVP reading will be inaccurate.
12. Turn stopcock off to patient and fill manometer with IV fluid.	Manometer must be vented to air on top for fluid to fill tubing.
13. Hold manometer at "X" on thorax and turn stopcock off to IV fluids, so system is patent from manometer to client.	Fluid in manometer will fall rapidly to a level equal to the amount of pressure in the central veins.
14. Take reading when fluid level stabilizes (Fig. 10); read at end expiration if level fluctuates.	End expiration is associated with constant intrapleural pressure. CVP is decreased with negative pressure breathing and shock, and increased by positive pressure breathing, straining, increased blood volume, and heart failure. Normal CVP is 2 to 8 cm H_2O (Alspach, 1991).
15. Turn stopcock off to manometer, leaving IV fluids in place at ordered fluid rate.	

Steps   Rationale

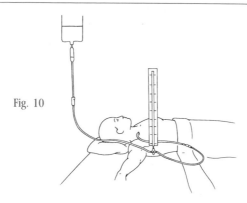

Fig. 10

16. Remove manometer from   Sterile cap prevents contamina-
    stopcock. Place sterile   tion of open ports and allows
    dead-end cap on upper port   for reuse without contamination.
    of stopcock and at connec-
    tor site of CVP manometer.

17. Wash hands.   Reduces transmission of micro-
                                   organisms.

18. Compare CVP reading with   Identifies physiologic changes
    any previous readings.   occurring in relation to fluid
                                   volume and blood pressure.

19. Record the CVP reading on   Abnormal values often require
    flow sheet. Report any ab-   immediate treatment.
    normal values to the nurse
    in charge or physician.

Nurse Alert

If fluids without medication are already infusing into the CVP
line, a stopcock may be carefully inserted at the connector site
and used for CVP measurement without adding another bottle of
fluids.

For frequent repeated measurements, the manometer may be
left in place on the bed.

If manometer is removed each time, care must be taken that the dead-end cap does not become contaminated—if it is contaminated, it should be disposed of and a new one obtained.

Client Teaching

Client should be instructed not to manipulate the stopcock or dead-end cap.

POSITIONING
AND
TRANSFER

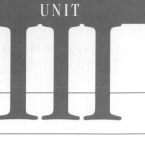

Proper Lifting

The nurse is at risk for injury to lumbar muscles in lifting. The rate of injuries in occupational settings has increased in recent years, and more than one half are back injuries resulting from improper lifting and bending techniques (Owen and Garg, 1991). Injury to the lumbar area affects the ability to bend forward, backward, and from side to side. In addition, the ability to rotate the hips and lower back is decreased.

As more clients are being discharged into the home setting for continuing care, it is necessary for the nurse to teach members of the client's family how to lift and transfer the client safely.

The purpose of this skill and all skills in this unit is to teach both the nurse and family members how to safely and correctly lift and transfer the client with impaired mobility.

Potential Nursing Diagnoses

Client data derived during the assessment reveal defining characteristics to support the following nursing diagnoses for clients requiring this skill:

Impaired skin integrity

High risk for injury

Steps	Rationale
1. Assess "basic four" lifting measures:	
a. Position of weight: The weight to be lifted should be as close to the lifter as possible.	Places the object to be lifted in the same plane as the lifter (Stamps, 1989).

Steps	Rationale

b. Height of object: The best height for lifting vertically is slightly above the level of the middle finger of a person with the arm hanging at the side (Owen and Garg, 1991).

c. Body position: The lifter should be positioned with the trunk erect so that multiple muscle groups work together.

d. Maximum weight: An object is too heavy if it is greater than 35% of the lifter's body weight.
    Determines need for assistance from additional personnel during lift.

2. Come close to object to be moved.
    Moves the lifter's center of gravity closer to the object.

3. Enlarge your base of support, placing feet apart.
    Maintains better body balance, reducing your risk of falling.

4. Lower your center of gravity to object to be lifted.
    Increases body balance and enables your muscle groups to work together in synchronized manner.

5. Maintain proper alignment of head and neck with vertebrae, keeping trunk straight.
    Reduces risk of injury to lumbar vertebrae and muscle groups (Owen and Garg, 1991).

Nurse Alert

Before lifting an object the nurse should decide if it can be safely lifted by one person. If the nurse feels that the object is too large or too heavy, additional personnel should be sought for assistance.

Client Teaching

Demonstrating correct lifting techniques is an excellent way for the nurse to teach the client and family how they can avoid injuring themselves when moving something.

Geriatric Considerations

The geriatric client may require reeducation on what he can and cannot safely lift. Objects that could be safely lifted in the early and middle adult years cannot usually be lifted in the later adult years.

Supported Fowler
Position

Correct positioning of a client is crucial for maintaining proper body alignment. Any client with impaired mobility is at risk of developing contractures, postural abnormalities, and pressure sores. The nurse has the primary responsibility to minimize this risk, which is done by changing the position of the client experiencing impaired mobility and decreased sensation at frequent intervals.

The supported Fowler position improves cardiac output and ventilation and facilitates urinary and bowel elimination. In this position the head of the client's bed is raised 45 to 60 degrees, and the client's knees are slightly elevated so no restriction of circulation to the lower extremities occurs. Proper alignment of the body when the client is in this position requires support that maintains comfort and reduces the risk of damage to body systems.

Potential Nursing Diagnoses

Client data derived during the assessment reveal defining characteristics to support the following nursing diagnoses in clients requiring these skills:

Impaired physical mobility
Impaired skin integrity
Altered peripheral tissue perfusion

Steps	Rationale
1. Wash hands and don gloves (if appropriate).	Reduces transmission of micro-organisms.
2. Position client supine with his head near headboard.	Prevents client from sliding toward foot of bed when head of bed is elevated.

Steps	Rationale
3. Elevate head of bed 45 to 60 degrees.	Increases client comfort, improves breathing, and increases his opportunity to socialize, relax, or watch television.
4. Rest client's head against mattress or on very small pillow.	Prevents flexion contracture of client's cervical vertebrae.
5. Use pillows to support client's arms and hands if he does not have voluntary control or use of arms and hands.	Prevents shoulder dislocation from downward gravitational pull of unsupported arms, promotes circulation by preventing venous pooling, reduces edema in arms or hands, and prevents flexion contractures of wrist.
6. Position pillow at client's lower back.	Supports lumbar vertebrae and decreases flexion of vertebrae.
7. Place small pillow or roll under client's thighs. If his lower extremities are paralyzed or he is unable to control lower extremities, use a trochanter roll in addition to a pillow under his thighs.	Prevents hyperextension of knees and occlusion of popliteal artery caused by pressure from body weight. Trochanter roll prevents external rotation of legs.
8. Place small pillow or roll under ankles.	Prevents prolonged pressure on heels from mattress.
9. Place footboard (Fig. 11) at bottom of client's feet.	Maintains feet in dorsiflexion. Reduces risk of foot-drop.

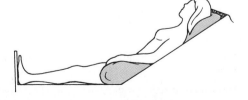

Fig. 11

Steps	Rationale
10. Remove gloves and wash your hands.	Reduces transmission of micro-organisms.
11. Record in nurse's notes client's new position.	Documents that procedure was performed.

Nurse Alert

Clients in the Fowler position are at risk of cervical flexion con-tractures if the pillow is too thick. Additional complications may include external rotation of the hips, foot-drop, and skin break-down at the sacrum and heels.

Client Teaching

The Fowler position provides an excellent opportunity for the nurse to implement client teaching in self-care (as with the newly diagnosed diabetic client), skin care, and knowledge about med-ications.

Geriatric Considerations

Elderly clients are at greater risk than are younger clients of skin breakdown because of increased capillary fragility, decreased muscle mass, and reduced skin moisture.

Supported Supine
Position

The supine position, also called the dorsal recumbent position, may be required after spinal surgery and administration of some spinal anesthetics. In this position the relationship of body parts is essentially the same as in proper standing alignment, except that the body is horizontal.

Potential Nursing Diagnoses

Client data derived during the assessment reveal defining characteristics to support the following diagnoses in clients requiring this skill:

Impaired physical mobility
Impaired skin integrity
Altered peripheral tissue perfusion

Steps	Rationale
1. Wash hands and don gloves (if appropriate).	Reduces transmission of microorganisms.
2. Place client flat in center of bed.	Prepares client for proper positioning.
3. Place small pillow or rolled towel under client's lumbar spine (Fig. 12).	Provides support to lumbar vertebrae.

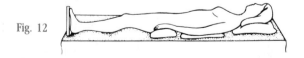

Fig. 12

Steps	Rationale
4. Place pillow under client's upper shoulders, neck, and head.	Maintains correct alignment and prevents flexion contracture of cervical vertebrae.
5. When necessary, place trochanter rolls or sandbags parallel with lateral surface of his thighs.	Reduces external rotation of hips.
6. Place small pillow or roll under client's ankles to elevate heels.	Raising heels from surface of bed reduces pressure on them.
7. Place footboard or footdrop stops against bottom of client's feet.	Maintains feet in dorsiflexion. Reduces risk of foot-drop.
8. Place pillows under pronated forearms, maintaining upper arms parallel with body (Fig. 13).	Reduces internal rotation of shoulders and prevents extension of elbows.

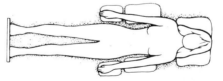

Fig. 13

9. Place hand rolls or towels in client's hands or use hand splints when available.	Reduces extension of fingers and abduction of thumb. Maintains thumb slightly adducted and in opposition to the fingers.
10. Remove gloves and wash your hands.	Reduces transmission of microorganisms.
11. Record in nurse's notes client's new position.	Documents that procedure was performed.

Nurse Alert

Clients in the supine position are at risk of internal rotation of the shoulders, external rotation of the hips, foot-drop, and pressure sores at the lumbar vertebrae, elbows, heels, and scapulae.

Client Teaching

While the client is supine, the nurse can teach him and his family the prescribed range-of-joint-motion exercises and skin care measures.

Pediatric Considerations

A child may be restrained in the supine position to maintain patency of an IV catheter or the integrity of postoperative drains. The nurse should incorporate time to hold and play with the child into her plan of care.

Geriatric Considerations

Elderly clients are at greater risk than are younger clients of skin breakdown because of increased capillary fragility, decreased muscle mass, and reduced skin moisture.

Supported Prone
Position

The primary therapeutic use of the prone position is to provide an alternative for clients who are immobilized or on prolonged bedrest. It is not a well-tolerated position, and frequent changes are required to relieve boredom and discomfort.

Potential Nursing Diagnoses

Client data derived during the assessment reveal defining characteristics to support the following diagnoses in clients requiring this skill:

Impaired physical mobility
Impaired skin integrity
Altered peripheral tissue perfusion

Steps	Rationale
1. Wash hands and don gloves (if appropriate).	Reduces transmission of micro-organisms.
2. Place client in supine position in center of flat bed.	Provides easy access to client and ease of repositioning client without working against gravity.
3. Roll client over arm positioned close to body with elbow straight and hand under hip. Position client on abdomen in center of flat bed.	Positions client so that alignment can be maintained.

Steps	Rationale
4. Turn client's head to one side and support with small pillow (Fig. 14). When excessive drainage from mouth is present, pillow may be contraindicated.	Reduces flexion or hyperextension of cervical vertebrae.

Fig. 14

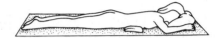

5. Place small pillow under client's abdomen below level of diaphragm.	Reduces pressure on breasts in some female clients, decreases hyperextension of lumbar vertebrae, and improves breathing by reducing pressure on diaphragm from mattress.
6. Position feet at right angles to legs, using pillow to elevate toes (Fig. 15).	Prevents foot-drop and reduces external rotation of legs and pressure on toes from mattress.

Fig. 15

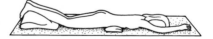

7. Remove gloves and wash your hands.	Reduces transmission of microorganisms.
8. Record in nurse's notes client's new position.	Documents that procedure was performed.

Nurse Alert

When placing a client in the prone position, the nurse should be sure that a pillow is under the client's lower legs to promote dorsiflexion of the ankles and knee flexion. Body alignment is poor when the ankles are continuously in plantar flexion and the lumbar spine remains hyperextended. In addition, the nurse must frequently assess the client's breathing patterns to detect any alterations that might result from the prone position.

Client Teaching

When the client is prone, the nurse can effectively teach his family about skin care or any dressing changes that may be required on the back.

Pediatric Considerations

Children placed prone usually do not tolerate the position well because of limited eye contact with their environment. When the prone position is required, the nurse should incorporate quiet play or stories into her plan of care.

Geriatric Considerations

Elderly clients may become disoriented when in the prone position because of decreased visual cues from their environment. The nurse can reduce this risk by placing a clock within the client's visual field, increasing the amount of time she spends with the client, and encouraging visitation by family.

Supported Side-Lying
(Lateral) Position

The side-lying position removes pressure from any bony prominences on the client's back and redistributes the major portion of
his body weight on the dependent hip and shoulder. In this position the client's trunk alignment should be the same as in proper
standing posture.

Potential Nursing Diagnoses

Client data derived during the assessment reveal defining characteristics to support the following diagnoses in clients requiring
this skill:

Impaired physical mobility
Impaired skin integrity
Altered peripheral tissue perfusion

Steps	Rationale
1. Wash hands and don gloves (if appropriate).	Reduces transmission of micro-organisms.
2. Place client in supine position in center of flat bed.	Provides easy access to client and ease of repositioning client without working against gravity.
3. Roll client onto his side.	Prepares him for proper positioning.
4. Place pillow under client's head and neck.	Maintains alignment. Reduces lateral flexion of neck. Decreases muscle strain on sterno-cleidomastoid muscle.
5. Bring shoulder blade forward.	Prevents client's weight from resting directly on shoulder joint.

Steps	Rationale
6. Position both arms in slightly flexed position: upper arm supported by a pillow level with shoulder.	Decreases internal rotation and adduction of shoulder, preventing dislocation. Supporting both arms in a slightly flexed position protects joints and improves ventilation because chest is able to expand more easily.
7. Place rolled pillow parallel to client's back.	Maintains support and alignment of vertebrae. Also keeps client from rolling back out of alignment and prevents rotation of spine.
8. Place one or two pillows under client's upper leg. Pillows should support leg evenly from groin to foot (Fig. 16).	Prevents internal rotation and adduction of thigh and reduces pressure to bony prominences of leg from mattress.

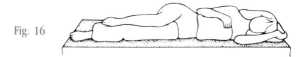

Fig. 16

9. Place supports, such as sandbags or foot-drop stops, at client's feet.	Maintains feet in dorsiflexion. Reduces risk of foot-drop.
10. Remove gloves and wash hands.	Reduces transmission of microorganisms.
11. Record in nurse's notes client's new position.	Documents that procedure was performed.

Nurse Alert

When placing a client in the side-lying position, the nurse should use caution to avoid lateral flexion of the neck, improper spinal alignment, internal rotation of the hips and shoulder joints, foot-drop, and pressure on the ilium, knees, and ankles.

Client Teaching

The side-lying position provides the nurse an excellent opportunity to teach the client (and family) about therapeutic measures that may be continued in the home.

Pediatric Considerations

The side-lying position is used with an unconscious, immobilized, or burned child. If the child is alert, the nurse should incorporate quiet diversional activities into her plan of care so this position will be maintained.

Geriatric Considerations

Elderly clients are at greater risk than are younger clients of skin breakdown caused by increased capillary fragility, decreased muscle mass, and reduced skin moisture.

Supported Sims'
(Semiprone) Position

The Sims' position is frequently used for an unconscious client to increase drainage of mucus from the mouth. In addition, it provides an alternative for clients who are immobilized or on bedrest. In this position the client's weight is placed on the anterior ilium and the humerus and clavicle.

Potential Nursing Diagnoses

Client data derived during the assessment reveal defining characteristics to support the following diagnoses in clients requiring this skill:

Impaired physical mobility
Impaired skin integrity
Altered peripheral tissue perfusion

Steps	Rationale
1. Wash hands and don gloves (if appropriate).	Reduces transmission of microorganisms.
2. Place client in supine position in center of flat bed.	Provides easy access to client and ease of repositioning client without working against gravity.
3. Position client in lateral position lying partially on abdomen.	Prepares client for proper positioning.
4. Place small pillow under head.	Maintains proper alignment and prevents lateral neck flexion.
5. Place a pillow under client's flexed arm. Pillow should extend from his hand to elbow.	Prevents internal rotation of shoulder.

Steps	Rationale
6. Place pillow under flexed leg, supporting leg level with hip (Fig. 17).	Prevents internal rotation of hip and adduction of leg. Prevents pressure on knees and ankles from mattress.

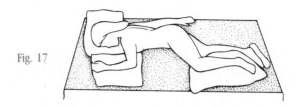

Fig. 17

Steps	Rationale
7. Place sandbags against client's feet.	Maintains feet in dorsiflexion. Reduces risk of foot-drop.
8. Remove gloves and wash hands.	Reduces transmission of micro-organisms.
9. Record in nurse's notes client's new position.	Documents that procedure was performed.

Nurse Alert

The nurse should be aware of potential trouble areas with the Sims' position: lateral flexion of the neck; internal rotation, adduction, or lack of support to the shoulders and hips; foot-drop; and potential pressure sores at the ears, ilium, humerus, clavicle, knees, and ankles.

Client Teaching

The Sims' position provides the nurse an opportunity to teach the family about range-of-joint motion and skin care. In addition, the nurse can demonstrate proper positioning measures.

Pediatric Considerations

The Sims' position is used with an unconscious, immobilized, or burned child. If the child is alert, the nurse should incorporate quiet diversional activities into her plan of care so the Sims' position will be maintained.

Geriatric Considerations

Because of the normal aging process, an elderly client's musculoskeletal system is at risk of joint deformities, loss of muscle mass, and skin breakdown. If degenerative joint disease (osteoarthritis) is also present, the client may require his position to be changed every hour instead of every 2 hours.

Assisting a Client
to Move Up in Bed

The nurse will frequently encounter a semi-helpless, helpless, or immobilized client whose position must be changed or who must be moved up in bed. Proper use of body mechanics can enable her (and a helper) to move, lift, or transfer such a client safely and at the same time avoid musculoskeletal injury to all involved.

Potential Nursing Diagnoses

Client data derived during the assessment reveal defining characteristics to support the following diagnoses in clients requiring this skill:

Impaired physical mobility
Impaired skin integrity
Activity intolerance

Steps	Rationale
1. Wash hands, and don gloves if appropriate.	Reduces transmission of micro-organisms.
2. Put bed in flat position with wheels on bed locked.	Provides easy access to client and allows positioning of client without working against gravity.
3. Face head of bed. (If two nurses are assisting client, they stand at opposite sides of bed.)	Facing direction of movement prevents twisting of your body when moving client.
4. Place your feet apart with foot nearer bed behind other foot.	Increases your balance. One foot behind other allows you to transfer your body weight as client is moved up in bed.

Steps	Rationale
5. If possible, ask client to flex his knees, bringing his feet as close to buttocks as possible.	Enables client to use his leg muscles during process of actually moving up in bed.
6. Instruct client to flex his neck, tilting chin toward chest.	Prevents hyperextension of neck when moving to head of bed.
7. Instruct client to assist in moving by using trapeze bar if available or by pushing on bed surface.	Reduces friction when client moves up in bed.
8. If client has limited upper-extremity strength or mobility, place his arms across his chest.	Prevents friction from arms dragging across bed surface during move.
9. Flex your knees and hips, bringing your forearms closer to level of bed.	Increases your balance and strength by bringing your center of gravity closer to client, the "object" to be moved.
10. Place your arm (that is closer to head of bed) under client's shoulder and your other arm under client's thighs.	Prevents trauma to client's musculoskeletal system because his shoulder and hip joints are supported. Also evenly distributes client's weight.
11. Instruct client to push with heels and elevate trunk while breathing out, then to move toward head of bed on count of 3.	Prepares client for actual move, thus reinforcing his assistance. Breathing out prevents Valsalva maneuver.
12. On count of 3, rock and shift your weight from back leg to front leg. At same time, client pushes with his heels and elevates his trunk (Fig. 18).	Enables you to improve your balance and overcome inertia. Shifting your weight counteracts client's weight. When client pushes with his heels and lifts his trunk, friction and workload are reduced.

Steps   Rationale

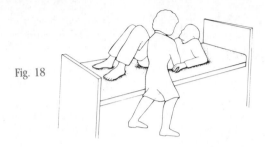

Fig. 18

13. Reassess client's body   Proper body alignment increases
    alignment. If poor, reposi-   client's comfort, promotes rest,
    tion client into proper posi-   and reduces hazards of immo-
    tion.   bility.

14. Remove gloves and wash   Reduces transmission of organ-
    hands.   isms.

15. Record client's new posi-   Documents that procedure was
    tion in nurse's notes.   performed.

Nurse Alert

The nurse must avoid dragging a client up in bed. This causes a
shearing force. The shearing force causes damage to the underlying tissue capillaries and reduces blood flow to the region. Shearing also causes abrasions to the skin, resulting in peripheral
thromboses, which further decreases blood flow to the area.

Client Teaching

This skill provides an excellent opportunity for the nurse to teach
a client and his family how to maintain proper body alignment
while moving him up in bed.

Pediatric Considerations

The nurse is usually able to pick up and reposition a child. However, when the child is in traction, additional assistance may be
needed to maintain alignment.

Geriatric Considerations

Elderly clients with degenerative joint disease (osteoarthritis) are at greater risk than are younger clients of shoulder joint dislocation while being moved. In addition, their decreased muscle mass and reduced skin elasticity and skin moisture increase their risk of skin breakdown from shearing force.

Assisting a Client to the Sitting Position

A partially immobilized or weak client will require nursing assistance to sit up in bed. The nurse can help such a client attain the sitting position while maintaining proper body alignment for herself and the client. Correct positioning techniques will reduce the risk of musculoskeletal injury to all persons involved.

Potential Nursing Diagnoses

Client data derived during the assessment reveal defining characteristics to support the following nursing diagnoses in clients requiring this skill:

Impaired physical mobility
Activity intolerance
Impaired skin integrity

Steps	Rationale
1. Wash hands and, if appropriate, don gloves.	Reduces transmission of microorganisms.
2. Place client in supine position.	Enables you to continually assess client's body alignment and administer additional care, such as suctioning or hygiene needs.
3. Remove all pillows.	Decreases interference while sitting client up in bed.
4. Face head of bed.	Reduces twisting of your body when moving client.

Steps	Rationale
5. Place your feet apart with foot nearer bed behind other foot.	Improves your balance and allows you to transfer your body weight as client is moved to sitting position.
6. Place hand that is farther from client under client's shoulders, supporting his head and cervical vertebrae.	Maintains alignment of client's head and cervical vertebrae and allows for even lifting of his upper trunk.
7. Place your other hand on bed surface.	Provides support and balance.
8. Raise client to a sitting position by shifting your weight from front leg to back leg.	Improves your balance, overcomes inertia, and transfers your weight in direction of move.
9. Push against bed with the hand that is on bed surface.	Divides activity of raising client to a sitting position between your arms and legs and protects your back from strain. By bracing one hand against mattress and pushing against it as you lift client, you transfer part of weight that would be lifted by your back muscles to your arm and onto mattress.
10. Remove gloves and wash hands.	Reduces transmission of microorganisms.
11. Record client's new position in nurse's notes.	Documents that procedure was performed.

Nurse Alert

The nurse must avoid dragging a client up in bed. Dragging against the bed linen causes shearing force. In addition, she should carefully observe the client for signs of development of postural hypotension (e.g., dizziness, fainting).

Client Teaching

This skill provides an opportunity for the client and family to learn appropriate body alignment for the sitting position.

Pediatric Considerations

Children are usually easy to move, and the nurse may be able to simply raise a child to the sitting position.

Geriatric Considerations

Elderly clients with degenerative joint disease (osteoarthritis) are at greater risk than are younger clients of shoulder joint dislocation while being moved. In addition, their decreased muscle mass and reduced skin elasticity and skin moisture increase the risk of skin breakdown from shearing force.

Assisting a Client to the Sitting Position on Edge of Bed

The partially immobilized or weak client will require nursing assistance to attain a sitting position on the edge of the bed. The nurse can help such a client sit up while at the same time (1) maintaining proper body alignment for herself and the client and (2) reducing the risk of musculoskeletal injuries to all persons involved. Frequently this is the first activity ordered for a client who has been on bedrest.

Potential Nursing Diagnoses

Client data derived during the assessment reveal defining characteristics to support the following nursing diagnoses in clients requiring this skill:

Impaired physical mobility
Activity intolerance
Impaired skin integrity

Steps	Rationale
1. Wash hands, and don gloves if appropriate.	Reduces transmission of microorganisms.
2. Place client in side-lying position, facing you on side of bed where he will be sitting. Put up side rail on opposite side.	Prepares client for move and protects him from falling.
3. Raise head of bed to highest level that client can tolerate.	Decreases amount of work needed by you and client to raise him to sitting position.

Steps	Rationale
4. Stand opposite client's hips.	Places your center of gravity nearer client.
5. Turn on a diagonal so you are facing client and far corner of bed.	Reduces twisting of your body because you are facing direction of movement.
6. Place your feet apart, with foot closer to head of bed in front of other foot.	Increases your balance and allows you to transfer your weight as client is brought to sitting position on edge of bed.
7. Place arm that is nearer head of bed under client's shoulders, supporting his head and neck.	Maintains alignment of client's head and neck as you bring him to sitting position.
8. Place your other arm over client's thighs (Fig. 19).	Supports client's hips and prevents him from falling backward during procedure.

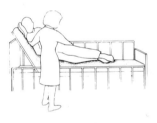

Fig. 19

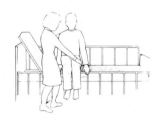

Fig. 20

9. Move client's lower legs and feet over edge of bed.	Decreases friction and resistance during the procedure.
10. Pivot toward your rear leg, allowing client's upper legs to swing downward (Fig. 20).	Allows gravity to work with you to lower client's legs.
11. At same time, shift your weight to rear leg and elevate client.	Allows you to transfer your weight in direction of motion.

Steps	Rationale
12. Remain in front of client until he regains balance.	Reduces client's risk of falling.
13. Lower the level of bed until client's feet are touching floor.	Supports client's feet in dorsal flexion and allows client to easily stand at side of bed.
14. Remove gloves and wash hands.	Reduces transmission of micro-organisms.
15. Record client's new position in nurse's notes.	Documents that procedure was performed.

Nurse Alert

A client who has been in bed for a long period is at risk of postural hypotension. The nurse should assess his vital signs before placing him in a sitting position. During the procedure, the nurse should assess for signs of dizziness, weakness, lightheadedness, or pallor. If these symptoms develop, stop the procedure. Once the client is stable and sitting on the edge of the bed, the nurse should reassess vital signs.

Client Teaching

This skill provides the client and family an opportunity to learn the basic mechanics of appropriate body alignment for the sitting position.

Pediatric Considerations

Children are usually easy to move, and the nurse may be able to independently lift a child up in bed.

Geriatric Considerations

Elderly clients with degenerative joint disease (osteoarthritis) are at greater risk than are younger clients of shoulder joint dislocation while being assisted to a sitting position in bed. In addition, because of underlying cardiovascular disease, they may be at increased risk of postural hypotension.

Transferring a Client from Bed to Chair

Transferring a client from bed to chair enables the nurse to change his surroundings as well as his position. If the client is able to tolerate transfer to a wheelchair, the nurse can move him out of his room into other surroundings and increase his opportunities for socialization. For clients who have been on bedrest, this is one of the first activities to be resumed.

Potential Nursing Diagnoses

Client data derived during the assessment reveal defining characteristics to support the following nursing diagnoses in clients requiring this skill:

Impaired physical mobility
Activity intolerance
Impaired skin integrity

Steps	Rationale
1. Wash hands, and don gloves if appropriate.	Reduces transmission of microorganisms.
2. Assist client to a sitting position on side of bed. Have chair positioned at a 45-degree angle to bed.	Prepares client for move.
3. Apply transfer belt if necessary.	Allows nurse to maintain stability of client during transfer and reduces risk of falling.
4. Ensure that client wears stable, nonskid shoes.	Decreases risk of slipping during transfer.
5. Place your feet apart.	Ensures better balance.

Steps	Rationale
6. Flex your hips and knees, aligning your knees with those of client (Fig. 21).	Flexion of hips and knees lowers your center of gravity to level of "object" being raised. Aligning your knees with client's knees allows for stabilization when he stands.

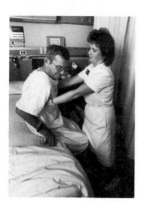

Fig. 21

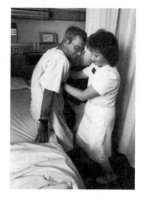

Fig. 22

7. Grasp transfer belt from underneath or reach through client's axillae and place hands on client's scapulae.	Reduces pressure on axillae and maintains client stability.
8. Rock client up to standing on count of 3 while straightening your hips and legs, keeping knees slightly flexed (Fig. 22).	Gives client's body momentum and requires less muscular effort to lift client. Uses correct body mechanics to raise client to standing position.
9. Maintain stability of weak or paralyzed leg with knee.	Ability to stand can often be maintained in paralyzed or weak limb with support of knee to stabilize.

Steps	Rationale
10. Pivot on foot that is farther from chair, moving client directly in front of chair (Fig. 23).	Maintains client's support while allowing adequate space for him to move.

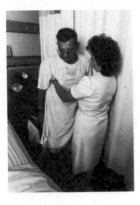

Fig. 23

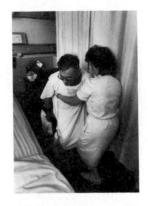

Fig. 24

Steps	Rationale
11. Instruct client to use armrests on chair for support.	Increases client's stability.
12. Flex your hips and knees while lowering client into chair (Fig. 24).	Prevents injury to you resulting from poor body mechanics.
13. Assess client for proper alignment.	
14. Remove gloves and wash hands.	Reduces transmission of microorganisms.
15. Record client's safe transfer to chair in nurse's notes.	Documents that procedure was performed.

Nurse Alert

Transfer of a client from bed to chair by one nurse requires assistance from the client and should not be attempted if the client is unable to help or to understand the nurse's instructions.

Client Teaching

This is an appropriate time to teach the client and his family the principles of safe-transfer technique and body alignment.

Pediatric Considerations

Because children often are easier to move, the nurse may be able to independently lift a child from bed to chair. However, once the child is in the chair, the nurse must reassess his body alignment to ensure proper positioning.

Geriatric Considerations

Physiologic changes of aging result in some sensory disturbances that make transferring an elderly client from bed to chair more difficult. First, the client may be increasingly susceptible to postural hypotension, dizziness, and the risk of fainting. Second, changes in his visual and hearing acuity may make it more difficult for him to accurately visualize the chair or understand instructions. Last, decreased balance and changes in the musculoskeletal system increase his risk of falling.

Crutch Walking

Crutches are often needed to increase a client's mobility. The use of crutches may be temporary (such as after ligament damage to the knee) or permanent (as with paralysis of the lower extremities). It is important that crutches be measured for the appropriate length and that clients be taught how to use them correctly.

Potential Nursing Diagnoses

Client data derived during the assessment reveal defining characteristics to support the following nursing diagnoses in clients requiring this skill:

Impaired physical mobility
High risk for injury

Equipment

Tape measure
Goniometer
Rubber crutch tips
Wooden crutches

Steps	Rationale
1. Wash hands.	Reduces transmission of micro-organisms.
2. Measure for crutch length: 3 to 4 finger widths from axilla to a point 15 cm (6 inches) lateral to client's heel is standard (Fig. 25).	Ensures that crutches are individualized to client's height.

Steps   Rationale

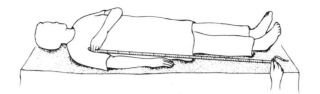

Fig. 25

3. Position crutch handgrips
   with elbows flexed at 20- to
   25-degree angle. Angle of
   elbow flexion should be
   verified by goniometer
   (Fig. 26).

Prevents client's body weight
from being supported by axil-
lae, which would result in nerve
damage.

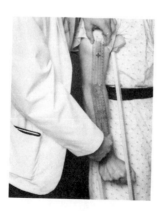

Fig. 26

4. Verify that distance between crutch pad and axilla
   is 3 to 4 finger widths (Fig.
   27).

Prevents axillary skin breakdown secondary to pressure
from crutch pad.

Steps   Rationale

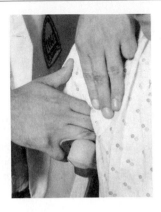

Fig. 27

5. Instruct client to assume   Improves balance by providing
   tripod stance. Tripod stance   wider base of support. No
   is formed when crutches   weight should be borne by axil-
   are placed 15 cm (6 inches)   lae.
   in front and 15 cm to side
   of each foot (Fig. 28).

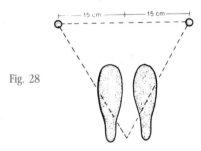

Fig. 28

6. Teach client one of four   Allows client to ambulate
   crutch-walking gaits.   safely. Specific type of gait
   (Darkened areas on Figs.   chosen depends on client's im-
   28 to 30 represent weight-   pairment and physician's order.
   bearing areas):

- Four-point alternating, or four-point gait, gives stability to client but requires weight bearing on both legs. Each leg is moved alternately with each crutch so three points of support are on floor at all times (Fig. 29).

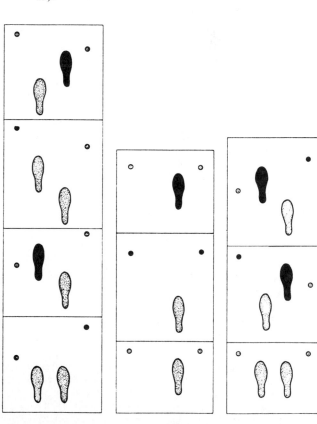

Fig. 29   Fig. 30   Fig. 31

Steps	Rationale

- Three-point alternating, or three-point gait, requires client to bear all weight on one foot. Weight is borne on uninvolved leg, then on both crutches, and the sequence is repeated. Affected leg does not touch ground during early phase of three-point gait. Gradually client progresses to touchdown and full weight bearing on affected leg (Fig. 30).
- Two-point gait requires at least partial weight bearing on each foot. Client moves each crutch at same time as opposing leg so crutch movements are similar to arm motion during normal walking (Fig. 31).
- Swing-through, or swing-to, gait is frequently used by paraplegics who wear weight-supporting braces on their legs. With weight on supported legs, the client places crutches one stride in front and then swings to or through them while they support his weight.

7. Teach client to ascend and descend on stairs:

Reduces risk of further damage to musculoskeletal system and risk of falling.

Steps	Rationale

Ascend
- Assume a tripod position.
- Transfer body weight to crutches (Fig. 32).
- Advance unaffected leg between crutches and stair.
- Shift weight from crutches to unaffected leg (Fig. 33).
- Align both crutches on stair (Fig. 34).

Descend
- Transfer body weight to unaffected leg (Fig. 35).
- Place crutches on stair and begin to transfer body weight to crutches, moving affected leg forward (Fig. 36).
- Align unaffected leg on stair with crutches (Fig. 37).

8. Teach client how to sit in chair and how to get up from chair:

Sitting
- Client positioned at center front of chair with posterior aspects of legs touching chair (Fig. 38).
- Client holds both crutches in hand opposite affected leg. If both legs are affected, crutches are held in hand on client's stronger side (Fig. 39).

Provides safe method of sitting in and getting up from chair. Reduces further damage to client's musculoskeletal system and the risk of falling.

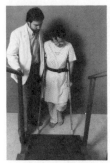
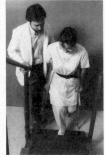
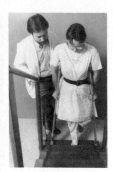

Fig. 32   Fig. 33   Fig. 34

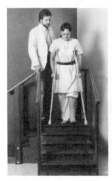
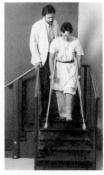
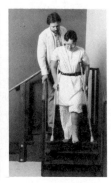

Fig. 35   Fig. 36   Fig. 37

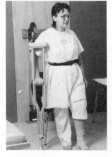
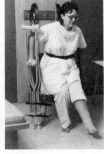
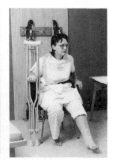

Fig. 38   Fig. 39   Fig. 40

Steps	Rationale
■ Client grasps arm of chair with other hand and lowers body into chair (Fig. 40).	

Getting up

- ■ Perform three steps above in reverse order.

9. Wash hands.	Reduces transmission of micro-organisms.
10. Record gait and procedures taught and client's ability to perform gaits in nurse's notes.	Documents teaching and client's learning.

Nurse Alert

The client with cognitive impairment or one who has received analgesics or tranquilizers may be unable to understand instructions or to ambulate safely with crutches.

Client Teaching

The nurse should instruct the client that, because of the potential for axillary skin breakdown and nerve damage, he must not lean on his crutches to support his body weight. Rubber crutch tips should be replaced as they wear out, and they should remain dry. Worn or wet crutch tips decrease surface tension and increase the risk of falling. The client should be given a list of medical suppliers in his community so he can obtain repairs as well as new rubber tips, handgrips, and crutch pads. In addition, advise him that he should have spare crutches and tips on hand.

Geriatric Considerations

The normal visual acuity and depth perception changes with aging may prevent the client from safely ascending or descending stairs with crutches.

Applying Elastic Stockings

Elastic stockings reduce the risk of thrombus formation. Available in toe-to-knee and toe-to-midthigh sizes, they promote venous return by maintaining pressure on the muscles of the lower extremities.

Potential Nursing Diagnoses

Client data derived during the assessment reveal defining characteristics to support the following nursing diagnosis in clients requiring this skill:

Altered peripheral tissue perfusion

Equipment

Talcum powder
Basin and water
Wash cloth and towel
Elastic support stockings in correct size

Steps	Rationale
1. Wash hands and don gloves, if appropriate.	Reduces transmission of micro-organisms.
2. After legs have been cleaned, apply a small amount of talcum powder to each leg and foot.	Reduces friction and allows for easier application of stocking.
3. Turn elastic stocking inside out down to foot by placing one hand into sock, holding toe of sock with other hand, and pulling (Fig. 41).	Allows easier application of stocking.

| Steps | Rationale |

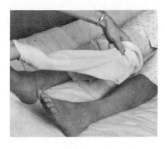

Fig. 41

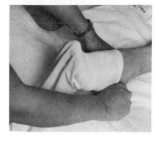

Fig. 42

4. Place client's toe into foot of elastic stocking, making sure that sock is smooth (Fig. 42).

   Wrinkles in sock can impede circulation to lower region of extremity.

5. Slide remaining portion of stocking over client's foot and heel, being sure that his toes are covered. Stocking will now be right side out (Fig. 43).

   Toes left uncovered are constricted by the elastic, and circulation in them can be reduced.

6. Slide stocking up over client's calf until it completely covers the leg. Be sure that it is smooth and contains no wrinkles (Fig. 44).

   Ridges impede venous return and can counteract overall purpose of elastic stocking.

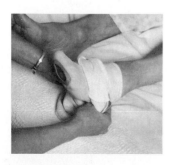

Fig. 43

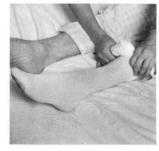

Fig. 44

Steps	Rationale
7. Instruct client not to roll the stockings partially down.	Rolling sock partially down will have a constricting effect and impede venous return.
8. Remove gloves and wash hands.	Reduces transmission of micro-organisms.
9. After 1 hour, observe stockings for wrinkles in binding, assess capillary refill in toes, and palpate pulses in feet.	Wrinkles increase pressure on skin and impair circulation. Assessment ensures that circulatory status in lower extremities has not been compromised.
10. Remove elastic stockings at least once every shift.	Enables you to clean and assess skin and vessels of the legs.
11. In nurses's notes, record removal and reapplication of elastic stockings, client's skin integrity, and adequacy of circulation to distal extremities.	Documents that procedure was performed.

Nurse Alert

Clients who wear elastic stockings must have the circulation to their distal extremities checked at least every 2 hours. The nurse evaluates the circulation by assessing capillary refill of the great toe. This is done by compressing the nail bed, observing the blanching, and noting the promptness of return to normal color (2 to 3 seconds). If capillary refill takes longer than 2 or 3 seconds and the toes are cold, the elastic stockings are impeding circulation and must be removed.

Client Education

This procedure enables the nurse to teach the client good foot care as well as application of elastic stockings for his return home.

Geriatric Considerations

Elastic stockings should not be used, or should be used only with caution, in clients who have chronic peripheral vascular disease, diabetes, or chronic venous leg ulcers.

PRESSURE
ULCERS

Risk Assessment and

Prevention

A pressure ulcer, or decubitus ulcer, is a lesion that develops in the skin as a result of prolonged, unrelieved pressure. Pressure, if not relieved, can cause irreversible tissue damage in as little as 90 minutes. These ulcers occur most often over bony prominences; however, they can occur in any area of the skin subjected to pressure. Such nonbony locations include the nares from nasogastric (NG) tubes or oxygen cannulae, the ears from oxygen cannulae, or the labia from tension of Foley catheters.

The pressure results in ischemia. Ischemia develops when the pressure on the skin is greater than the pressure inside the small peripheral blood vessels supplying blood to the skin. Normally the skin responds to this ischemia with a reddened area (regional hyperemia) that develops when the pressure is relieved. The regional hyperemia should resolve in a matter of minutes following pressure relief.

Pressure ulcers pose serious threats to a client's health. The break in the skin eliminates the body's first line of defense against infection. Ulcers that invade the subcutaneous tissues result in the loss of protein-rich and electrolyte-rich body fluids from the wound.

Optimum nursing care for the treatment of pressure ulcers comprises early identification of the at-risk client and implementation of prevention strategies. Three at-risk populations are (1) clients with a neurologic impairment that decreases sensation, (2) chronically ill clients, and (3) long-term care clients. These clients require continuous assessment of the skin and potential pressure sites (Fig. 45 on pages 124-125), meticulous hygiene, turning, and other aggressive measures to prevent pressure ulcer formation.

Potential Nursing Diagnoses

Client data derived during the assessment reveal defining characteristics to support the following nursing diagnoses for clients requiring this skill:

  Impaired physical mobility
  Impaired skin integrity
  High risk for impaired skin integrity
  Altered peripheral tissue perfusion

Equipment

Risk assessment tool
Devices to measure existing areas of skin breakdown
Documentation records
Pressure relief devices

Steps	Rationale
1. Assess client's risk for decubitus ulcer formation:	Determines need to administer preventive care in addition to use of topical agents for existing ulcers.
a. Paralysis or immobilization caused by restrictive devices	Client unable to turn or reposition self independently.
b. Sensory loss	Client feels no discomfort from pressure.
c. Circulatory disorders	Disorders reduce perfusion of skin's tissue layers.
d. Fever	Causes increase in metabolic demands of tissues. Accompanying diaphoresis leaves skin moist.
e. Anemia	Decreased hemoglobin reduces oxygen-carrying capacity of blood and amount of oxygen available to tissues.

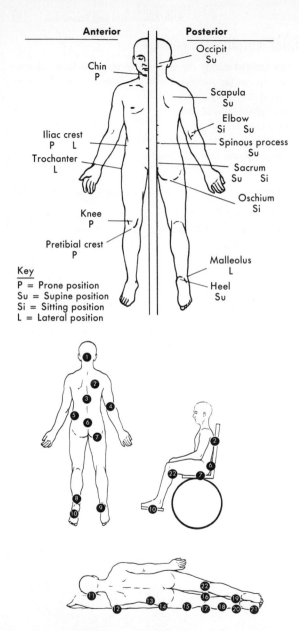

Anterior | Posterior

Chin
P

Occipit
Su

Scapula
Su

Elbow
Si   Su

Iliac crest
P   L

Spinous process
Su

Trochanter
L

Sacrum
Su   Si

Oschium
Si

Knee
P

Pretibial crest
P

Malleolus
L

Heel
Su

Key
P = Prone position
Su = Supine position
Si = Sitting position
L = Lateral position

Fig. 45

Steps	Rationale
f. Malnutrition	Inadequate nutrition can lead to weight loss, muscle atrophy, and reduced tissue mass. Less tissue is available as a pad between skin and underlying bone. A normal adult requires 0.8 to 1 g/kg/day of protein. Stable clients during acute illness require 1.5 g/kg/day, whereas stressed clients (e.g., those in the ICU) may need up to 2 to 3 g/kg/day (Arbiet and Way, 1988).
g. Incontinence	Skin becomes exposed to moist environment containing bacteria. Moisture causes skin maceration.
h. Heavy sedation and anesthesia	Client is not mentally alert; does not turn or change position independently. Sedation can also alter sensory perception.
i. Elderly	Skin is less elastic and drier; tissue mass is reduced.
j. Dehydration	Results in decreased elasticity and turgor.

Key for Fig. 45

Pressure ulcer sites

1. Occipital bone
2. Scapula
3. Spinous process
4. Elbow
5. Iliac crest
6. Sacrum
7. Ischium
8. Achilles tendon
9. Heel
10. Sole
11. Ear

12. Shoulder
13. Anterior iliac spine
14. Trochanter
15. Thigh
16. Medial knee
17. Lateral knee
18. Lower leg
19. Medial malleolus
20. Lateral malleolus
21. Lateral edge of foot
22. Posterior knee

Steps	Rationale
k. Edema	Edematous tissues are less tolerant of pressure, friction, and shear force.
l. Existing pressure ulcers	Limits surfaces available for position changes, placing available tissues at increased risk.
2. Assess condition of client's skin over regions of pressure (see Fig. 45):	
a. Redness, warmth	May indicate that tissue was under pressure. Hyperemia is normal physiologic response to hypoxemia in tissues.
b. Pallor and mottling	Persistent hypoxia in tissues that were under pressure—an abnormal physiologic response.
c. Absence of superficial skin layers	Represents early pressure ulcer formation.
3. Assess client for additional areas of potential pressure, specifically:	High-risk clients have multiple sites besides bony prominences for pressure necrosis:
a. Nares	NG tube, oxygen cannulae
b. Tongue, lips	Oral airway, ET tube
c. Ears	Oxygen cannulae, pillow
d. IV sites (especially long-term access sites)	Stress on catheter at exit site
e. Drainage tubes	Stress against tissue at exit site
f. Foley catheter	Pressure against labia, especially with edema
4. Observe client for preferred positions when in bed or chair.	Weight of body will be placed on certain bony prominences. The presence of contractures may result in pressure being exerted in unexpected places. This phenomenon can best be assessed through observation.

Steps	Rationale
5. Observe ability of client to initiate and assist with position changes.	Potential for friction and shear pressure increases when client is completely dependent on nurse for position changes.
6. Calculate "Risk Score" (Table 2).	Risk score will depend on the instrument used.
7. Assess client's and support persons' understanding of risks for pressure ulcers.	Provides opportunity for beginning prevention education.
8. Wash hands and don gloves.	Prevents transmission of infection.
9. Close room door or bedside curtain.	Maintains client privacy.
10. Assist client to change of position:	
a. Supine b. Prone c. Side-lying	See Unit III for specifics. Avoid positions that place client directly on an area of existing ulceration.
d. 30-degree oblique	Achieved with one pillow under the shoulder and one pillow under the leg on the same side. Protects sacrum and trochanters.
11. Observe area that had been under pressure for redness. Initial flushing is expected.	Early indication of pressure indicates need for more frequent position change. Delayed flushing may represent skin under stress from a poor hyperemic response, placing the client at high risk.
12. Palpate an area of redness or mottling.	Brisk capillary refill is an expected response; sluggish or completely absent capillary refill is an abnormal response. Skin should be gently palpated for texture.

Text continued on p. 133.

Table 2   Braden scale for predicting pressure sore risk

	1 Point	2 Points	3 Points	4 Points
Sensory Perception Ability to respond meaningfully to pressure-related discomfort	Completely Limited: Unresponsive (does not moan, flinch, or gasp) to painful stimuli because of diminished level of consciousness or sedation. OR Limited ability to feel pain over most of body surface.	Very Limited: Responds only to painful stimuli. Cannot communicate discomfort except by moaning or restlessness. OR Has a sensory impairment that limits the ability to feel pain or discomfort over half of body.	Slightly Limited: Responds to verbal commands but cannot always communicate discomfort or need to be turned. OR Has some sensory impairment that limits ability to feel pain or discomfort in 1 or 2 extremities.	No Impairment: Responds to verbal commands. Has no sensory deficit that would limit ability to feel or voice pain or discomfort.

	Constantly Moist:	Very Moist:	Occasionally Moist:	Rarely Moist:
Moisture Degree to which skin is exposed to moisture	Skin is kept moist almost constantly by perspiration, urine, etc. Dampness is detected every time patient is moved or turned.	Skin is often, but not always, moist. Linen must be changed at least once a shift.	Skin is occasionally moist, requiring an extra linen change approximately once a day.	Skin is usually dry; linen requires changing only at routine intervals.

	Bedfast:	Chairfast:	Walks Occasionally:	Walks Frequently:
Activity Degree of physical activity	Confined to bed.	Ability to walk severely limited or nonexistent. Cannot bear own weight and/or must be assisted into chair or wheelchair.	Walks occasionally during day, but for very short distances, with or without assistance. Spends majority of each shift in bed or chair.	Walks outside the room at least twice a day and inside room at least once every 2 hours during waking hours.

Continued.

Instructions: Score client in each of the six subscales. Maximum score is 23, indicating little or no risk. A score of ≤16 indicates "at risk"; ≤9 indicates high risk.

Copyright 1988. Used with permission of Barbara Braden, Ph.D., R.N.

Table 2   Braden scale for predicting pressure sore risk—cont'd

	1 Point	2 Points	3 Points	4 Points
Mobility Ability to change and control body position	Completely Immobile: Does not make even slight changes in body or extremity position without assistance.	Very Limited: Makes occasional slight changes in body or extremity position but unable to make frequent or significant changes independently.	Slightly Limited: Makes frequent though slight changes in body or extremity position independently.	No Limitations: Makes major and frequent changes in position without assistance.

Nutrition	Very Poor:	Probably Inadequate:	Adequate:	Excellent:
Usual food intake pattern	Never eats a complete meal. Rarely eats more than a third of any food offered. Eats 2 servings or less of protein (meat or dairy products) per day. Takes fluids poorly. Does not take a liquid dietary supplement. OR Is NPO and/or maintained on clear liquids or IVs for more than 5 days.	Rarely eats a complete meal and generally eats only about half of any food offered. Protein intake includes only 3 servings of meat or dairy products per day. Occasionally will take a dietary supplement. OR Receives less than optimal amount of liquid diet or tube feeding.	Eats over half of most meals. Eats a total of 4 servings of protein (meat, dairy products) each day. Occasionally will refuse a meal, but will usually take a supplement if offered. OR Is on a tube-feeding or TPN regimen that probably meets most of nutritional needs.	Eats most of every meal. Never refuses a meal. Usually eats a total of 4 or more servings of meat and dairy products. Occasionally eats between meals. Does not require supplements.

Continued.

Table 2 Braden scale for predicting pressure sore risk—cont'd

	1 Point	2 Points	3 Points	4 Points
Friction and Shear	Problem: Requires moderate to maximal assistance in moving. Complete lifting without sliding against sheets is impossible. Frequently slides down in bed or chair, requiring frequent repositioning with maximal assistance. Spasticity, contractions, or agitation leads to almost constant friction.	Potential Problem: Moves feebly or requires minimal assistance. Skin probably slides to some extent against sheets, chair, restraints, or other devices during a move. Maintains relatively good position in chair or bed most of the time, but occasionally slides down.	No Apparent Problem: Moves in bed and in chair independently and has sufficient muscle strength to sit up completely during move. Maintains good position in bed or chair at all times.	

Steps	Rationale

13. Monitor length of time any area of redness persists.
  ■ Determine appropriate turning interval.
  ■ Turning interval of less than 1½ to 2 hours may not be realistic, therefore use of a pressure relief device would be recommended.
	It is safe to assume redness will persist for 50% of the time hypoxia actually lasted.
	EXAMPLE: Previous turning interval 2 hours:
	  ■ Redness lasts 15 minutes.
	  ■ Hypoxia therefore lasted approximately 30 minutes.
	  ■ Recommended turning interval should be:
	    Turning interval − hypoxia time = suggested interval
	  ■ In this example, interval would be:
	    2 hours − 30 minutes = 1½ hours

14. Remove gloves and wash hands.	Prevents spread of microorganisms.
15. Record appearance of tissues under pressure.	Baseline observations coupled with subsequent inspections reveal success of prevention program.
16. Record positions used, turning intervals, and other prevention measures used.	Documents care provided.

Nurse Alert

The nurse should pay special attention to body regions that receive the greatest amount of pressure in specific positions: **sitting:** ischial tuberosities and sacrum; **supine:** back of skull, elbow, sacrum, ischial tuberosities, and heels; **prone:** elbows, knees, and toes; **side-lying:** knees and greater trochanters.

Clients who have experienced prolonged ($\geq$ 3 hours) surgical or testing procedures should be considered at risk.

Teaching Considerations

When teaching the alert client to change position for pressure relief, suggest using television programming/commercial intervals or use of a watch with hourly alarm intervals.

Pediatric Considerations

The pediatric client is at risk for skin breakdown when nutritional and electrolyte impairments, fever, circulatory disorders, and incontinence are present. Also, the pediatric client with orthopedic immobilization is at risk for pressure ulcers at the cast or traction site.

Geriatric Considerations

Many older adult clients are being cared for in their homes by family members or older adult spouses. In addition to the risks listed in Step 1, family members need to understand that consistency must be practiced for pressure ulcer assessment and prevention.

Treatment of Pressure Ulcers

Various topical agents have been used in treating pressure ulcers. Some of these agents (e.g., astringents, alkaline soap products) have proven harmful. Beneficial agents include enzymes, antiseptics, oxidizing agents, and dry dextranomer beads.

The agent of choice depends on the depth of the ulcer. Deeper ulcers may derive greater benefit from enzyme application.

Local treatment of pressure ulcers also includes using various dressings. The occlusive dressings are a group of dressings that are widely marketed and are being used with increasing frequency to treat pressure ulcers. These dressings (including transparent dressings, hydrocolloid dressings, and hydrogels) may be used in combination with topical agents or by themselves.

Potential Nursing Diagnoses

Client data derived during the assessment reveal defining characteristics to support the following nursing diagnoses in clients requiring this skill:

Impaired skin integrity

Equipment

Wash basin, soap, water, cleansing agent or prescribed topical agents, ordered dressings, skin protectant, cotton-tipped applicators, hypoallergenic tape or adhesive dressing sheet (Hypofix), disposable and sterile gloves, measuring device

Steps	Rationale
1. Wash hands and don gloves.	Reduces transmission of blood-borne pathogens. Gloves should be worn when handling items soiled by body fluids.

Table 3   Pressure ulcer stages*

Stage	Appearance
Stage 1	
Stage 2	
Stage 3	
Stage 4	
Stage 5	

*Stages describe layers of tissue visually involved. It is important to remember that even at the early stages (1 and 2), what is seen is only a small part of the damaged, swollen tissue underneath.

Nonblanchable erythema of the intact skin; may be soft or indurated; edge is usually irregular.

Partial-thickness skin loss involves epidermis and/or dermis. Ulcer is superficial and presents clinically as an abrasion, blister, or shallow crater.

Full-thickness skin loss involves damage or necrosis of subcutaneous tissue that may extend to the fascia. Ulcer presents clinically as a deep crater, with or without undermining of adjacent skin.

Full-thickness skin loss occurs with extensive destruction or necrosis through subcutaneous layers into muscle and bone. Ulcer edge appears to "roll over" into the defect and is a tough fibrinous ring.

Lesion is covered by a tough membranous layer that may be rigidly adherent to the ulcer base. Stage is difficult to determine until eschar has sloughed or has been surgically removed.

Steps	Rationale
2. Close room door or bedside curtains.	Maintains client's privacy.
3. Position client comfortably with area of decubitus ulcer and surrounding skir easily accessible.	Area should be accessible for cleansing of ulcer and surrounding skin.
4. Assess pressure ulcer and surrounding skin to determine ulcer stage (Table 3).	
a. Note color, moisture, and appearance of skin around ulcer.	Skin condition may indicate progressive tissue damage. Retained moisture causes maceration.
b. Measure two perpendicular diameters.	Provides an objective measure of wound size. May determine type of dressing chosen. Surface area = length (L) × width (W).
c. Measure depth of pressure ulcer using a sterile cotton-tipped applicator or other device that will allow a measurement of wound depth.	Depth measure is important for determining wound volume. Although surface area adequately represents tissue loss in stage 1 and 2 ulcers, volume more adequately represents tissue loss in the deeper stage 3 through 4 wounds.
	Volume = 2 (L × D) + 2 (W × D) + (L + D)
d. Measure depth (D) of skin undermined by lateral tissue necrosis. Use a sterile cotton-tipped applicator and gently probe under skin edges.	Undermining represents the loss of underlying tissues to a greater extent than that of the skin. Undermining may indicate progressive tissue necrosis.
5. Wash skin surrounding ulcer gently with warm water and soap. Rinse area thoroughly with water.	Cleansing of skin surface reduces number of resident bacteria. Soap can be irritating to skin.

Steps	Rationale
6. Gently dry skin thoroughly by patting lightly with towel.	Retained moisture causes maceration of skin layers.
7. Apply sterile gloves.	Aseptic technique must be maintained during cleansing, measuring, and application of dressings. (Check institutional policy regarding use of clean or sterile gloves.)

8. Cleanse ulcer thoroughly with normal saline or cleansing agent.
  a. Use irrigating syringe for deep ulcers.
  b. Cleansing may be accomplished in the shower with a hand-held shower head.
  c. Whirlpool treatments may be used to assist with wound cleansing and debridement.
	Removes debris of digested material from wound. Previously applied enzymes may require soaking for removal.

9. Apply topical agents, if prescribed (Table 4):	

Enzymes

▪ Keeping gloves sterile, place small amount of enzyme ointment in palm of hand.	It is not necessary to apply thick layer of ointment. A thin layer absorbs and acts more effectively. Excess medication can irritate surrounding skin. Apply only to necrotic areas.
▪ Soften medication by rubbing briskly in palm of hand.	Makes ointment easier to apply to ulcer.
▪ Apply thin, even layer of ointment over necrotic areas of ulcer. Do not apply enzyme to surrounding skin.	Proper distribution of ointment ensures effective action. Enzyme can cause burning, paresthesia, and dermatitis to surrounding skin.

Table 4 Treatment options by ulcer stage

Ulcer Stage	Ulcer Status	Dressing	Comments*	Expected Change	Adjuvants
1	Intact	None	Allows visual assessment.	Resolves slowly without epidermal loss over 7 to 14 days.	■ Turning schedule. ■ Support hydration. ■ Nutritional support. ■ Silicone-based lotion to decrease shear. ■ Pressure relief mattress/chair cushion.
		Film, adherent Hydrocolloid	Protects from shear. May not allow visual assessment.		
2	Clean	Composite	Viasorb, film+telfa, Exudry. Limits shear.		■ See Stage 1. ■ Manage incontinence.
		Hydrocolloid	Change every 7 days if occlusive seal.		
		Hydrogel sheet	Absorbent; requires secondary dressing of gauze or adherent film.	Heals through reepithelialization and epithelial budding.	

3	Clean	Hydrocolloid	See Stage 2.		■ See Stages 1 and 2.
		Hydrogel	Apply ¼-inch thick; cover with gauze or hydrocolloid.	Heals through granulation and reepithelialization.	■ Electrical stimulation.
		Exudate absorbers Calcium alginate Wound pastes	Change when strikethrough is noted on secondary dressing. Cover with gauze or hydrocolloid.	(NOTE: does not become a Stage 2 ulcer as it heals.)	■ Evaluate pressure relief needs.
		Gauze, fluffy	Use with normal saline.		
		Growth factors	Use with gauze.		

*As with all occlusive dressings, wounds should not be clinically infected.

Continued.

Table 4   Treatment options by ulcer stage—cont'd

Ulcer Stage	Ulcer Status	Dressing	Comments*	Expected Change	Adjuvants
3	Eschar	Adherent film	Will facilitate softening of eschar.	Eschar will lift at the edges as healing progresses.	■ See previous stages.
		Hydrocolloid	Will facilitate softening of eschar.	Cross-hatching central area of eschar with a small blade will facilitate release from center.	■ Surgical consultation for debridement.
		Gauze with ordered solution	Absorb drainage and control odor if Dakins is used.		
		None	Rarely, if eschar is dry and intact, no dressing is used, thus allowing eschar to act as physiologic cover.		

Stage		Dressing			
4	Clean	Hydrogel	See Stage 3—Clean.	Heals through granulation and reepithelialization.	Surgical consultation for closure.
		Hydrocolloid and hydrocolloid paste/beads	See Stage 3—Clean, critical to treat areas of undermining.	Surface may close more rapidly than base because of contraction, leaving wound cavity.	See Stages 1, 2, 3—Clean.
		Calcium alginate	See Stage 3—Clean.		
		Gauze	Pack deeply undermined ulcers. Use with gauze.		
		Growth factors	See Stage 3—Eschar.		
5	Eschar		See Stage 3—Eschar.	See Stage 3—Eschar.	See Stage 3—Eschar.

*As with *all* occlusive dressings, wounds should *not* be clinically infected.

Steps	Rationale
■ Moisten gauze dressing in saline and apply directly over ulcer.	Protects wound. Keeping ulcer surface moist reduces time needed for healing. Skin cells normally live in moist environment.
■ Cover moistened gauze with single piece of dry gauze and tape securely in place.	Prevents bacteria from entering moist dressing.

Antiseptics

■ Deep ulcers: apply antiseptic ointment to dominant gloved hand and spread ointment in and around ulcer. (Avoid spread of contamination if area is infected.)	Antiseptic ointment causes minimal tissue irritation. All surfaces of wound must be covered to effectively control bacterial growth.
■ Apply sterile gauze pad over ulcer and tape securely in place.	Protects ulcer and prevents removal of ointment during turning or repositioning.

Dextranomer Beads

■ Hold container of beads approximately 1 inch (2.5 cm) above ulcer site and lightly sprinkle 5 mm-diameter layer over wound.	Layer of insoluble powder is needed to absorb wound exudate.
■ Apply gauze dressing over ulcer.	Holds beads in place and protects wound.

Hydrocolloid Beads/Paste

■ Fill ulcer defect to approximately half of the total depth with hydrocolloid beads or paste.	Hydrocolloid beads/paste will assist in absorbing wound drainage. Highly draining wounds are best treated with hydrocolloid beads/granules.

Steps	Rationale
■ Cover with hydrocolloid dressing; extend dressing 1 to 1½ inches beyond edges of wound.	Dressing maintains wound humidity. May be left in place up to 7 days.

Hydrogel Agents

■ Cover surface of ulcer with hydrogel using sterile applicator or gloved hand.	Maintains wound humidity while absorbing excess drainage. May be used as a carrier for topical agents.
■ Apply dry, fluffy gauze over gel to completely cover ulcer.	Holds hydrogel against wound surface, is absorbent.

Calcium Alginates

■ Pack wound with alginate using applicator or gloved hand.	Maintains wound humidity while absorbing excess drainage.
■ Apply dry gauze, foam, or hydrocolloid over alginate.	Holds alginate against wound surface.
10. Reposition client comfortably off pressure ulcer.	Avoids accidental removal of dressings.
11. Remove gloves and dispose of soiled supplies. Wash hands.	Prevents transmission of microorganisms.
12. Record appearance of ulcer and treatment (type of topical agent used, dressing applied, and client's response) in nurse's notes.	Baseline observations and subsequent inspections reveal progress of healing. Documents care.
13. Report any deterioration in ulcer's appearance to nurse in charge or physician.	Deterioration of condition may indicate need for additional therapy.

Nurse Alert

Early ulcers tend to have irregular borders; with time, borders become smooth and rounded. If wound is large, irrigating with plain sterile water from an irrigating syringe may be helpful.

Teaching Considerations

All individuals participating in client's wound care should be taught the correct method to administer ulcer care.

Geriatric Considerations

Medicare regulations limit reimbursement for some types of pressure relief equipment used for Stages 3, 4, and 5 pressure ulcers.

MEDICATIONS

Administering Oral
Medications

The most desirable route to administer medications is by mouth. Oral medications are available in various liquid and solid forms, with each type requiring special considerations when given to a client. For example, enteric-coated tablets should never be crushed, cough syrups should never be followed by liquids, and sublingual medications should be placed under the client's tongue. Unless the client has impaired gastrointestinal functioning or is unable to swallow, an oral medication is the safest and easiest to give.

Potential Nursing Diagnoses

Client data derived during the assessment reveal defining characteristics to support the following nursing diagnoses in clients requiring this skill:

Knowledge deficit

Altered health maintenance

Equipment

Medication cards, Kardex, or record form

Medication cart or tray

Disposable medication cups

Glass of water or juice

Drinking straw

Steps	Rationale
1. Assess for any contraindications for oral medication administration, including difficulty in swallowing, nausea or vomiting, bowel inflammation or reduced peristalsis, recent gastrointestinal surgery, reduced or absent bowel sounds, and gastric suction. Obtain history of allergies, medication history, diet history, and NPO order.	Alterations in gastrointestinal functioning interfere with drug distribution, absorption, and excretion.
2. Determine client's preference and tolerance for fluids to accompany medications.	Facilitates medication administration and increases client's fluid intake.
3. Gather equipment listed on previous page.	Facilitates efficient and accurate medication administration.
4. Check accuracy and completeness of each medication card, form, or printout with physician's written medication order, looking at client's name, drug name and dosage, route of administration, and time for administration. Report any discrepancy in order to charge nurse or physician.	Physician's order is most reliable resource and the only legal record of drugs client is to receive. NOTE: Check all orders at least every 24 hours.
5. Wash hands.	Removal of microorganisms minimizes their transfer from your hands to medications and equipment.
6. Arrange medication tray and cups in medicine room or move medication cart to position outside client's room.	Organization of equipment saves time and reduces error.

Steps	Rationale
7. Unlock medicine drawer or cart. (Narcotics are generally stored in a double-locked box separate from medicine drawers or carts).	Medications are safeguarded when locked in cabinet or cart.
8. Prepare medications for one client at a time. Keep medication tickets or forms for each client together.	Prevents preparation errors.
9. Select correct drug from stock or unit dose drawer and compare with medication card or form.	Reading label against transcribed order reduces error.
10. Calculate correct dosage. Take time. Double check calculations.	Calculation will be more accurate when information from drug labels is at hand.
11. To administer tablets or capsules from bottle, pour required number into bottle cap and transfer to medication cup. *Do not touch medicines with your fingers.* Extra tablets or capsules may be returned to bottle.	Aseptic technique maintains cleanliness of drugs.
12. To prepare unit dose tablets or capsules, place packaged tablet or capsule directly into medicine cup. Do not remove wrapper.	Wrappers maintain cleanliness and identification of medications.
13. All tablets or capsules to be given to client at same time may be placed in one cup except for those requiring preadministration assessments such as pulse rate or blood pressure.	Keeping medications that require preadministration assessments separate from others will make it easier to withhold those drugs if necessary.

Steps	Rationale
14. If client has difficulty swallowing, grind tablets in mortar with pestle. Continue grinding until a smooth powder remains. Mix in a small amount of soft food.	Large tablets can be difficult to swallow. Ground tablets mixed with small amounts of palatable soft food are usually easy to swallow.
15. To pour liquids, remove bottle cap and place it upside down.	Prevents contamination.
■ Hold bottle with label against palm of hand while pouring.	Spilled liquid will not soil or fade label.
■ Hold medication cup at eye level and fill to desired mark. Scale should be even with fluid at bottom of meniscus. (Fig. 46).	Ensures accuracy of measurement.

Fig. 46
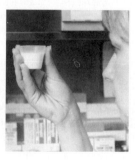

| 16. When preparing narcotic, check narcotic record for previous drug count, remove required volume of drug, record necessary information on form, and sign form. | Controlled substance laws require careful monitoring of dispensed narcotics. |

Steps	Rationale
17. Compare medication card or form with prepared drug and container.	Reading label a second time reduces error.
18. Return stock containers or unused unit-dose medications to shelf or drawer and read labels third time.	Reduces administration error.
19. Place medications and cards, forms, or printouts together on tray or cart.	Drugs are labeled at all times for identification.
20. Do not leave drugs unattended.	You are responsible for safe-keeping of drugs.
21. Take medications to client at correct time.	Medications are administered within 30 minutes before or 30 minutes after prescribed time to ensure intended therapeutic effect.
22. Identify client by comparing name on card, form, or printout with name on client's identification band. Ask client to state his name.	Identification bands are made at time of client's admission and are most reliable source of identification. Replace any missing ID bands.
23. Perform any necessary preadministration assessment.	Determines whether medications should be given at that time.
24. Explain purpose of medication and its action to client.	Client's understanding of purpose of medication will improve his compliance with drug therapy.
25. Assist client to sitting or side-lying position.	Prevents aspiration during swallowing.
26. Administer drugs properly. Offer client choice of water or juice with drugs to be swallowed. Client may wish to hold solid medications in hand or cup before placing in mouth.	Choice of therapy promotes client comfort. Client can become familiar with medications by seeing each drug and then will be able to recognize correct drugs.

Steps	Rationale
27. If client is unable to hold medications, place medication up to his lips and gently introduce drugs into his mouth.	Prevents contamination of medications.
28. If tablet or capsule falls to floor, discard it and repeat preparation.	Prevents contamination.
29. Stay with client until he has completely swallowed each medication. If uncertain whether medication was swallowed, ask client to open his mouth.	You are responsible for ensuring that client receives ordered dose. If left unattended, client may not take dose or may save drugs, causing risk to his health.
30. Wash your hands.	Reduces spread of microorganisms.
31. Record each drug administered on medication record.	Prompt documentation prevents errors such as repeated doses.
32. Return medication cards, forms, or printouts to appropriate file for next administration time.	These are used as reference for when next dose is due. Loss of card may lead to administration error.
33. Discard used supplies, replenish stock (e.g., cups and straws), and clean work area.	Clean working space assists other staff in completing duties efficiently.
34. Return within 30 minutes to evaluate client's response to medications.	By monitoring client's response, you will assess drug's therapeutic benefit and be able to detect onset of side effects or allergic reactions.

Nurse Alert

If the client begins coughing during drug administration, stop immediately. Aspiration of medication or fluid can easily occur.

Client Teaching

Clients may require extensive instruction on how to take prescribed medications correctly. They should understand the purpose of each medication, its action and potential side effects, and the correct time and frequency of its administration. They should particularly understand what can happen if they arbitrarily increase or omit a dose or cease taking the medication entirely. They should also know whether to take medications before or after meals. When teaching a client about medications, be sure to allow sufficient time for client to ask questions.

When attempting to establish medication schedules, consider the client's home environment and daily routines. Clients with visual alterations may be unable to read printed labels and thus require large-print instructions. Include family members in the teaching in case a client becomes too ill to self-administer drugs reliably.

Pediatric Considerations

Children unable to swallow or chew solid medications should be given only liquid preparations. Generally it is safe to administer solid drug forms to children 5 years or older. Pediatric preparations are usually colorful and pleasant tasting. However, a child may enjoy a "chaser" of juice, carbonated soft drink, or frozen juice bar. A bad-tasting drug can be mixed in small amounts of jam, syrup, or honey. Oral medications are most easily administered to infants by spoon, plastic cup or dropper, or small plastic syringe.

Geriatric Considerations

Elderly clients often have multiple medications prescribed. It can be quite helpful to set specific time schedules convenient with their daily routines so they do not forget to take a dose. Many elderly clients have mobility and sensory limitations that prohibit safe drug preparation and administration, and family members or friends should be available for assistance.

Preparing an Injectable Medication from an Ampule or Vial

An ampule is a clear glass container with a constricted neck. It contains a single dose of a medication in liquid form. The nurse must snap off the ampule's neck to gain access to the medication. When withdrawing the medication, the nurse uses aseptic technique (preventing the needle from touching the ampule's outer surface). Fluid can be aspirated easily into the syringe by simply drawing back on the syringe plunger.

A vial is a single-dose or multidose glass container with a rubber seal at the top. A metal cap protects the sterile seal until the vial is ready for use. Vials contain liquid and/or dry forms of medication. The vial is a closed system, and air must be injected into it to permit easy withdrawal of the solution. Failure to inject air before withdrawing the solution leaves a vacuum within the vial that makes withdrawal difficult.

Potential Nursing Diagnoses

This procedure may be performed by nurses caring for clients with various nursing diagnoses.

Equipment

Syringe and needle of desired size
Ampule or vial of prescribed medication
Alcohol swab or 2- × 2-inch gauze pad
Metal file (optional)
Extra sterile needle

Steps	Rationale
1. Wash hands.	Reduces transmission of micro-organisms.

2. Prepare medication:

Ampule

a. Tap top of ampule lightly and quickly with finger (Fig. 47).

Dislodges any fluid that collects above neck. All solution moves into lower chamber.

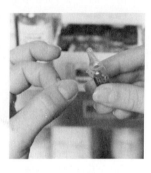

Fig. 47

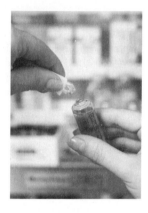

Fig. 48

b. Place small gauze pad or alcohol swab around neck of ampule.

Protects fingers from trauma as glass is broken.

c. Snap neck of ampule away from your hands (Fig. 48). (If neck does not break, use a file to score one side of it.)

Prevents shattering glass toward your fingers or face.

d. Hold ampule either inverted or right side up. Insert needle into center of ampule opening. Do not allow needle tip or shaft to touch rim of ampule.

Broken rim of ampule is considered contaminated.

Steps	Rationale

NOTE: Ampule may be held inverted as long as needle tip or shaft does not touch its rim.

e. Aspirate medication into syringe by pulling back on plunger (Fig. 49).

Withdrawal of plunger creates a negative pressure within barrel that pulls fluid into syringe.

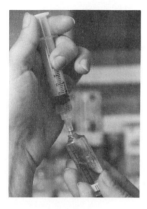

Fig. 49

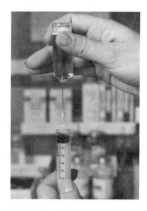

Fig. 50

f. Keep needle tip below surface of liquid. If holding ampule upright, tip it to bring all fluid within reach of needle (Fig. 50).

Prevents aspiration of air bubbles.

g. If air bubbles are aspirated, do not expel air into ampule.

Air pressure will force fluid out of ampule, and medication will be lost.

h. To expel excess air bubbles, remove needle from ampule. Hold syringe with needle pointing up. Draw back slightly on plunger and push it upward to eject air. *Do not eject fluid.*

Withdrawing plunger too far will pull it from barrel. Holding syringe vertically allows fluid to settle in bottom of barrel. Pulling back on plunger allows fluid within needle to enter barrel.

Steps	Rationale
i. If syringe contains excess fluid, use sink for disposal. Hold syringe vertically with needle tip up and slanted slightly toward sink. Slowly eject excess fluid into sink. Recheck fluid level by holding syringe vertically.	Medication is safely dispersed into sink. Rechecking fluid level ensures proper dosage.

Vial

a. Remove metal cap to expose rubber seal.	Vial comes packaged with cap to prevent contamination of seal.
b. With alcohol swab, wipe off surface of rubber seal.	Removes dust or grease but does not sterilize surface.
c. Remove needle cap. Pull back on plunger to draw into syringe amount of air equivalent to volume of medication to be aspirated (Fig. 51).	Prevents buildup of negative pressure when aspirating medication. You must first inject air into vial.

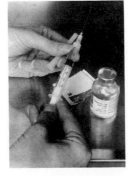

Fig. 51

Steps	Rationale
d. Insert tip of needle, with bevel pointing up, through center of rubber seal (Fig. 52).	Center of seal is thinner and easier to penetrate. Keeping bevel up and using firm pressure prevents cutting rubber core from seal.

Fig. 52

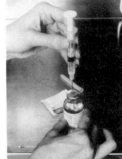

e. Inject air into vial, not allowing plunger to back up.	Air must be injected first before aspirating fluid. Plunger may be forced backward by air pressure within vial.
f. Invert vial while keeping firm hold on syringe and plunger. Hold vial between thumb and middle finger of non-dominant hand. Grasp end of barrel and plunger with thumb and forefinger of dominant hand.	Inverting vial allows fluid to settle in lower half of container. Position of hands prevents movement of plunger and permits easy manipulation of syringe.
g. Keep tip of needle below fluid level.	Prevents aspiration of air.

Steps	Rationale

h. Allow air pressure to gradually fill syringe with medication. Pull back slightly on plunger if necessary (Fig. 53). | Positive pressure within vial forces fluid into syringe.

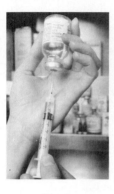

Fig. 53

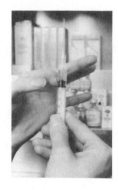

Fig. 54

i. Tap side of barrel carefully to dislodge any air bubbles. Eject any air remaining at top of syringe into vial. | Forcefully striking barrel while needle is inserted in vial may bend needle. Accumulation of air displaces medication and causes dosage errors.

j. Once correct volume is obtained, remove needle from vial by pulling back on barrel of syringe. | Pulling plunger rather than barrel causes separation from barrel and loss of medication.

k. To expel excess air bubbles, remove needle from vial by pulling back on barrel. Hold syringe with needle pointing up and tap it to dislodge bubbles. Draw back slightly on plunger and push plunger upward to eject air. *Do not eject fluid* (Fig. 54). | Withdrawing plunger too far will pull it from barrel. Holding syringe vertically allows fluid to settle in bottom of barrel. Pulling back on plunger allows fluid within needle to enter barrel.

Steps	Rationale
1. Label vial if any medication remains. Note amount of solution and concentration of drug.	Ensures accurate drug administration when successive doses are given.
3. Cover needle with its sheath or cap. Change needle on syringe.	Prevents contamination of needle and protects nurse from needle stick. Changing needle is required if nurse suspects medication is on needle shaft. New needle prevents tracking medication through skin and subcutaneous tissues.
4. Dispose of soiled supplies in proper containers.	Prevents transmission of infection.
5. Wash hands.	Reduces transmission of microorganisms.

Nurse Alert

Be sure that air pressure does not force the plunger out of the syringe barrel. This causes contamination of the syringe.

Use caution when snapping off the neck of an ampule. Shattering of glass can injure your hands and fingers. If you suspect that the ampule has not broken cleanly, discard and begin with a fresh ampule.

Mixing Two Types
of Insulin

Frequently clients with diabetes mellitus receive a combination of different types of insulin to control their blood glucose levels. Regular, rapid-acting insulin is also called unmodified insulin. This type of insulin is in a clear solution.

Other types of insulin are cloudy solutions. The cloudiness is caused by the addition of protein, which slows the absorption of the drug. These types of insulin are intermediate or long-lasting types.

When mixing two kinds of insulin, the nurse must follow two simple guidelines (Fig. 55):

1. Regular insulin can be mixed with any other type of insulin.
2. The Lente insulins can be mixed with each other but should not be mixed with other types of insulin, except regular.

Steps	Rationale
1. Wash hands.	Reduces transmission of infection.
2. Take insulin syringe and aspirate volume of air equivalent to dosage to be withdrawn from modified insulin (cloudy vial).	Air must be introduced into vial to create pressure needed to withdraw solution.
3. Inject air into vial of modified insulin (cloudy vial). Be sure needle does not touch solution.	Prevents cross-contamination.

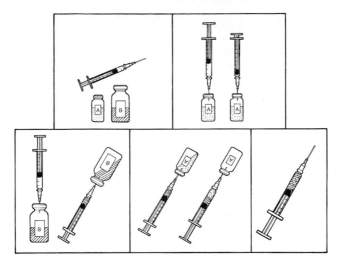

Fig. 55

Steps	Rationale
4. Withdraw needle and syringe from vial and then aspirate air equivalent to dosage to be withdrawn from unmodified regular insulin (clear vial).	Air is injected into vial to withdraw desired dosage.
5. Insert needle into vial of unmodified regular insulin (clear vial), inject air, and then fill syringe with proper insulin dosage.	First portion of dosage has been prepared.
6. Withdraw needle and syringe from vial by pulling on barrel. Check dosage.	Prevents accidental pulling of plunger, which may cause loss of medication. Ensures correct dosage prepared.
7. Determine at which point on syringe scale combined units of insulin should measure.	Prevents accidental withdrawal of too much insulin from second vial.

Steps	Rationale
8. Insert needle into vial of modified insulin (cloudy vial). Be careful not to push plunger and expel medication into vial. Invert vial and carefully withdraw desired amount of insulin into syringe.	Positive pressure within vial of modified insulin allows fluid to fill syringe without need to aspirate.
9. Withdraw needle and expel any excess air or fluid from syringe.	Air bubbles should not be injected into tissues. Air or excess fluid causes incorrect dosage.
10. Dispose of soiled supplies in proper receptacle.	Controls spread of infection.
11. Wash hands.	Reduces transmission of microorganisms.

Administering Subcutaneous and Intramuscular Injections

Injecting medication is an invasive procedure involving deposition of medication through a sterile needle inserted into body tissues. Aseptic technique must be maintained because a client is at risk of infection once the needle penetrates the skin. The characteristics of tissues influence the rate of drug absorption and onset of drug action. Thus, before injecting a drug, the nurse should know the volume of medication to administer, the characteristics of the drug, and the location of anatomic structures underlying injection sites.

For subcutaneous injections, medication is deposited into the loose connective tissue under the dermis. Because the subcutaneous tissue is not as richly supplied with blood vessels, drug absorption is somewhat slower than with intramuscular injections. Subcutaneous tissues contain pain receptors, so only small doses of water-soluble, nonirritating medications should be given by this route.

The intramuscular route provides faster drug absorption because of a muscle's vascularity. The danger of tissue damage is less when medications enter deep muscle. Muscles also are less sensitive to irritating and viscous drugs. However, there is a risk of inadvertently injecting into a blood vessel if the nurse is not careful.

Potential Nursing Diagnoses

This procedure may be performed by nurses caring for clients with various nursing diagnoses.

Equipment

Syringe (size varies according to volume of drug to be administered)

Needle (size varies according to type of tissue and size of client;
intramuscular—20 to 23 gauge and 1 to 1½ inches in length
[adult]; 25 to 27 gauge and ½ to 1 inch in length [child] [Wha-
ley and Wong, 1991]; subcutaneous—25 to 27 gauge and ½
to ⅞ inch in length)

Antiseptic swab (e.g., alcohol)

Medication ampule or vial

Medication card or form

Steps	Rationale
1. Wash hands and don clean gloves.	Reduces transmission of micro-organisms.
2. Assemble equipment and check medication order for route, dose, and time.	Ensures accuracy of order.
3. Prepare medication from ampule or vial as described in Skill 5-2.	Ensures that medication is sterile.
4. Check client's identification band and ask client's name. Assess for allergies.	Ensures that correct client receives correct drug.
5. Explain procedure to client and proceed in calm manner.	Helps client anticipate nurse's actions.
6. Select appropriate injection site. Palpate site for edema, masses, or tenderness. Avoid areas of scarring, bruising, abrasion, or infection (Fig. 56).	Injection sites should be free of lesions that might interfere with drug absorption. Sufficient muscle mass is needed to ensure accurate intramuscular injection into proper tissue.

Steps   Rationale

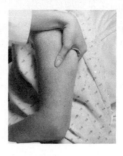

Fig. 56

- When administering hep-
  arin subcutaneously, use
  abdominal injection sites.
- For intramuscular injection, palpate muscles to
  determine their firmness
  and size.

7. In cases of repeated daily
   insulin injections, do not
   use same injection site. Rotate within a single anatomic region and then
   change anatomic site. Do
   not reuse same site within
   3-week period.

8. Assist client to comfortable
   position depending on site
   chosen:

NOTE: Anticoagulants may cause
local bleeding and bruising
when injected into areas such as
arms and legs, which are involved in muscular activity.

Rotation of site prevents subcutaneous scarring and lipodystro-
phy, which can interfere with
drug absorption.

Subcutaneous Injection Sites

Arm—client sitting or standing
Abdomen—client sitting or
supine
Leg—client sitting in bed or
chair

Provides easy access to site
with client in relaxed position.

Steps	Rationale

Intramuscular Injection Sites

Thigh (vastus lateralis)—client lying supine with knee slightly flexed
Ventrogluteal—client lying on side, back, or abdomen with knee and hip on side to be injected flexed
Dorsogluteal—client prone with feet turned inward, or on side with upper knee and hip flexed and placed in front of lower leg
Upper arm (deltoid)—client sitting or lying flat with lower arm flexed but relaxed across abdomen or lap

Helping client assume position that reduces strain on muscle will minimize discomfort of injection.

9. Ask client to relax his arm or leg, whichever site is chosen. Talk with him about subject of interest.

Minimizes discomfort during injection. Distraction helps reduce anxiety.

10. Relocate site using anatomic landmarks.

Accurate injection requires insertion in correct anatomic site to avoid injuring underlying nerves, bones, or blood vessels.

11. Clean the site with antiseptic swab. Apply swab at center of site and rotate outward in circular direction for about 5 cm (2 inches) (Fig. 57).

Mechanical action of swab removes secretions containing microorganisms.

12. Hold swab between third and fourth fingers of your nondominant hand.

Swab will remain readily accessible when time to withdraw needle.

13. Remove needle cap from syringe by pulling cap straight off.

Prevents needle from touching sides of cap and becoming contaminated.

Steps   Rationale

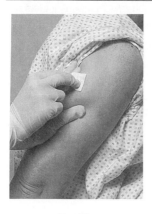

Fig. 57

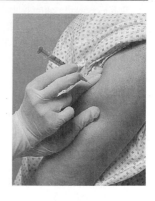

Fig. 58

14. Hold syringe between thumb and forefinger of your dominant hand as though it were a dart. (Most nurses hold syringe palm up for subcutaneous injections and palm down for intramuscular injections because of different angles of insertion [Fig. 58]).

Quick smooth injection requires proper manipulation of syringe parts.

15. Inject syringe:

Subcutaneous

- For average-sized client, with your nondominant hand either spread skin tightly across injection site or pinch skin.

Needle penetrates tight skin more easily than loose skin. Pinching skin elevates subcutaneous tissue.

- For obese client, pinch skin at site and inject needle below tissue fold.

Obese clients have fatty layer of tissue above subcutaneous tissue.

Steps	Rationale
■ Inject needle quickly and firmly at a 45-degree angle. (Then release skin if pinched.)	Quick, firm insertion minimizes client anxiety and discomfort.

Intramuscular

Steps	Rationale
■ Position nondominant hand at proper anatomic landmarks and spread skin tightly. Inject needle quickly at a 90-degree angle.	Speeds insertion and reduces discomfort.
■ If muscle mass is small, grasp body of muscle and inject medication.	Ensures that medication reaches muscle tissue.
■ If giving irritating preparation, use Z-track method. When using this technique the nurse draws up 0.5 ml of air in the syringe to create an air lock. Pull overlying skin and subcutaneous tissues 2.5 to 3.5 cm (1 to 1½ inches) laterally to side. Hold skin back and inject needle quickly.	An air lock clears the needle of medication to prevent tracking of medication through the tissues and skin. Z-track method creates zig-zag path through tissues that seals needle track to avoid tracking medication through sensitive subcutaneous tissues.
16. Once needle enters site, with your nondominant hand grasp lower end of syringe barrel. Move your dominant hand to end of plunger. Avoid movement of syringe (Fig. 59).	Properly performed injection requires smooth manipulation of syringe parts. Movement of syringe may displace needle and cause discomfort.
■ If using Z-track, keep tight hold of skin with nondominant hand. Use dominant hand to carefully move toward plunger.	Skin must remain pulled until drug is injected.

Steps   Rationale

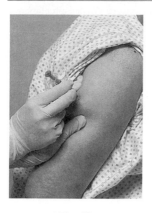

Fig. 59

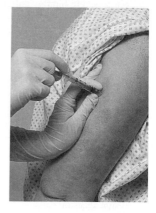

Fig. 60

17. Slowly pull back on plunger to aspirate medication. If blood appears in syringe, withdraw needle, dispose of syringe, and repeat medication preparation. If no blood appears, inject medication slowly.
    NOTE: Some agencies recommend not aspirating subcutaneous heparin injections.

Aspiration of blood into syringe indicates intravenous placement of needle. Subcutaneous and intramuscular medications are not for intravenous use. Slow injection reduces pain and tissue trauma.
NOTE: Heparin is an anticoagulant that is typically given in small subcutaneous doses. The drug may cause bruising when aspirated. The drug is not harmful if given intravenously.

18. Withdraw needle quickly while placing antiseptic swab just above injection site (Fig. 60).
    ■ When using Z-track, keep needle inserted after injecting drug for 10 seconds. Then release skin after withdrawing needle.

Support of tissues around the injection site minimizes discomfort during needle withdrawal.

Allows medication to disperse evenly. Tissue planes slide across one another to create zigzag path that seals medication into muscle tissues.

Steps	Rationale
19. Massage site lightly, unless contraindicated as for heparin.	Massage stimulates circulation and thus improves drug distribution and absorption.
20. Assist client to a comfortable position.	Gives client sense of well-being.
21. Discard unsheathed needle and attached syringe into appropriately labeled receptacles.	Prevents injury to client and hospital personnel. Recapping needle can cause needle stick and is no longer considered safe practice.
22. Remove gloves and wash hands.	Controls spread of infection.
23. Chart medication in medication sheet or nurse's notes.	Documents administration of drug and prevents future drug errors.
24. Return to evaluate client's response to medication within 15 to 30 minutes.	Parenteral drugs are absorbed and act more quickly than do oral medications. Your observations determine efficacy of drug action.

Nurse Alert

The needle of the syringe must remain sterile before insertion. If blood appears in the syringe during aspiration, immediately withdraw it and start over. Document and report any sudden localized pain or burning at the injection site, which may indicate nerve injury.

Client Teaching

The insulin-dependent client may have to learn how to self-administer injections if family members are not available. It may be necessary to teach the client aseptic principles, the basic pharmacology of insulin, the selection and rotation of injection sites, and injection techniques.

Pediatric Considerations

When it is essential to deliver a prescribed volume of solution to a child, draw up 0.2 ml of air into the syringe after preparing the drug dose. Air acts as dead space to clear the needle bore of medication. Give parents the option of helping to restrain their child during an injection. Some parents do not wish to be looked on as the ones causing the child discomfort. It may help to keep the needle out of the child's line of vision to minimize anxiety. Never surprise a child. Be sure that he knows he is to receive an injection. The vastus lateralis is the preferred injection site for children. The dorsogluteal muscle should not be used for children unless the muscle is fully developed. After the injection, comfort the child.

Geriatric Considerations

The elderly client's muscle mass may be reduced. It is therefore important to choose a proper-sized needle. Remember also that the elderly client may be unable to tolerate more than 2 ml of an intramuscular injection.

Adding Medications to an Intravenous Fluid Container

The safest method for administering intravenous (IV) medications is to add the drugs to large-volume fluid containers (usually with dextrose and water solution or normal saline). Then the medication infuses slowly, the risk of side effects is minimized, and therapeutic blood levels are maintained. Drugs added to IV fluid containers include electrolytes, vitamins, and minerals. The primary risk involved with infusing drugs by this method is fluid overload.

Potential Nursing Diagnoses

This procedure may be performed by nurses caring for clients with various nursing diagnoses.

Equipment

Prepared medication in syringe
IV fluid container (bag or bottle, 500 or 1000 ml volume)
Alcohol or antiseptic swab
Label to attach to IV bag or bottle

Steps	Rationale
1. Wash hands.	Reduces transmission of micro-organisms.
2. Verify physician's order.	Client's overall physical condition determines type of solution, medication, and dosage.
3. Explain procedure to client.	Reduces client anxiety.
4. Check client's identification by reading his ID band and asking his name.	Ensures that correct client gets prescribed medication.

Steps	Rationale
5. Add medication to new container:	
a. Locate medication injection port on IV fluid bag.	The medication injection port is self-sealing to prevent introduction of microorganisms after repeated use.
b. Wipe off port with alcohol or antiseptic swab.	Reduces risk of introducing microorganisms into bag during needle insertion.
c. Carefully insert needle of syringe through center of injection port and depress plunger (Fig. 61).	Injection of needle into sides of port may produce leak and lead to contamination of fluid.

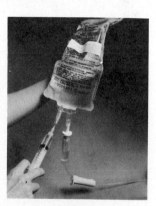

Fig. 61

d. Withdraw syringe and mix solution by holding bag and turning it gently from end to end.	Allows medication to be distributed evenly throughout bag.
e. Hang bag and check infusion rate.	Prevents rapid infusion of fluid.
f. Complete medication label and stick it upside down on bag.	Label can be easily read during infusion. It alerts nurses to drug in bag.
g. Wash hands.	Reduces transmission of microorganisms.

Steps	Rationale
6. Add medication to existing container:	
a. Wash hands.	Reduces transmission of microorganisms.
b. Check volume of solution remaining in container.	Proper volume is needed to dilute medication adequately.
c. Close off IV infusion clamp.	Prevents medication from directly entering client's circulation during injection.
d. Wipe off medication port with alcohol or antiseptic swab.	Mechanically removes microorganisms that could enter container during needle insertion.
e. Insert syringe needle through port and inject medication (Fig. 62).	Injection port is self-sealing and prevents fluid leaks.

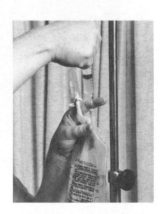

Fig. 62

f. Lower container from IV pole and mix gently.	Ensures that medication is evenly distributed throughout bag.
g. Rehang and regulate infusion to desired rate.	Prevents rapid infusion of fluid.
h. Label container with name and dosage of medication.	Alerts other nurses to drug in bag.
i. Wash hands	Reduces transmission of microorganisms

Nurse Alert

Be aware of the signs and symptoms of fluid overload in case you discover that an excess amount of fluid has infused too quickly. These include tachycardia, bounding pulse, jugular venous distention, and shortness of breath.

Client Teaching

To prevent unnecessary anxiety, the nurse should explain to the client that medications are being added to an existing IV line.

Pediatric Considerations

Infants and children are very susceptible to fluid overload, so infusions must be frequently monitored. IV infusions in children are usually hung with a volume control device or infusion pump.

Geriatric Considerations

Although the conditions of renal and heart failure are not limited to the elderly population, it is especially important to consider these clients' risk for fluid overload.

Administering a Medication by Intravenous Bolus

Administering concentrated medications directly into a vein by the bolus technique is the most dangerous method of drug administration. These drugs act rapidly because they enter the client's circulation directly. Serious side effects can occur within seconds. Therefore it is imperative that the nurse time the administrations carefully to prevent too rapid an infusion. Drugs may be given intravenously through a heparin lock or an existing IV infusion line. IV drugs are often given by bolus in emergency situations when rapid actions are desired. The technique is also used to avoid mixing medications that are incompatible.

Potential Nursing Diagnoses

This procedure may be performed by nurses caring for clients with various nursing diagnoses.

Equipment

Heparin Lock

Prepared medication in syringe with small-gauge (25 or 26) needle
Syringe containing 1 ml of 1:1000 heparin solution (optional) or 9 ml normal saline
Alcohol or antiseptic swab
Watch with second hand or digital readout
Sterile 21- and 25-gauge needles
Medication card or form

Intravenous Infusion Line

Prepared medication in syringe with small-gauge (25 or 26) needle
Alcohol or antiseptic swab
IV line tubing with injection port
Watch with second hand or digital readout
Medication card or form

Steps	Rationale
1. Wash hands and don clean gloves.	Reduces transmission of infection.
2. Verify physician's order.	Client's overall physical condition determines type of solution, medication, and dosage.
3. Explain procedure to client.	Reduces any anxiety client may have.
4. Check client's identification by reading identification band and asking client's name.	Ensures that correct client receives correct medication.

Heparin Lock

5. Verify placement of needle within vein.	Ensures that medication enters vein and not surrounding tissue.
6. Clean heparin lock's rubber diaphragm with antiseptic swab.	Prevents introduction of microorganisms during needle insertion.
7. Insert 25-gauge needle of syringe containing prepared drug through center of diaphragm (Fig. 63).	Prevents damage to diaphragm and subsequent leakage.
8. Inject medication bolus slowly over several minutes. (Each medication has recommended rate for bolus administration. Check agency policy.) Use watch to time administration.	Rapid injection could prove fatal to client.

Steps   Rationale

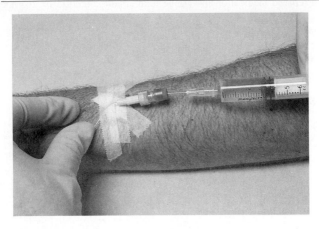

Fig. 63

9. After administering bolus, withdraw syringe. Insert 25-gauge needle of syringe containing diluted heparin (heparin flush) or normal saline solution. Inject this.

Maintains patency of heparin-lock needle by inhibiting clot formation. Dilution of heparin solution prevents systemic anti-coagulation of client.

10. Observe client closely for any adverse reactions.

IV medications act rapidly.

11. Dispose of unsheathed needle and attached syringe in proper receptacle.

Prevents accidental injury from needle sticks.

12. Remove gloves and wash hands.

Reduces transmission of microorganisms.

13. Record drug administered in medication record.

Prompt documentation prevents drug errors.

Intravenous Infusion Line

1. Determine if IV fluids are infusing at proper rate.

Infusion must be at prescribed rate for therapeutic effect.

Steps	Rationale
2. Wash hands and don clean gloves.	Reduces transmission of micro-organisms.
3. Select injection port of tubing closest to needle insertion site.	Allows for easier fluid aspiration to obtain blood return.
4. Clean off injection port with antiseptic swab.	Prevents introduction of micro-organisms during needle insertion.
5. Insert small-gauge needle containing prepared drug through center of port.	Prevents damage to port's diaphragm and subsequent leakage.
6. Occlude IV line by pinching tubing just above injection port. Pull back gently on syringe's plunger to aspirate for blood return (Fig. 64).	Ensures that medication is being delivered into bloodstream.

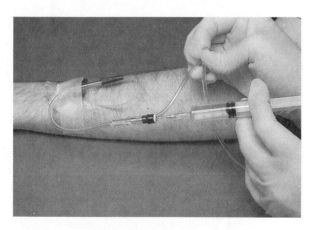

Fig. 64

Steps	Rationale
7. After noting blood return, inject medication slowly over several minutes, (usually not more than 1 ml per minute, unless an emergency. Check agency policy.) Use a watch to time administration (Fig. 65).	Allows slow infusion of fluids. Rapid injection could prove fatal to client.

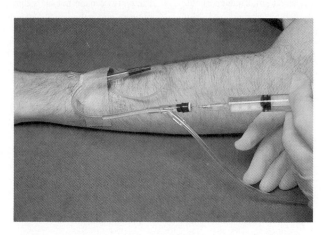

Fig. 65

8. After injecting medication, withdraw syringe and recheck infusion rate.	Injection of bolus may alter rate of fluid infusion. Rapid infusion can cause circulatory overload.
9. Dispose of unsheathed needle and attached syringe in proper receptacles.	Prevents accidental needle sticks and reduces transfer of infection.
10. Observe client closely for adverse reactions.	IV bolus medications act rapidly.
11. Remove gloves and wash your hands.	Reduces transfer of microorganisms.
12. Record drug administered in medication record.	Prompt documentation prevents drug errors.

Nurse Alert

Watch the IV site during drug infusion. The sudden development of swelling indicates infiltration. Then it is imperative to stop the injection. It is also imperative to know each drug's side effects and to watch the client for any reaction.

Client Teaching

The nurse may wish to inform the client of the anticipated effects of a medication. For example, an analgesic can bring rapid pain relief, and knowing that may encourage the client, learning that his discomfort will soon be lessened.

Pediatric Considerations

Remember, an infant's veins are small and fragile. Rapid injection can cause infiltration.

Geriatric Considerations

An elderly client's veins are generally more fragile than are those of a younger client, and infiltration may occur if fluid is forced too rapidly.

Administering an
Intravenous Medication
by "Piggyback" or
Small-Volume Container

Administering IV medications through piggyback or small-volume containers engenders less risk of causing sudden drug side effects. Medications infuse slowly over several minutes. This technique also avoids infusing large volumes of fluid in clients who have fluid restrictions and mixing drugs with others that may be incompatible. It is important that the existing IV line be infusing properly to ensure proper drug distribution.

Potential Nursing Diagnoses

This procedure may be performed by nurses caring for clients with various nursing diagnoses.

Equipment
Infusion through Adjacent Line

Medication prepared in a 50- or 100-ml infusion bag with IV infusion tubing set
Main IV infusion line
Needle (21- or 23-gauge)
Needle-lock device
Alcohol or antiseptic swab

Infusion through Volutrol

Volutrol (plastic graduated container that is part of a main IV line
  and hangs between main IV bag or bottle and infusion tubing)
Syringe with prepared medication
Alcohol or antiseptic swab
Medication label

Steps	Rationale
1. Review physician's orders for name of drug and dosage.	Ensures safe and accurate drug administration.
2. Wash hands and don gloves.	Reduces transmission of micro-organisms.
3. Check client's identification band and ask client's name.	Ensures that correct client receives right medication.

Piggyback Infusion through Adjacent Line

a. Prepare secondary infusion line, being sure tubing is completely filled with medication-fluid mixture.	Prevents introduction of air into main IV line.
b. Check infusion rate of main IV line.	Checking infusion rate determines patency of system. Any obstruction to flow will interfere with medication delivery.
c. Hang secondary fluid bag at or above level of main fluid bag.	Height of fluid bag regulates rate of fluid flow to client.
d. Connect needle to the end of secondary line tubing. Clean injection port to main IV line with an antiseptic swab.	Prevents introduction of micro-organisms during needle insertion.

Steps	Rationale
e. Insert needle of secondary line through injection port of main IV line. Regulate flow rate of medication solution (usually 30 to 60 min.). If available, use needle-less or needle-lock devices to secure needle of secondary piggyback line through injection port of mainline (Fig. 66).	Provides direct route for slow intermittent medication infusion. For optimal therapeutic effect, drug should infuse within 30 to 60 minutes. Needle-lock devices prevent piggyback needle from slipping out of injection port, which increases the risk of needlestick injury to health care workers.

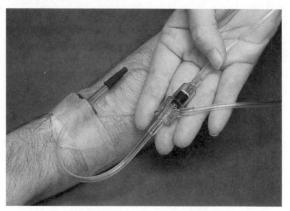

Fig. 66

f. Observe client for signs of adverse reactions.	IV medications act rapidly.
g. After medication has infused, turn off flow regulator on secondary IV line. Leave needle, tubing, and secondary bag hanging for future drug administration.	Secondary line is route for microorganisms to enter main line. Repeated changes of tubing or needle increase risk of infection transmission.

Steps	Rationale
Infusion through Volutrol	
a. Check infusion rate of IV line.	Determines patency of system. Obstruction to flow interferes with medication delivery.
b. Fill Volutrol with desired amount of fluid (50 to 100 ml) by opening clamp between Volutrol and main IV bag (Fig. 67).	Small volume of fluid dilutes IV medication and reduces risk of rapid dose infusion.
c. Clean off injection port on top of Volutrol.	Prevents introduction of micro-organisms during needle insertion.

Fig. 67

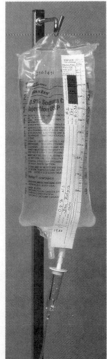
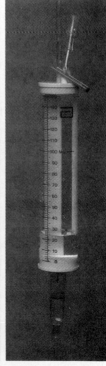

Steps	Rationale
d. Insert syringe needle into port and inject medication. Gently rotate Volutrol between your hands.	Mixes medication within Volutrol to ensure equal distribution.
e. Recheck IV infusion rate (medication should infuse in 30 to 60 minutes).	For optimal therapeutic effect, drug should infuse within 30 to 60 minutes.
f. Observe client for signs of adverse reactions.	IV medications act rapidly.
g. After medication has infused, refill Volutrol with IV solution and monitor flow rate as ordered.	Keeps IV line patent.
4. Wash hands.	Reduces transmission of microorganisms.
5. Record drug administered in medication record.	Prompt documentation prevents drug errors.

Nurse Alert

Know the potential side effects of a medication. Drugs can act rapidly.

Client Teaching

Explain the purpose and actions of a medication to the client.

Pediatric Considerations

Pediatric doses are small. Be sure that the child receives the medication in the Volutrol as well as that in the tubing. An infant or child may not receive as much infusion as an adult because of the risk of fluid overload.

Geriatric Considerations

The veins of an elderly client are fragile. Infiltration at the IV site can develop easily. Observe the site periodically during any intermittent drug infusion.

Topical Skin

Applications

Various pharmacologic preparations can be applied to the client's skin for several purposes: maintaining hydration of skin layers, protecting skin surfaces, reducing local skin irritation, creating local anesthesia, or treating infections, abrasions, or irritations.

Although each preparation is applied in a specific manner, the nurse should be aware that these applications can create both systemic and local effects. These preparations should be applied with gloves and applicators. When an open wound is present, use of sterile techniques is crucial.

Application of these preparations enables the nurse to assess the client's skin thoroughly and document any changes in the client's skin integrity.

Potential Nursing Diagnoses

This procedure may be performed by nurses caring for clients with various nursing diagnoses.

Equipment

Ordered topical agent (e.g., cream, lotion, aerosol, spray, powder)
Medication ticket or form
Small sterile gauze dressings
Disposable or sterile gloves (optional)
Cotton-tipped applicator or tongue blade
Basin with warm water, washcloth, towel, and nondrying soap
Gauze dressings, plastic wrap, tape

Steps	Rationale
1. Review physician's order for name of drug, strength, time of administration, and site of application.	Ensures that drug will be administered safely and accurately.
2. Wash hands.	Reduces transmission of infection.
3. Arrange supplies at client's bedside.	Topical agents usually are not premeasured in medication room.
4. Close room curtain or door.	Provides for client privacy.
5. Check client's identification by reading ID bracelet and asking client's name.	Ensures that correct client receives prescribed medication.
6. Position client comfortably. Remove gown or bed linen, keeping unaffected areas draped.	Provides for easy access to area being treated. Promotes client comfort.
7. Inspect condition of client's skin thoroughly. Wash any affected area, removing all debris and crustations. (Use mild nondrying soap.)	Provides baseline to determine change in skin's condition following therapy. Skin should be clean for a proper assessment. Removal of debris enhances penetration of topical drug through skin. Cleaning removes microorganisms resident in debris.
8. Pat skin dry or allow area to air dry.	Excess moisture can interfere with even application of topical agent.
9. If skin is excessively dry and flaking, apply topical agent while skin is still damp.	Retains moisture within skin layers.

Steps	Rationale
10. Don gloves if indicated.	Sterile gloves are used when applying agents to open, noninfected skin lesions. Disposable gloves prevent cross-contamination of infected or contagious lesions.

11. Apply topical agent:

Cream, Ointment, and Oil-based Lotion

■ Place 1 to 2 teaspoons of medication in palm and soften by rubbing briskly between hands.	Softening a topical agent makes it easier to apply to skin.
■ Once medication is thin and smooth, smear it evenly over skin surface using long, even strokes that follow direction of hair growth.	Ensures even distribution of medication. Prevents irritation of hair follicles.
■ Explain to client that skin may feel greasy after application.	Ointments often contain oils.

Antianginal (Nitroglycerine) Ointment

■ Apply desired number of inches of ointment over paper measuring guide (Fig. 68).	Ensures correct dosage of medication. Medication is applied to back of guide. This ensures that name and dosage of medication is readable once applied to client's skin.

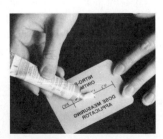

Fig. 68

Steps	Rationale
■ Don disposable glove if desired. Apply ointment to skin surface by holding edge or back of paper wrapper and placing ointment and wrapper directly on skin. Do not rub or massage ointment into skin (Fig. 69).	Drug can be absorbed through your fingertips, causing serious systemic effects. Medication is designed to absorb slowly over several hours and should not be massaged.

Fig. 69

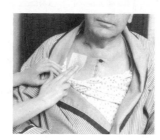

■ Cover ointment and paper with plastic wrap and tape securely (optional).	Prevents soiling of clothing.

Aerosol Spray

■ Shake container vigorously.	Mixes contents and propellant to ensure distribution of fine, even spray.
■ Read label for distance recommended to hold spray away from area (usually 6 to 12 inches).	Proper distance ensures that fine spray hits skin surface. Holding container too close results in thin, watery distribution.
■ If neck or upper chest is to be sprayed, ask client to turn face away from spray.	Prevents inhalation of spray.

Steps	Rationale
■ Spray medication evenly over affected site (in some cases spray is timed for certain number of seconds).	Entire affected area of skin should be covered with thin spray.

Suspension-based Lotion

Steps	Rationale
■ Shake container vigorously.	Mixes powder throughout liquid to form well-mixed suspension.
■ Apply small amount of lotion to small gauze dressing or pad and apply to skin by stroking evenly in direction of hair growth.	Method leaves protective film of powder on skin after water base of suspension dries. Prevents irritation to hair follicles.
■ Explain to client that area will feel cool and dry.	Water evaporates to leave thin layer of powder.

Powder

Steps	Rationale
■ Be sure that skin surface is thoroughly dry.	Minimizes caking and crusting of powder.
■ Fully spread apart any skin folds such as between toes or under arms.	Fully exposes skin surface for application.
■ Dust skin site lightly with dispenser so area is covered with fine, thin layer of powder.	Thin layer of powder is more absorbent and reduces friction by increasing area of moisture evaporation.
12. Cover skin area with dressing if ordered by physician.	May help prevent agent from being rubbed off skin.
13. Assist client to comfortable position, reapply gown, and cover with bed linen as desired.	Provides for client's sense of well-being.
14. Dispose of soiled supplies in proper receptacle and wash hands.	Keeps client's environment neat and reduces transmission of infection.

Nurse Alert

When applying nitroglycerine pastes, the nurse should avoid markedly hairy regions that might alter drug absorption. Antianginal creams are ordered in inches and can be measured in small sheets of paper marked in ½-inch markings.

Assess the client for allergy to topical agents. Avoid patting or rubbing skin when applying creams, ointments, or lotions. This can cause skin irritation.

Client Teaching

Assess the client's knowledge of action and purposes of medication. Determine if the client is physically able to apply medication. Caution the client against using too much of a medication because a buildup on the skin interferes with drug absorption. Be sure that the client knows the signs of local reaction to a topical agent.

Pediatric Considerations

When applying topical agents to a young child's skin, it is often necessary to cover the affected area with a dry dressing. Otherwise he may try to rub the medication off.

Geriatric Considerations

The elderly client's skin can be thin and fragile. Apply any topical agent carefully to avoid breaks in the skin. To prevent tape burns, use tape sparingly.

Administering an Eye
Medication

The eye is a very sensitive organ. The cornea, or anterior portion of the eyeball, is richly supplied with sensitive pain fibers. The nurse should avoid instilling drops directly onto the corneal surface so that the client's discomfort is minimal. It is also important that the nurse use caution in administering eye medications so the applicator does not accidentally touch the eye's surface. Injury can occur easily.

Eye medications are given to dilate the pupil for examination of internal eye structures, to paralyze lens muscles for measurement of lens refraction, to relieve local irritation, to treat eye disorders, and to lubricate the cornea and conjunctiva.

Potential Nursing Diagnoses

Client data derived during the assessment reveal defining characteristics to support the following nursing diagnoses in clients requiring this skill:

Sensory/perceptual alterations

Knowledge deficit regarding drug administration

Equipment

Medication bottle with sterile eye dropper or ointment tube

Medication card or form

Cotton ball or tissue

Wash basin with warm water

Eye patch (optional)

Gloves

Steps	Rationale
1. Review physician's order for name of drug, dose, time of administration, and route.	Ensures safe and accurate administration of drug.
2. Wash your hands and don gloves.	Reduces transfer of microorganisms.
3. Check client's identification band and ask client's name.	Ensures that correct client receives right medication.
4. Explain procedure to client.	Reduces client's anxiety.
5. Ask client to lie supine with neck slightly hyperextended.	Provides easy access to eye for medication instillation. Also minimizes drainage of medication through tear duct.
6. If crusts or drainage are present along eyelid margins or inner canthus, gently wash away. Soak any crusts that have dried and are difficult to remove by applying damp washcloth or cotton ball over eye for a few minutes. Always wipe clean from inner to outer canthus.	Crusts or drainage harbor microorganisms. Soaking allows easy removal and prevents pressure from being applied directly over eye. Cleansing from inner to outer canthus avoids entrance of microorganisms into lacrimal duct.
7. Hold cotton ball or clean tissue in nondominant hand on client's cheekbone just below lower eyelid.	Cotton or tissue absorbs medication that escapes eye.
8. With tissue or cotton resting below lower lid, gently press downward with thumb or forefinger against bony orbit.	Technique exposes lower conjunctival sac. Retraction against bony orbit prevents pressure and trauma to eyeball and prevents fingers from touching eye.
9. Ask client to look at ceiling.	Action retracts sensitive cornea up and away from conjunctiva and reduces stimulation of blink reflex.

Steps	Rationale

10. Instill eyedrops:

a. With dominant hand resting on client's forehead, hold filled medication eye dropper approximately 1 to 2 cm (0.5 to 0.75 inches) above conjunctival sac (Fig. 70).

Helps prevent accidental contact of eyedropper with eye structures, thus reducing risk of injury to eye and transfer of infection to dropper. Ophthalmic medications are sterilized.

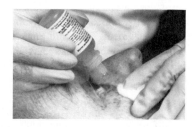

Fig. 70

b. Drop prescribed number of medication drops into conjunctival sac.

Conjunctival sac normally holds 1 to 2 drops. Applying drops to sac provides even distribution of medication across eye.

c. If client blinks or closes eye or if drops land on outer lid margins, repeat procedure.

Therapeutic effect of drug is obtained only when drops enter conjunctival sac.

d. When administering drugs that cause systemic effects, protect your finger with gloves or clean tissue and apply gentle pressure to client's nasolacrimal duct for 30 to 60 seconds.

Prevents overflow of medication into nasal and pharyngeal passages. Prevents absorption into systemic circulation.

e. After instilling drops, ask client to close eye gently.

Helps to distribute medication. Squinting or squeezing of eyelids forces medication from conjunctival sac.

Steps	Rationale
11. Instill eye ointment:	
a. Holding ointment applicator above lid margin, apply thin stream of ointment evenly along inside edge of lower eyelid on conjunctiva.	Distributes medication evenly across eye and lid margin.
b. Ask client to look down.	Reduces blink reflex during ointment application.
c. Apply thin stream of ointment along upper lid margin on inner conjunctiva.	Distributes medication evenly across eye and lid margin.
d. Have client close eye and rub lid lightly in circular motion with cotton ball.	Further distributes medication without traumatizing eye.
12. If excess medication is on eyelid, gently wipe it from inner to outer canthus.	Promotes comfort and prevents trauma to eye.
13. If client had eye patch, apply clean one by placing it over affected eye so entire eye is covered. Tape securely without applying pressure to eye.	Clean eye patch reduces chance of infection.
14. Remove gloves, wash hands, and dispose of supplies.	Reduces transmission of microorganisms.
15. Record drug, concentration, number of drops, time of administration, and eye (left, right, or both) that received medication.	Timely documentation prevents drug errors (e.g., repeated or missed doses).

Nurse Alert

To avoid systemic side effects of certain medications, be sure to occlude the nasolacrimal duct (at the inner canthus) after administration.

Client Teaching

It may be necessary to instruct a client who is to receive an eye medication on self-administration techniques. A client with glaucoma will usually receive medications for life for control of this disease. Family members should also be taught proper administration techniques, especially after eye surgery occurs and the client's vision is blurred, causing him difficulty in assembling supplies and handling applicators.

Warn the client against touching eye structures with the applicator. He should also know that preparations are sterile and should never be used if prescribed for another family member. It is common for certain medications to cause temporary blurring of vision; warn the client about this phenomenon.

Pediatric Considerations

A child can easily be frightened when receiving an eye medication. Talk gently to the infant or young child and be sure to restrain his head to prevent movement during instillation. A sudden twist of the head can cause the applicator to strike the eye accidentally. It is also helpful to have the hand that holds the dropper rest on the child's forehead so the hand moves synchronously with the head.

Geriatric Considerations

An elderly client with severe visual alterations will be unable to read labels of prepared medications. Certain clients may learn to recognize containers by their size and shape. However, a family member should be familiar with dose schedules and instillation techniques. A client with motor tremors may not be able to administer drugs safely.

Using Metered Dose Inhalers

Metered dose inhalers (MDIs) are becoming more popular. Medications administered through inhalers are dispersed through aerosol spray, mist, or fine powder to penetrate airways. Although these medications are designed to produce local effects (e.g., bronchodilator or to liquefy secretions), the medication is absorbed rapidly through the pulmonary circulation and can create systemic effects. For example, isoproterenol (Isuprel) is a bronchodilator, but it can also cause cardiac arrhythmias.

Clients with chronic lung disease often depend on MDIs to control their airway symptoms. MDIs are advantageous to clients because (1) medications can be delivered to the airways in high concentrations and (2) systemic side effects are usually avoided.

Potential Nursing Diagnoses

Client data derived during the assessment reveal defining characteristics to support the following nursing diagnoses in clients requiring this skill:

Ineffective airway clearance
Ineffective breathing patterns
Knowledge deficit regarding use of inhalant

Equipment

Metered dose inhaler with medication canister
Aerochamber (optional)
Tissues (optional)
Water for rinsing mouth, especially after use of steroid inhalers

Steps	Rationale
1. Allow client an opportunity to manipulate inhaler and canister. Explain and demonstrate how canister fits into inhaler.	Client must be familiar with how to use equipment.
2. Explain what a metered dose is and warn client about overuse of inhaler, including drug side effects.	Client must not arbitrarily decide to administer excessive inhalations—serious side effects can result. If drug is given in recommended doses, side effects are uncommon.
3. Explain steps used to administer an inhaled dose of medication (demonstrate steps when possible):	Simple, step-by-step explanations allow client to ask questions at any point during procedure. You cannot demonstrate actual depression of canister without self-administering a dose.
■ Remove cap and hold inhaler upright, grasping it with thumb and first two fingers.	
■ Shake inhaler.	Mixes medication evenly within solution so that aerosol drug concentration is even.
■ Tilt head back slightly and breathe out.	Maximizes airway exposure to medication from inhaler.
■ Position inhaler in one of the following ways:	
(1) Open mouth with inhaler 0.5 cm (1 to 2 inches) away from mouth (Fig. 71).	Avoids rapid influx of inhaled medication and subsequent airway irritation.

 Fig. 71

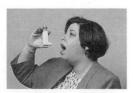

Steps	Rationale
(2) Attach spacer to mouthpiece of inhaler (Fig. 72).	Eliminates rapid influx of particles from inhaled drugs, which reduces irritant properties and tendency to cough. Spacer is recommended for young children (National Heart, Lung, and Blood Institute, 1991).

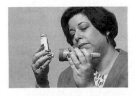

Fig. 72

(3) Place mouthpiece of inhaler or spacer in mouth.

■ Press down on inhaler to release medication (one puff) while inhaling slowly (Fig. 73).

Medication is distributed to airways during inhalation. Inhaling by mouth rather than by nose draws medication more effectively into airways.

Fig. 73

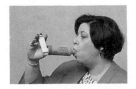

■ Breathe in slowly for 2 to 3 seconds.

As client inhales, particles of medication are delivered to airway (National Heart, Lung, and Blood Institute, 1991).

■ Hold breath for approximately 10 seconds.

Allows tiny drops of aerosol spray to reach deeper branches of airways.

Steps	Rationale
▪ Repeat puffs as ordered, waiting 1 minute between puffs.	Allows tiny drops of aerosol spray to reach deeper branches of airways.
4. If two MDIs are prescribed, wait 5 to 10 seconds between inhalations.	Allows maximal airway effect from first puff of medication. Therefore airways are more open for second delivery of medication.
5. Explain that client may feel gagging sensation in throat caused by droplets of medication on pharynx or tongue.	Results when inhalant is sprayed and inhaled incorrectly.
6. Instruct client in removing medication canister and cleaning inhaler in warm water.	Accumulation of spray around mouthpiece can interfere with proper distribution during use.
7. Ask if client has any questions.	Provides opportunity to clarify misconceptions or misunderstandings.
8. Have client demonstrate use of inhaler.	Return demonstration provides feedback for measuring client's learning.
9. Instruct client against repeating inhalations before next scheduled dose.	Drugs are prescribed at intervals during day to provide constant bronchodilation and minimize side effects.
10. Record in nurse's notes content or skills taught and client's ability to use inhaler.	Provides continuity to teaching plan so other members of nursing staff will not teach same material.

Nurse Alert

The client may gag or swallow medication if unable to inhale while spray is administered. The client's need for bronchodilator more frequently than every 4 hours can signal worsening of respiratory conditions, and the client's physician needs to be notified.

Clients who use steroid inhalers are at risk for topical *Candida* infection in the mouth and posterior pharynx. The nurse should observe for patchy white areas in the client's mouth.

Client Teaching

Instruct the client on proper use of an inhaler and the common side effects to expect. Explain the common signs and symptoms of xanthine and sympathomimetic drug overuse: tachycardia, palpitations, headache, restlessness, and insomnia. Instruct the client to clean the inhaler properly so as to avoid transmission of microorganisms. Instruct client to inspect mouth daily for signs of *Candida* infection; that is, patchy white lesions in mouth.

Pediatric Considerations

Children may not be able to learn how to use an inhaler until they reach school age. They also may need to pinch their nose shut during inhalation to gain the drug's effects.

Geriatric Considerations

Elderly clients with hand tremors or weakness in the ability to grasp objects may not be able to use an inhaler.

Instilling Vaginal
Medication

Vaginal medications come in cream and suppository forms and are used to treat localized infection or inflammation. It is important to avoid embarrassing the client when administering these preparations. Often the client prefers to learn how to self-administer the medication. Because the discharge that is symptomatic of vaginal infections can be foul smelling, it is important to offer the client good perineal hygiene.

Potential Nursing Diagnoses

Client data derived during the assessment reveal defining characteristics to support the following nursing diagnoses in clients requiring this skill:

   Pain
   Body-image disturbance
   Sexual dysfunction

Equipment

Medication ticket or form

Vaginal Suppository

Suppository
Clean disposable gloves
Lubricating jelly
Clean tissues
Suppository inserter (optional)
Perineal pad (optional)

Vaginal Cream

Cream
Plastic applicator
Clean disposable gloves
Paper towel
Perineal pad (optional)

Steps	Rationale
1. Review physician's order for name of drug, dosage, and route of administration.	Ensures safe and accurate administration of drug.
2. Wash hands and don clean gloves.	Reduces risk of transferring microorganisms.
3. Explain procedure to client.	Reduces client anxiety.
4. Check client's identification band and ask client's name.	Ensures that correct client receives right medication.
5. Have client lie in dorsal recumbent position.	Provides easy access to and good exposure of vaginal canal. Dependent position of client allows suppository to dissolve in vagina without escaping through orifice.
6. Keep abdomen and lower extremities draped.	Minimizes client embarrassment.
7. Don disposable gloves.	Prevents transmission of infection between nurse and client.

Suppository

1. Remove suppository from foil wrapper and apply liberal amount of water-soluble lubricant to smooth or rounded end. Lubricate gloved index finger of dominant hand.	Reduces friction against mucosal surfaces during insertion.
2. With nondominant gloved hand gently retract labial folds.	Exposes vaginal orifice.

Steps	Rationale
3. Insert rounded end of suppository along posterior wall of vaginal canal to length of index finger (7.5 to 10 cm [3 to 4 inches]) (Fig. 74).	Ensures equal distribution of medication along walls of vaginal cavity.

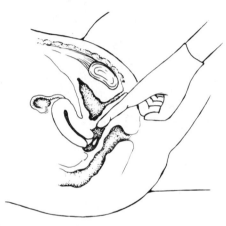

Fig. 74

4. Withdraw finger and wipe away any remaining lubricant from around orifice and labia.	Maintains client comfort.
5. Instruct client to remain on her back for at least 10 minutes.	Allows medication to melt and be absorbed into vaginal mucosa.
6. Offer perineal pad before client resumes ambulation.	Provides for client comfort.
7. Remove gloves by pulling them inside out and discard them in appropriate receptacle.	Prevents spread of microorganisms.
8. Wash hands. NOTE: Follow same procedure when using suppository inserter.	Reduces transfer of microorganisms.

Steps	Rationale
9. Record in medication record drug administered.	Prompt documentation prevents drug errors.

Vaginal Cream

Steps	Rationale
1. Fill cream applicator, following package directions.	Dosage is prescribed by volume in applicator.
2. With your nondominant gloved hand, gently retract labial folds.	Exposes vaginal orifice.
3. With your dominant gloved hand, insert applicator approximately 7.5 cm (3 inches). Push applicator plunger to deposit medication.	Allows for equal distribution of medication along walls of vaginal cavity.
4. Withdraw plunger and place it on a paper towel. Wipe off any residual cream from labia or vaginal orifice.	Residual cream on applicator may contain microorganisms.
5. Instruct client to remain flat on her back for at least 10 minutes.	Cream will be distributed and absorbed evenly in vaginal cavity rather than being lost through vaginal orifice.
6. Wash applicator with soap and warm water. Store it for future use.	Vaginal cavity is not sterile. Soap and water will assist in removing bacteria and residual cream.
7. Offer client a perineal pad before she resumes ambulation.	Provides client comfort.
8. Remove gloves and turn them inside out. Dispose of them in appropriate receptacle.	Disposing of gloves in this way reduces transfer of microorganisms.
9. Wash your hands.	Reduces transmission of microorganisms.
10. Record in medication record drug administered.	Prompt documentation prevents drug errors.

Nurse Alert

If suppository fails to dissolve and solid form is expelled, check expiration date on package.

Client Teaching

Clients often prefer to learn how to self-administer vaginal preparations. Using a step-by-step approach, allow the client to do a demonstration of the technique. It is important that she insert the suppository or cream correctly into the vaginal canal.

Geriatric Considerations

An elderly woman may have difficulty assuming a position that allows for self-administration of vaginal preparations. Arthritic conditions of the hips, knees, or upper extremities can make self-administration painful and difficult.

SKILL 5-12

Inserting a Rectal

Suppository

A variety of drugs are available in suppository form and create local as well as systemic effects. Aminophylline suppositories act systemically to dilate the respiratory bronchioles. A Dulcolax suppository acts locally to promote defecation. Suppositories are safe to administer. The nurse should be concerned primarily with placing the suppository correctly against the rectal mucosal wall, past the internal anal sphincter, so the suppository will not be expelled. Clients who have had rectal surgery or are experiencing rectal bleeding should not be given a suppository.

Potential Nursing Diagnoses

Client data derived during the assessment reveal defining characteristics to support the following nursing diagnoses in clients requiring this skill:

Alteration in health maintenance related to mobility restriction (client unable to self-administer drug)

Knowledge deficit regarding drug therapy

Constipation

Equipment

Medication ticket or form
Rectal suppository
Lubricating jelly
Clean disposable gloves
Tissue

Steps	Rationale
1. Review physician's order for name of drug, dosage, and route of administration.	Ensures that drug will be administered safely and accurately.
2. Wash hands and don gloves.	Reduces transfer of microorganisms.
3. Explain procedure to client.	Reduces client anxiety.
4. Check client's identification band and ask client's name.	Ensures that correct client receives right medication.
5. Ask client to assume a side-lying (Sims) position with upper leg flexed upward.	Exposes anus and helps client relax external anal sphincter.
6. Keep client draped with only anal area exposed.	Draping client maintains privacy and facilitates relaxation.
7. Remove suppository from its foil wrapper and lubricate rounded end with jelly. Lubricate gloved index finger of your dominant hand.	Lubrication reduces friction as suppository enters rectum.
8. Ask client to take slow deep breaths through his mouth and to relax anal sphincter.	Forcing suppository through a constricted sphincter causes pain.
9. Retract client's buttocks with your nondominant hand. With your gloved index finger, insert suppository gently through anus, past internal anal sphincter, and against rectal wall: 10 cm (4 inches) in adults, 5 cm (2 inches) in children and infants (Fig. 75).	Suppository must be placed against rectal mucosa for eventual absorption and therapeutic action.

Steps	Rationale

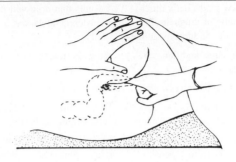

Fig. 75

10. Withdraw your finger and wipe off client's anal area.

   Provides client comfort.

11. Instruct client to remain flat or on his side for 5 minutes.

   Prevents expulsion of the suppository.

12. If suppository contains a laxative or fecal softener, place call light within client's reach so he can obtain assistance to reach a bedpan or toilet.

   Being able to call for assistance provides client with sense of control over elimination.

13. Discard gloves by turning them inside out and dispose of them in appropriate receptacle.

   Disposing of gloves in this way reduces transfer of microorganisms.

14. Wash your hands.

   Reduces transfer of microorganisms.

15. Record in medication record drug administered.

   Prompt documentation prevents drug errors.

Nurse Alert

Although it is unusual, a client may experience a vagal reflex response (slowing of the heart rate) as a result of excessive rectal stimulation.

Client Teaching

Clients may prefer learning how to self-administer rectal suppositories. This can be difficult unless the nurse is clear as to how to insert the suppository past the internal anal sphincter. A client must be familiar with the sensation felt as the sphincter relaxes over the insertion finger.

Pediatric Considerations

The rectal route is chosen only when children are unable to take food or liquid by mouth and when it is unlikely that they have large amounts of stool. The rectum must be empty for effective drug absorption.

Geriatric Considerations

An elderly client may have mobility restrictions that prohibit self-administration of suppositories.

INFECTION
CONTROL

Handwashing

Nosocomial infections are infections that result from then delivery of health services or occur in a health care facility. They are associated with diagnostic or therapeutic procedures and often involve extended stays, thus increasing the cost of health care to both the client and the health care worker.

Using masks, protective eyewear, gloves, and specialized gowns assists in reducing the risk of transmission of blood-borne pathogens (CDC, 1988; Pugliese and Lampinen, 1989). Along with these aids to infection control, the nurse must remember that handwashing is the most important and basic technique in preventing and controlling infection (CDC, 1988). However, the ideal duration of handwashing is not known. The Centers for Disease Control (CDC) and the Public Health Service note that washing times of at least 10 to 15 seconds will remove most transient microorganisms from the skin (Garner and Favero, 1985). If hands are visibly soiled, more time may be needed. Agency policies often recommend that staff members wash hands for 1 to 2 minutes after working in high-risk areas (e.g., trauma units and emergency rooms). Routine handwashing may be performed with bar, liquid, or granule soap or soap-impregnated tissue.

Potential Nursing Diagnoses

Client data derived during the assessment reveal defining characteristics to support the following nursing diagnoses:

High risk for infection

Equipment

Sink with warm running water
Soap or disinfectant in foot-operated dispenser (or bar soap)
Paper towels
Orange stick (optional)

Steps	Rationale
1. Push wristwatch and long uniform sleeves up above your wrists. Remove jewelry.	Provides complete access to fingers, hands, and wrists. Rings increase number of microorganisms on hands (Jacobson et al, 1985).
2. Keep your fingernails short and filed.	Most microbes on hands come from beneath the nails (McGinley et al, 1988).
3. Inspect surface of your hands and fingers for any breaks or cuts in skin and cuticles. Report such lesions when caring for highly susceptible clients.	Open cuts or wounds can harbor high concentrations of microorganisms. Such lesions may serve as portals of exit, increasing client's exposure to infection, or as portals of entry, increasing your risk of acquiring an infection.
4. Stand in front of sink, keeping hands and uniform away from sink surface. (If hands touch sink during handwashing, repeat the process.) Use a sink where it is comfortable to reach faucet.	Inside of sink is a contaminated area. Reaching over sink increases risk of touching edge, which is contaminated.
5. Turn on water. Press foot pedals with foot to regulate flow and temperature. Push knee pedals laterally to control flow and temperature. Turn on hand-operated faucets by covering faucet with paper towel.	When hands come in contact with faucet, they are considered contaminated. Organisms spread easily from hands to faucet.
6. Avoid splashing water against your uniform.	Microorganisms travel and grow in moisture.
7. Regulate flow of water so temperature is warm.	Warm water is more comfortable. Hot water opens pores of skin, causing irritation.

Steps	Rationale
8. Wet hands and forearms thoroughly under running water. Keep hands and forearms lower than elbows during washing (Fig. 76).	Hands are the most contaminated parts to be washed. Water flows from least to most contaminated area.

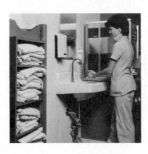

Fig. 76

Steps	Rationale
9. Apply 1 ml of regular or 3 ml of antiseptic liquid soap to hands and lather thoroughly. If bar soap is used, hold it throughout the lathering period. Soap granules and leaflet preparations may be used.	Bacterial counts drop significantly on hands when using 3 to 5 ml of antimicrobial soap (Larsen, 1987).
10. Wash hands using plenty of lather and friction for 10 to 15 seconds. Interlace fingers and rub palms and back of hands with circular motion (Fig. 77).	Soap cleanses by emulsifying fat and oil and lowering surface tension. Friction and mechanical rubbing loosen and remove dirt and transient bacteria. Interlacing fingers and thumbs ensures that all surfaces are cleansed. Antimicrobial soap must be in contact with skin for at least 10 seconds (Garner, 1985).
11. If areas underlying fingernails are soiled, clean them with fingernails of other hand and additional soap or a clean orange wood stick.	Mechanical removal of dirt and sediment under nails reduces microorganisms on hands.

Steps   Rationale

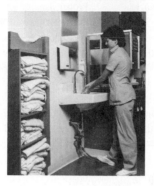

Fig. 77

Do not tear or cut skin under or around nail.

12. Rinse hands and wrists   Rinsing mechanically washes
    thoroughly, keeping hands   away dirt and microorganisms.
    down and elbows up.

13. Repeat Steps 9 through 11   The greater the likelihood that
    but extend actual period of   hands will be contaminated, the
    washing for 1-, 2-, and   greater the need for thorough
    3-minute handwashings.   handwashing.

14. Dry hands thoroughly, wip-   Dry from cleanest area (finger-
    ing from fingers down to   tips) to least clean area (wrists)
    wrists and forearms (Fig.   to avoid contamination.
    78).   Drying hands prevents chapping
                                    and roughened skin.

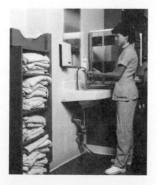

Fig. 78

Steps	Rationale
15. Discard paper towel in proper receptacle.	Proper disposal of contaminated objects prevents transfer of microorganisms.
16. Turn off water with foot and knee pedals. To turn off a hand faucet, use a clean, dry paper towel.	Wet towel and wet hands allow transfer of pathogens by capillary action.
17. Keep hands and cuticles well lubricated with hand lotion or moisturizer between washings.	Dry, chapped skin cracks easily, creating portal of entry for infection.

Nurse Alert

If the nurse has an open lesion or wound on the hand, some agencies have policies prohibiting contact with clients.

Care of a Client
in Isolation

The nurse must observe special precautions when caring for clients who either have greater susceptibility to infection or are carriers of microorganisms that can be easily transmitted to other persons. Occasionally, protective isolation or isolation precautions keep the affected client within the confines of the room. The nurse uses protective coverings such as a mask, gown, or gloves, depending on how the organism is transmitted and how susceptible the client is to infection. Staying within a confined area and being cared for by nurses covered in protective clothing are factors that can cause a person to feel socially isolated. Whenever the nurse cares for the client in isolation, it is important to maintain therapeutic communication and provide a personalized approach to care.

Potential Nursing Diagnoses

Client data derived during the assessment reveal defining characteristics to support the following nursing diagnoses in clients requiring this skill:

High risk for infection
Impaired social isolation

Equipment

The selection of equipment depends on the type of care to be administered to the client (e.g., supplies for administering medications, supplies for hygiene, supplies for bedmaking).

Steps	Rationale
1. Refer to physician's orders for type of isolation in which client is to be placed.	Type of isolation category influences type of protective clothing worn and precautions followed.
2. Refer to policy and procedure manual or infection control policy of institution for precautions to follow.	Each institution may require guidelines that vary from CDC recommendations.
3. Review laboratory test results to determine type of microorganisms for which client is being isolated.	Allows you to know what microorganism is infecting client and medium in which it was identified (e.g., sputum, blood, wound). This information will enable you to be appropriately cautious when handling infected exudate or drainage.
4. Consider types of care measures or procedures to be performed while in client's room.	Helps you anticipate needs for supplies, time your organization while in room, and coordinate your activities.
5. Prepare all necessary equipment and supplies.	Prevents need to leave and reenter room several times, increasing risk of infection.
6. Wash hands.	Reduces transmission of microorganisms.
7. Apply gown, mask, and gloves as appropriate:	Protective garments prevent transmission of organisms from nurse to client and protect nurse from contact with infectious pathogens.
a. Apply gown, being sure it covers all outer garments. Pull sleeves down to wrist. Tie securely at neck and waist (Fig. 79).	
b. Apply disposable gloves. If worn with gown, bring cuffs over edge of gown sleeves.	

Steps	Rationale

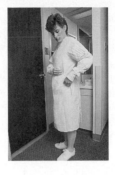

Fig. 79

   c. Apply surgical mask around mouth and nose; tie securely.

8. Enter client's room. Arrange supplies and equipment. (If equipment will be removed from room for reuse, place on paper towel.)

Prevents contamination of items.

9. Assess vital signs:
   a. Place clean paper towel on bedside table. Place additional piece of paper on top.
   b. Place watch on towel for easy visibility.
   c. If equipment remains in room, proceed to assess vital signs by routine procedures. Avoid contact of stethoscope or blood pressure cuff with infective material.
   d. Write vital sign results on piece of paper.

Helps avoid contact of clean items with contaminated environment in isolation room.

Steps	Rationale
e. If stethoscope is to be reused, clean diaphragm or bell with alcohol. Set aside on clean surface.	
10. Administer medications.	
a. Give oral medication in wrapper or cup.	Supplies are handled and discarded to minimize transfer of microorganisms.
b. Dispose of wrapper or cup in plastic-lined receptacle.	
c. Administer injection while wearing gloves.	
d. Discard syringe and uncapped needle into special container. If reusable syringe (e.g., Carpuject) is used, dispose of inner cartridge and needle in special container.	
e. Place reusable syringe on clean towel for eventual removal and disinfection.	Prevents added contamination of syringe.
11. Provide hygiene.	
a. Avoid allowing gown to become wet.	Moisture on gown provides path for microorganisms to spread to your uniform.
b. Assist client in removing gown; discard in special linen bag.	
c. Remove linen from bed; if excessively soiled, avoid contact with your gown. Dispose in special linen bag.	Linen soiled by client's body fluids is disposed of to prevent contact with clean items.
d. Provide clean bed linen and set of towels.	

Steps	Rationale
e. Change gloves if they become excessively soiled and further care is necessary.	
12. Collect specimens.	Specimens of blood and body fluids are placed in well-constructed containers with secure lids to prevent leaks during transport.
a. Place specimen containers on clean paper towel in client's bathroom.	
b. Collect necessary specimens using appropriate technique. Transfer specimen to container by minimizing contact of gloved hands with outer surface of container.	Each type of body excretion or exudate must be collected in specific manner to prevent contamination by resident flora. Containers will be handled by laboratory personnel and should remain clean on outside.
c. Verify that specimen container is sealed tightly and outer surface of container is not soiled. Transfer container to clean, leak-proof bag.	Prevents spillage and contamination of its outer surface.
d. Label specimen container with client's name. Send to laboratory (warning labels may be used, depending on hospital policy).	Properly labeled specimens are essential so that correct laboratory results are reported for correct client.
13. Dispose of linen and trash bags as they become full.	Soiled linen or refuse should be totally contained to prevent exposure of personnel to infective material.

Steps	Rationale

a. Use single bags to contain soiled articles if they are impervious to moisture and are sturdy.

b. Tie bags securely at top (Fig. 80).

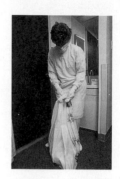

Fig. 80

14. Resupply room as needed by having another caregiver hand over supplies at door.

Limited trips of personnel into and out of room reduces your and client's exposure to microorganisms.

15. Leave isolation room

a. Untie gown at waist. Remove gloves by grasping cuff of one glove and pulling it off, turning glove inside out. With your ungloved hand, tuck finger inside cuff of remaining glove and pull off, turning inside out (Figs. 81 and 82).

Gloves are removed first because they are most likely to be contaminated and should not be used to touch hair around mask.

b. Untie or pull off mask from around your ears and dispose of it in receptacle.

Steps   Rationale

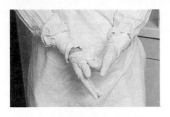

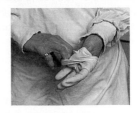

Fig. 81   Fig. 82

c. Untie neck strings of
   gown. Allow gown to
   fall from shoulders. Remove hands from
   sleeves without touching
   outside of gown. Hold
   gown inside at shoulder
   seams and fold inside
   out. Discard in laundry
   bag.

d. Wash your hands for   Mechanically removes any tran-
   minimum of 10 seconds.   sient microorganisms contacted.
                                Clean hands may touch clean
e. Retrieve wristwatch and   watch and stethoscope.
   stethoscope, taking care
   not to touch them. Note
   vital sign values on paper.

f. Tell client when you
   plan to return to room.
   Ask whether client re-
   quires any personal care
   items.

g. Leave room, closing   Room should remain closed,
   door securely.   especially when airborne infec-
                                tion is being isolated.

16. Record vital signs and other   Documents care provided.
    procedures according to
    guidelines for each skill in
    nurse's notes.

Nurse Alert

Be sure that you are familiar with the specific guidelines for each isolation category. It is important to know what type of infection the client has and in what manner the infective organisms are transmitted.

Client Teaching

Explain the purpose for and importance of isolation techniques. Clients must understand that the precautions used are for everyone's safety. If the client understands isolation practices, he can help enforce procedures when visitors enter the room.

Pediatric Considerations

Preschoolers may view isolation as a form of punishment. Older children should be given a thorough explanation of procedures to minimize fears and fantasies. Show children the different forms of protective clothing. Young children can play "dress up" with masks and gloves. If possible, allow children to see your face before applying a mask.

Geriatric Considerations

Elderly clients may be more at risk of sensory deprivation than are younger clients because of normal aging processes. They will consistently need meaningful sensory stimuli while in isolation. Some simple actions to take might include turning on the lights when entering the room, raising the head of the bed and repositioning the client, opening window shades or curtains, and sitting down to have a relaxed discussion.

Protective Eyewear

Using protective eyewear such as goggles, a face shield, or a face mask prevents transmission of pathogens by way of the health care worker's mucous membranes (e.g., around the eye, nasal, and oral cavities). This protection is recommended when health care workers are in areas where suctioning, dressing changes, or hygiene care can cause the splattering of blood and/or body fluids on the health care worker (Pugliese and Lampinen, 1989).

Potential Nursing Diagnoses

Client data derived during the assessment reveal defining characteristics to support the following nursing diagnoses:

High risk for infection

Equipment

Plastic face shield
or
Plastic eye goggles

Steps	Rationale
1. Wash hands.	Reduces transmission of micro-organisms.
2. Apply protective eyewear.	

Goggles

■ Secure goggles comfortably over eyes. Tighten as needed.	Goggles reduce the risk of blood/body fluid droplet transmission to the mucous membranes of the eyes only.

Steps	Rationale

Face Shield

■ Secure shield over top of the head. Move shield over the face and adjust as needed to protect the worker's facial mucous membranes.

Face shields offer more protection to the mucous membranes of the face. During procedures resulting in the splattering of droplets of blood and body fluids, this type of protection is recommended.

3. After procedure is completed, either leave protective goggles or shield at the client's bedside or discard in appropriate receptacle. Do not wear goggles or shield outside the client's room.

Protective shields may be worn more than once for nonsterile procedures.
Proper disposal reduces transmission of pathogens.
Wearing protective eye shields outside the client's room increases risk of transmission of pathogens.

4. Wash hands.

Reduces transmission of microorganisms.

Nurse Alert

These protective devices are designed to reduce the risk of transmission of blood-borne pathogens to the nurse; they are not ordered by physicians. It is a nursing judgment to wear these shields. In certain agencies, wearing these face protectors is mandatory in high-risk situations (e.g., in trauma units, when caring for a client with AIDS and a respiratory infection, and in operating rooms).

Donning a Mask

A mask may be worn for several reasons: as a precaution to reduce air-droplet transmission of microorganisms while caring for a client in isolation, when assisting with a sterile procedure, or when preparing sterile supplies for a sterile field. A special high-filtration mask should be worn to protect the nurse from infectious respiratory diseases such as tuberculosis. The type of mask used is determined by hospital policy. The nurse should apply the mask snugly around face and nose; otherwise it is ineffective in controlling air-droplet nuclei. A surgical mask is always applied before the nurse performs a surgical handwash. When a mask becomes moist, it should be changed. Moisture promotes the spread of microorganisms.

Potential Nursing Diagnoses

Client data derived during the assessment reveal defining characteristics to support the following nursing diagnoses:

High risk for infection

Equipment

Clean disposable mask

Steps	Rationale
Application of Mask	
1. Find top edge of mask (mask usually has a thin metal strip along edge). Newer masks recommended by the CDC have elastic headbands. Check agency policy for proper mask use.	Pliable metal fits snugly against bridge of nose.

Steps	Rationale
2. Hold mask by top two strings or loops. Tie two top ties at the top of the back of your head, with ties *above* your ears (alternative: slip loops over each ear) (Fig. 83). NOTE: High-filtration masks are secured by two rubber bands.	Position of ties at top of head provides tight fit. Ties overlapping ears may cause irritation.

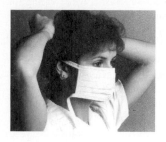

Fig. 83   Fig. 84

3. Tie two lower ties snugly around your neck, with mask well under chin (Fig. 84).	Prevents escape of microorganisms through sides of mask as you talk or breathe.
4. Gently pinch upper metal band around the bridge of your nose.	Prevents microorganisms from escaping around nose.

Removal of Mask

1. If you have gloves on, remove them and wash your hands.	Prevents contamination of hair, neck, and face from contact with soiled gloves.
2. Untie both ties and fold mask in half with inner surfaces together.	Avoids contact with contaminated inner surface.
3. Dispose of mask in receptacle.	Reduces spread of infection.

Client Teaching

When caring for a client in isolation, explain the purpose of a mask. The mask may add to a client's feeling of becoming depersonalized.

Pediatric Considerations

If a child is awake in the operating room, allow him to see your face, if possible, before applying the mask.

Surgical

Handwashing

Nurses who work in sterile areas such as operating rooms or labor and delivery rooms must practice surgical handwashing. The technique requires greater effort than routine handwashing. During a surgical scrub the nurse washes a wider area, from fingertips to elbows. Usually the duration of a scrub is from 5 to 10 minutes to ensure that all skin surfaces are thoroughly cleaned. For maximal cleansing and removal of bacteria the nurse removes all jewelry from her fingers and arms and keeps her fingernails short, clean, and free of polish.

Potential Nursing Diagnoses

Client data derived during the assessment reveal defining characteristics to support the following nursing diagnoses in clients requiring this skill:
    High risk for infection

Equipment

Deep sink with foot pedals or knee controls
Antimicrobial soap (e.g., CHG or iodophor)
Disposable hand brushes and nail file
Orange stick or disposable nail file

Steps	Rationale
1. Check hands and fingers for cuts or abrasions.	Areas of inflammation or breaks in skin can harbor microorganisms.
2. Remove all jewelry.	Harbors microorganisms.

Steps	Rationale
3. Apply a face mask, making certain to cover your nose and mouth snugly.	Prevents escape of microorganisms into air, which can contaminate hands.
4. Adjust water flow to lukewarm temperature.	Hot water removes protective oils from the skin and increases skin's sensitivity to soap.
5. Wet your hands and forearms liberally, keeping hands above level of elbows during entire procedure. NOTE: Your scrub dress or uniform must be kept dry.	Water runs by gravity from fingertips to elbows. Hands become cleanest part of upper extremity. Keeping hands elevated allows water to flow from least to most contaminated area.
6. Dispense a liberal amount of soap (2 to 5 ml) into hands and lather hands and arms to 5 cm (2 inches) above elbows.	Washing wide area reduces risk of contaminating overlying gown that you will apply.
7. Clean nails under running water with orange stick or file (Fig. 85). Discard file.	Removes dirt and organic material that harbor large numbers of microorganisms.
8. Wet brush and apply antimicrobial soap. Scrub fingernails, hand, arm in following manner (Fig. 86)	Loosens resident bacteria that adhere to skin's surface. Methodical scrub covers all skin surfaces.

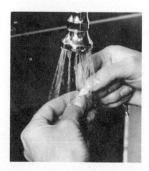

Fig. 85

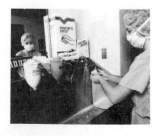

Fig. 86

Steps	Rationale
a. Scrub nails of hand 15 strokes.	
b. Using circular motion, scrub palm of hand and anterior surface of fingers 10 strokes.	
c. Scrub side of thumb 10 strokes and posterior aspect of thumb 10 strokes.	
d. Scrub sides and back of each finger 10 strokes each area.	
e. Scrub back of hand 10 strokes	
9. Rinse brush thoroughly. Reapply soap.	Rinsing of brush removes microorganisms and avoids contamination of arms.
10. Mentally divide arms into thirds. Scrub each surface of lower forearm with circular motion for 10 strokes; scrub middle and upper forearm in same manner. Discard brush.	Scrubbing loosens resident bacteria that adhere to skin's surface.
11. With arms flexed, rinse thoroughly from fingertips to elbow in one motion, allowing water to run off at elbow (Fig. 87).	

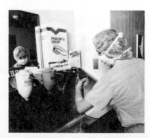

Fig. 87

Steps	Rationale
12. Repeat steps 8 through 11 for other arm.	
13. Keeping arms flexed, discard second brush. Turn off water with foot pedal.	Prevents contamination of hands.
14. Use sterile towel to dry one hand thoroughly, moving from fingers to elbow. Dry in a rotating motion. NOTE: If you wish to apply sterile gloves for use in a regular clinical area you need not use brushes or dry your hands with sterile towels. Thorough lathering and friction performed twice according to procedure will ensure clean hands. In this situation you may use clean paper towels for drying.	Dry from cleanest to least clean area. Drying prevents chapping and facilitates donning of gloves.
15. Repeat drying method for other hand, using different area of towel or a new sterile towel.	Prevents contamination of hand.
16. Keep hands higher than elbows and away from your body.	Prevents accidental contamination.
17. Proceed into operating room or labor and delivery area, keeping hands from contacting any object.	If your hands touch any object, scrub must be repeated.

Nurse Alert

Throughout the procedure and afterwards the nurse must not allow an unsterile object to touch her hands or lower arms.

Open Gloving

The nurse applies sterile gloves by the open method when preparing to work with certain types of sterile equipment and when performing sterile procedures such as dressing changes or catheter insertion. The gloves provide a barrier between the nurse's hands and the objects she contacts. She is able to freely touch objects in a sterile field without concern of contamination. When wearing sterile gloves, she should always remain conscious of which objects are sterile and which are not. A glove becomes contaminated whenever it contacts a nonsterile object.

Potential Nursing Diagnoses

This procedure may be performed by nurses caring for clients with various nursing diagnoses.

Equipment

Package of sterile gloves of proper size

Steps	Rationale
1. Wash hands thoroughly.	Reduces numbers of microorganisms residing on surfaces of hands.
2. Remove outer package wrapper by carefully peeling apart sides.	Prevents inner glove package from accidentally opening and touching contaminated objects.
3. Grasp inner package and lay it on a clean flat surface just above waist level. Open package, keeping gloves on wrapper's inside surface.	Sterile object held below your waist is considered contaminated. Inner surface of glove package is considered sterile.

Steps	Rationale
4. If gloves are not prepowdered, take packet of powder and apply lightly to hands over a sink or wastebasket.	Powder allows gloves to slip on easily. (Some physicians do not use powder for fear of promoting growth of microorganisms.)
5. Identify right and left glove. Each glove has a cuff approximately 5 cm (2 inches) wide. Glove your dominant hand first.	Proper identification of gloves prevents contamination by improper fit. Gloving of dominant hand first improves your dexterity with procedure.
6. With thumb and first two fingers of your nondominant hand, grasp edge of cuff of glove for dominant hand. Touch only the glove's inside surface (Fig. 88).	Inner edge of cuff will lie against your skin and thus is not considered sterile. NOTE: Left hand dominant in photo.
7. Carefully pull glove over your dominant hand, leaving a cuff and being sure that cuff does not roll up your wrist. Be sure also that thumb and fingers are in proper spaces (Fig. 89).	If glove's outer surface touches your hand or wrist, it is contaminated.
8. With your gloved dominant hand, slip your fingers underneath second glove's cuff (Fig. 90).	Cuff protects your gloved fingers. Sterile touching sterile prevents glove contamination.

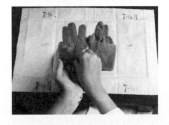

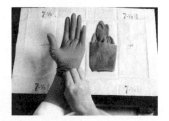

Fig. 88   Fig. 89

Steps   Rationale

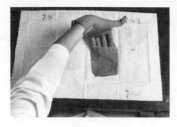

Fig. 90

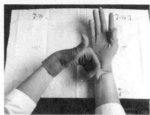

Fig. 91

9. Carefully pull second glove
   over your nondominant
   hand. Do not allow fingers
   and thumb of gloved dominant hand to touch any part
   of your exposed nondominant hand. Keep thumb of
   dominant hand abducted
   back (Fig. 91).

Contact of gloved hand with
exposed hand results in contamination.

10. Once second glove is on,
    interlock your hands. Cuffs
    usually fall down after ap-
    plication. Be sure to touch
    only sterile sides (Fig. 92).

Ensures smooth fit over fingers.

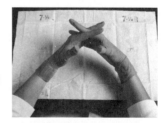

Fig. 92

Nurse Alert

If the outer (clean) surface of a glove touches a nonsterile object,
such as a portion of your arm or the table surface, remove and
repeat gloving.

Client Teaching

Explain to the client why gloves are used during a procedure. At
times the client may perceive the use of gloves as the nurse's re-
luctance to touch him.

HYGIENE

Tepid Sponging

A common form of therapeutic bath is tepid sponging. Tepid sponging is used when a client has a high fever. The procedure promotes the controlled loss of body heat through evaporation and conduction. Because cooling occurs slowly, temperature fluctuations are avoided. The use of tepid water prevents chilling, which can cause an elevation in body temperature from muscular shivering.

Parents of small children should learn how to safely administer tepid sponge baths in the home setting. Young children are at risk of having a seizure when fevers become high. The nurse in a health care setting can begin tepid sponging while pursuing additional orders from a physician for temperature control.

Potential Nursing Diagnoses

Client data derived during the assessment reveal defining characteristics to support the following nursing diagnoses in clients requiring this skill:

  Hyperthermia
  Knowledge deficit regarding fever management

Equipment

Bath basin
Waterproof pads
Tepid water (37° C [98.6° F])
Bath blanket
Bath thermometer
Ethyl alcohol (optional)
Washcloths
Thermometer
Disposable gloves

Steps	Rationale
1. Wash hands and apply gloves if appropriate.	Reduces transmission of micro-organisms.
2. Explain to client that purpose of tepid sponging is to cool body slowly. Describe in brief the steps of procedure.	Procedure can be uncomfortable because of cool water application. Anxiety over procedure can increase body temperature.
3. Close room curtain or door.	Maintains client privacy.
4. Measure client's temperature and pulse.	Provides baseline to measure effects of sponging.
5. Place waterproof pads under client and remove gown.	Pads prevent soiling of bed linen. Removing gown provides access to all skin surfaces.
6. Keep bath blanket over body parts not being sponged. Close windows and door to prevent drafts in room.	Bath blanket prevents chilling.
7. Check water temperature.	Tepid water prevents chilling.
8. Immerse washcloths in water and apply wet cloths under each axilla and over groin. If using tub, immerse client for 20-30 minutes.	Axilla and groin are areas containing large superficial blood vessels. Application of sponges promotes cooler temperature of the body's core by conduction. Immersion provides more effective heat loss.
9. Gently sponge an extremity for 5 minutes. Note client's response. Opposite extremity may be covered by a cool washcloth.	Prevents sudden temperature decrease and minimizes risk of developing chills.
10. Dry extremity and reassess client's pulse and body temperature. Observe client's response to therapy.	Client's response to therapy is monitored to prevent sudden temperature change.

Steps	Rationale
11. Continue sponging other extremities, back, and buttocks for 3 to 5 minutes each. Reassess temperature and pulse every 15 minutes.	Exposure of all body parts to sponging facilitates drop in body temperature.
12. Change water and reapply sponges to axilla and groin as needed.	Water temperature rises as result of exposure to client's warm body surface.
13. When body temperature falls to slightly above normal (38° C or 100° F), discontinue procedure.	This prevents a temperature drift to a subnormal level.
14. Dry extremities and body parts thoroughly. Cover client with a light bath blanket or sheet.	Drying and covering client prevent chilling. Excessively heavy covering may increase body temperature.
15. Dispose of equipment and change bed linen if soiled.	Controls transmission of infection.
16. Measure client's body temperature.	Indicates response to therapy.
17. Record in nurse's notes time that procedure was started and terminated, vital sign changes, and client's response, such as the presence of chills.	Communicates care provided in an accurate and timely fashion.

Nurse Alert

If the client begins to shiver, discontinue the procedure. Shivering causes elevation in body temperature.

Client Teaching

Teach parents of small children how to perform a tepid bath in the home. Temperatures above 39° C or 102° F generally indicate the need for sponging. Adding alcohol to the water should be done only after instructions by the pediatrician. Adding alcohol to the water increases the risk of alcohol poisoning by inhalation.

Pediatric Considerations

A child's temperature can rise suddenly because his temperature regulation mechanisms are immature. Often the only warning sign is warm skin. It may be easier to immerse an infant or small child in a tub of tepid water than to actually sponge him. Exposure of all body parts simultaneously improves heat loss. Immersion also reduces the infant's tendency to cry, which can increase body temperature. The child's head and shoulders should always be firmly supported during immersion.

Geriatric Considerations

The elderly client may have altered circulatory and heat conservation mechanisms. Peripheral vasoconstriction and muscular contraction (the shivering response) do not always occur normally following a drop in the environmental temperature. During sponging it is especially important to monitor an elderly client's body temperature because a decrease can occur quickly.

Female
Perineal Care

Perineal care in women involves thorough cleaning of the external genitalia. The procedure can usually be performed during the bath. Most women prefer washing their perineal areas themselves if they are physically able. Perineal care prevents and controls the spread of infection, prevents skin breakdown, promotes comfort, and maintains cleanliness.

When a nurse provides perineal hygiene for the client, the nurse must wear gloves to reduce the risk of transmission of microorganisms, such as HIV or herpes, from perineal drainage.

Potential Nursing Diagnoses

Client data derived during the assessment reveal defining characteristics to support the following nursing diagnoses in clients requiring this skill:

High risk for infection
Knowledge deficit regarding basic hygiene care
Impaired skin integrity related to drainage or incontinence

Equipment

Washbasin
Bath blanket
Soap dish with soap
Waterproof pad or bedpan
Disposable or cloth washcloths (two or three)
Toilet tissue
Disposable gloves
Bath towel
Disposable bag

Steps	Rationale
1. Explain procedure and its purpose to client.	Helps minimize anxiety during a procedure that is often embarrassing both to you and client.
2. Pull curtain around client's bed or close room door. Assemble supplies at bedside.	Maintains client's privacy.
3. Raise bed to comfortable working position.	Facilitates good body mechanics, which helps protect you from injury.
4. Wash hands and don gloves.	Reduces transmission of microorganisms.
5. Lower side rail. Assist client to a dorsal recumbent position.	Provides easy access to genitalia.
6. Position waterproof pad under client's buttocks or place bedpan under client.	Prevents bedclothes from becoming wet.
7. Drape client by placing bath blanket with one corner between client's legs, one corner pointing toward each side of bed, and one corner at client's chest. Wrap bath blanket around client's far leg by bringing corner around leg and tucking it under hip. Drape near leg in same way (Figs. 93 and 94).	Prevents unnecessary exposure of body parts and maintains client's warmth and comfort during procedure.

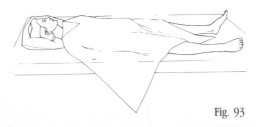

Fig. 93

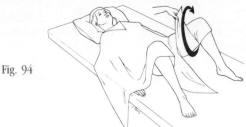

Fig. 94

Steps	Rationale
8. Raise side rail. Fill washbasin with water that is approximately 41° to 43° C (105° to 109.4° F).	Rail maintains client's safety from accidental fall. Proper water temperature prevents burns to perineum.
9. Place washbasin and toilet tissue on overbed table. Place disposable or regular washcloths in washbasin.	
10. Lower side rail and help client flex her knees and spread her legs (a client with knee or hip disease may keep her legs straight).	Provides full exposure of genitalia.
11. Fold lower corner of bath blanket up between client's legs onto her abdomen.	Keeping client draped until procedure begins minimizes anxiety.
12. Wash and dry client's upper thighs.	Buildup of perineal secretions can soil surrounding skin surfaces.
13. Wash labia majora. Using your nondominant hand, retract labia from thigh. With dominant hand, wash carefully in skin folds. ■ Wipe from perineum toward anus. Repeat on opposite side using different section of washcloth. Rinse and dry area thoroughly.	Skinfolds may contain body secretions that harbor infection and cause body odor. Reduces chance of transmitting microorganisms to urinary meatus.

Steps	Rationale
14. Separate labia with your nondominant hand. With other hand, wash downward from pubic area toward anus in one smooth stroke. Use different section of washcloth for each stroke. Pay particular attention to areas around labia minora, clitoris, and vaginal orifice (Fig. 95).	Reduces chance of transmitting microorganisms to urinary meatus.

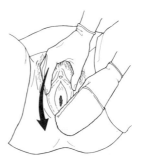

Fig. 95

15. If client is on a bedpan, pour warm water over her perineal area. Dry perineal area thoroughly.	Rinsing removes soap and microorganisms more effectively than wiping. Retained moisture harbors microorganisms.
16. Fold center corner of bath blanket back between client's legs over perineum. Help client off bedpan, lower her legs, and assist her to side-lying position.	Bath blanket prevents unnecessary exposure of body parts. Side-lying position provides easy visualization of anal area.
17. Clean anal area by wiping off any excess fecal material with toilet tissue. Wash area by wiping from vagina toward anus with one stroke. Discard washcloth. Repeat with clean cloth until skin is clear (Fig. 96).	Cleaning prevents transmission of microorganisms.

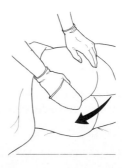

Fig. 96

Steps	Rationale
18. Rinse area well and dry with towel. Remove blanket and dispose of all soiled bed linen.	Retained moisture can cause maceration of skin. Properly disposing of equipment reduces spread of microorganisms.
19. Remove gloves and dispose of them in proper receptacle.	Moisture and body excretions on gloves can harbor microorganisms.
20. Assist client to comfortable position and cover her with sheet.	Making client comfortable minimizes emotional stress of procedure.
21. Raise side rail and lower bed to proper height. Return client's room to condition it was in before procedure.	Side rail protects client from fall. Clean environment promotes client's comfort.
22. Wash your hands.	Reduces transmission of microorganisms.
23. Record in nurse's notes and report any observations (e.g., amount and character of discharge, condition of genitalia).	Timely recording ensures accurate documentation of care.

Nurse Alert

The presence of foul-smelling discharge may indicate an infection and require a physician's attention.

Women with urinary or fecal incontinence or who are recovering from rectal or perineal surgery, surgery involving the lower urinary tract, or childbirth require special attention with perineal care. Care needs to be offered frequently.

Client Teaching

Adolescent girls should learn basic perineal hygiene and understand why they are predisposed to urinary tract infections.

Pediatric Considerations

A common problem among infants is diaper rash, created by the hot humid environment under the diaper. Airing and cooling are the most effective ways to promote healing. Change diapers as soon as they become wet. Remove excess clothing and occlusive diaper coverings.

Geriatric Considerations

Elderly women commonly have atrophy of the external genitalia along with a reduction in hair growth over the perineum.

Male
Perineal Care

A male client requires special attention during perineal care, especially if he is uncircumcised. The foreskin causes secretions to accumulate easily around the crown of the penis near the urethral meatus. Penile cancer occurs more frequently in uncircumcised males and is believed to be related to cleanliness. Bacteria that collect under the foreskin act on desquamated cells to produce smegma, a substance irritating to the glans penis and prepuce.

As with the female client, the nurse should wear gloves when providing perineal care to the male. In addition, the male client requires perineal hygiene as a routine part of the bath, but also whenever urinary incontinence occurs and as a part of Foley catheter care.

Potential Nursing Diagnoses

Client data derived during the assessment reveal defining characteristics to support the following nursing diagnoses in clients requiring this skill:

High risk for infection
Knowledge deficit regarding basic hygiene care

Equipment

Washbasin
Bath blanket
Soap dish with soap
Waterproof pad or bedpan
Disposable or cloth washcloths (two or three)
Toilet tissue
Disposable gloves
Bath towel
Disposable bag

Steps	Rationale
1. Explain procedure and its purpose to client.	Helps minimize anxiety during a procedure that is often embarrassing to both you and client.
2. Pull curtain around client's bed or close room door. Assemble supplies at the bedside.	Maintains client privacy.
3. Raise bed to comfortable working position.	Facilitates good body mechanics and safety.
4. Wash hands and don gloves.	Reduces transmission of microorganisms.
5. Lower side rail. Assist client to a supine position.	Provides easy access to genitalia.
6. Position waterproof pad under client's buttocks or place bedpan under client.	Prevents bedclothes from becoming wet.
7. Drape client by placing bath blanket with one corner between his legs, one corner pointing toward each side of body, and one corner over his chest.	Prevents unnecessary exposure before beginning procedure.
8. Raise side rail. Fill washbasin with water that is approximately 41° to 43° C (105° to 109.4° F).	Rail maintains client's safety. Proper water temperature prevents burns to perineum.
9. Place washbasin and toilet tissue on overbed table. Place disposable or regular washcloths in washbasin.	Equipment placed within your reach prevents accidental spills.
10. Lower side rail and lower top corner of bath blanket below client's perineum.	Towel prevents moisture from collecting in inguinal area.

Steps	Rationale
11. Gently raise penis and place bath towel underneath it. Gently grasp shaft of penis. If client is uncircumcised, retract foreskin. Defer procedure if client has an erection.	Gentle handling of penis reduces the chance of client having an erection. Secretions capable of harboring microorganisms collect underneath foreskin.
12. Wash the tip of penis at urethral meatus first. Using a circular motion, clean from meatus outward. Do not allow soap to get into meatus. Discard washcloth and repeat until penis is clean. Rinse and dry gently (Fig. 97).	Cleaning moves from area of least contamination to area of most contamination, preventing entrance of microorganisms into urethra.

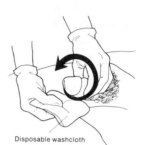

Fig. 97

Disposable washcloth

13. Return foreskin to its natural position.	Tightening of foreskin around shaft of penis can cause localized edema and discomfort.
14. Wash shaft of penis with gentle but firm downward strokes. Pay special attention to underlying surface of penis. Rinse and dry penis thoroughly. Instruct client to spread his legs apart slightly.	Vigorous massage of penis can lead to erection, which can embarrass client and nurse. Spreading legs provides easy access to scrotal tissues.
15. Gently clean scrotum. Lift testicles carefully and wash underlying skinfolds. Rinse and dry.	Pressure on scrotal tissues can be very painful to client.

Steps	Rationale
16. Fold bath blanket back over client's perineum and assist client in turning to a side-lying position.	Bath blanket maintains client's comfort and minimizes anxiety during procedure. Side-lying position provides access to anal area.
17. Clean anal area by wiping off any excess fecal material with toilet tissue. Wash area by wiping from perineum toward anus with one stroke. Discard washcloth. Repeat with a clean cloth until skin is clear.	Prevents transmission of microorganisms.
18. Rinse area well and dry with towel.	Retained moisture can promote skin breakdown.
19. Remove gloves and dispose of them in proper receptacle.	Moisture and body excretions on gloves can harbor microorganisms.
20. Assist client to a comfortable position and cover him with sheet.	Making client comfortable minimizes emotional stress of procedure.
21. Raise side rail and lower bed to proper height. Return client's room to its condition before procedure.	Side rail protects client from falling. Clean environment promotes client comfort.
22. Remove blanket and dispose of all soiled bed linen.	Reduces transfer of microorganisms.
23. Wash hands.	Reduces transmission of microorganisms.
24. Record procedure in nurse's notes and report any observations (e.g., amount and character of discharge, condition of genitalia).	Timely recording ensures accurate documentation of care.

Nurse Alert

If a male client has an erection because of manipulation of the shaft of the penis, simply defer the procedure until later to avoid embarrassing him. Thorough rinsing is necessary to remove soap, which can be very irritating to the urinary meatus.

Client Teaching

During perineal care the nurse can instruct the young male client on testicular self-examinations. Testicular cancer is the most common form of solid tumor in males between ages of 15 and 35.

Pediatric Considerations

In an infant the prepuce is normally tight for the first several months and should not be retracted for cleaning. Accidental tearing of the membranes may occur.

Geriatric Considerations

In elderly clients the testes diminish in size. This is a normal process of aging.

Nail and

Foot Care

The nurse provides routine nail and foot care to prevent infection, foot odors, and injury to soft tissue. Often a client is unaware of a foot or toenail problem until pain or discomfort develops. The integrity of the feet and toenails is important to maintaining normal function of the feet so a person can stand and walk comfortably. The most common fingernail, foot, and toenail problems result from abuse or poor care such as biting nails or trimming them improperly, exposure to harsh chemicals, and wearing ill-fitting shoes. Disease, poor nutrition, and the physiologic processes of aging also impair integrity of the nails.

Potential Nursing Diagnoses

Client data derived during the assessment reveal defining characteristics to support the following nursing diagnoses in clients requiring this skill:

Impaired skin integrity

Pain

Knowledge deficit regarding nail and foot care

Equipment

Washbasin
Emery board or nail file
Bath towel, face towel
Lotion
Washcloth
Disposable bath mats
Emesis basin
Paper towels
Nail clippers

Disposable gloves
Orange stick

Steps	Rationale
1. Explain procedure to client.	Promotes client's participation in care procedures.
2. Obtain physician's order if agency policy requires it.	During cutting, client's skin may accidentally be broken. Certain clients are more at risk of infection.
3. Wash hands and don gloves.	Reduces transmission of micro-organisms.
4. Arrange equipment on overbed table. Pull curtain around bed or close room door.	Easy access to equipment prevents delays. Maintaining client's privacy reduces anxiety.
5. Assist client to bedside chair if possible. Place disposable bath mat on floor under client's feet. Place call light within client's reach.	Chair makes it easier for client to immerse feet in basin. Call light within reach ensures his safety.
6. Fill washbasin with water at 43° to 44° C (109° to 110° F).	Warm water softens nails, reduces inflammation of skin, and promotes circulation.
7. Place basin on bath mat and help client place his feet in basin.	
8. Adjust overbed table to low position and place it over client's lap.	Easy access prevents accidental spills.
9. Fill emesis basin with water at 43° to 44° C (109° to 110° F) and place on paper towel on overbed table.	Warm water softens nails and thickened epidermal cells.
10. Instruct client to place his fingers in basin with his arms in a comfortable position.	Allows client to retain position.

Steps	Rationale
11. Allow client's toenails and fingernails to soak for 10 to 20 minutes. Rewarm water in 10 minutes.	Softening of cuticles promotes easy removal of dead cells.
12. Clean gently under fingernails with orange stick. Remove emesis basin and dry fingers thoroughly.	Orange stick can be used to remove debris that harbors microorganisms. Thorough drying impedes fungal growth and prevents maceration of tissues.
13. With nail clippers, clip fingernails straight across and even with tops of fingers. Shape nails with an emery board or nail file (Fig. 98).	Cutting straight across prevents splitting of nail margins and formation of sharp nail spikes that can irritate lateral nail margins. Filing prevents cutting nail too close to nail bed.
14. Push the cuticle back gently with orange stick.	Reduces incidence of inflamed cuticles.
15. Move overbed table away from client.	
16. Put on disposable gloves and scrub callused areas of client's feet with washcloth.	Gloves prevent transmission of fungal infections to you. Friction removes dead skin layers.
17. Clean gently under client's toenails with orange stick. Remove feet from basin and dry them thoroughly.	Removal of debris and excess moisture reduces chances of infection.
18. Clean and trim toenails straight across (see Step 13). Do not file corners of toenails.	Shaping corners of toenails may damage tissue.

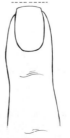

Fig. 98

Steps	Rationale
19. Apply lotion to client's feet and then assist him back to bed and into a comfortable position.	Lotion lubricates dry skin by helping to retain moisture.
20. Make sure that call light is within reach. Raise side rail.	Call light and side rail provide for client safety.
21. Clean and return equipment and supplies to proper place. Dispose of soiled linen. Wash your hands.	Controls transmission of micro-organisms.
22. Record procedure in nurse's notes and report any pertinent observations (e.g., breaks in skin or areas of inflammation).	Accurate documentation is timely and descriptive.

Nurse Alert

Clients with diabetes may have peripheral neuropathies that cause reduced sensation. Therefore, test the water temperature carefully. Take extra care in trimming the nails of clients with diabetes mellitus or peripheral vascular disease. Agency policy usually requires that a podiatrist cut the nails of the diabetic client. These clients tend to have poor wound-healing capabilities, and a slight cut could lead to serious infection.

Client Teaching

During nail care, instruct the client on proper techniques so routine care can be performed at home. Educate the client about safe use of home remedies for foot and nail care. Moleskin should be used to protect areas of the feet with corns or calluses. Moleskin does not cause local pressure, as do corn pads. Chemical preparations used to remove corns can cause burns and ulcerations. Clients should be warned against cutting off corns or calluses because the risk of infection is great. Wrapping lamb's wool around toes can effectively reduce irritation to the skin.

Clients should also be taught about proper footwear. Socks

can be worn to absorb perspiration. Footwear must always be clean to avoid infection. Women should be advised against wearing tight nylons or garters, which can constrict circulation. A person's shoes must not fit too tightly. It is recommended that a ¾-inch space between the great toe and the widest part of the shoe be present when a person stands. Clients should not try to cut hardened or hypertrophied nails. Referral to a podiatrist is a safer measure.

Pediatric Considerations

Infants and young children require routine trimming of fingernails and toenails to prevent cuts in the skin. Soaking is usually unnecessary. A child with short, ragged fingernails may be a habitual nail biter. The presence of uncut nails with dirt accumulated under the edges is a sign of poor hygiene practices.

Geriatric Considerations

Elderly clients are more likely to have foot or toenail problems because poor vision, uncoordination, obesity, or inability to bend over can impede their performance of proper care. It is common for an elderly person to have dry feet and fissures of the feet and toes resulting from reduced sebaceous gland secretion and dehydration of tissue cells. The elderly are also more likely to suffer from conditions such as diabetes, heart or renal failure, and cerebrovascular accidents, all of which can contribute to foot and nail problems.

Care of

Contact Lenses

Contact lens care is important to maintaining a client's optimal visual acuity and preventing corneal irritation or infection. Clients generally prefer to care for their own lenses whenever possible. However, illness may necessitate the nurse's assistance. Contact lens care includes cleaning, proper application and removal, and storage. Clients usually have a preferred method of caring for their lenses. When it becomes necessary for the nurse to assist with lens care, the client's preferences should be considered.

There are two major types of contact lenses: rigid and soft. Rigid lenses are thick and approximately 6 to 11 mm in diameter. Soft lenses are approximately 12.5 to 16.5 mm in diameter, large enough to cover the cornea completely. Soft lenses are flimsy because they consist primarily of water, 30% to 79% by weight (Carden, 1985). Both types are available as in clear (untinted) or tinted forms.

Potential Nursing Diagnoses

Client data derived during the assessment reveal defining characteristics to support the following nursing diagnoses in clients requiring this skill:

    Pain
    Altered visual perception
    Knowledge deficit regarding contact lens care

Equipment

1. Prepare equipment and supplies for removal of lenses:
    a. Contact lens storage container
    b. Suction cup (optional)

      c. Sterile saline solution
      d. Bath towel
2. Prepare equipment and supplies for cleansing and insertion:
      a. Lenses in storage container
      b. Thermal disinfecting kit (optional)
      c. Surfactant cleaner
      d. Rinsing solution
      e. Sterile lens disinfectant and/or enzyme solution
      f. Sterile wetting solution for rigid lenses
      g. Cotton ball or cotton-tipped applicator
      h. Bath towel
      i. Emesis basin
      j. Glass of warm tap water

Steps	Rationale
1. Discuss procedure with client.	Client can assist in planning by explaining technique that may aid removal and insertion. Client may be anxious as nurse retracts eyelids and manipulates lenses.
2. Have client assume supine or sitting position in bed or chair.	Provides easy access for nurse while retracting eyelids and manipulating lens.
3. Lens removal	

Removing Soft Lenses

a. Wash hands.	Reduces transmission of microorganisms.
b. Place towel just below client's face.	Catches lens if one should accidentally fall from eye.
c. Add a few drops of sterile saline to client's eye.	Lubricates eye to facilitate lens removal.
d. Tell client to look straight ahead.	Eases tipping of lens during removal.
e. Using middle finger, retract lower eyelid.	Exposes lower edge of lens.

Steps	Rationale
f. With pad of index finger of same hand, slide lens off cornea onto white of eye.	Positions lens for easy grasping. Use of finger pad prevents injury to cornea and damage to lens.
g. Pull upper eyelid down gently with thumb of other hand and compress lens slightly between thumb and index finger.	Causes soft lens to double up. Air enters underneath lens to release suction.
h. Gently pinch lens and lift out.	Protects lens from damage. Avoid lens edges from sticking together.
i. If lens edges stick together, place lens in palm and soak thoroughly with sterile saline. Gently roll lens with index finger in back-and-forth motion. If gentle rubbing does not separate edges, soak lens in sterile solution.	Assists in returning lens to normal shape.
j. Clean and rinse lens (see "Cleansing and Disinfecting Contact Lenses"). Place lens in proper storage case compartment: *R* for right lens and *L* for left lens. Be sure lens is centered.	Ensures proper lens will be reinserted into correct eye. Proper storage prevents cracking or tearing.
k. Repeat Steps c through j for other lens. Secure cover over storage case.	Proper storage prevents damage to lens.
l. Dispose of towel and wash hands.	Reduces transmission of infection.

Removing Rigid Lenses

a. Wash hands.	Reduces transmission of microorganisms.
b. Place towel just below client's face.	Catches lens if one should accidentally fall from eye.

Steps	Rationale
c. Be sure lens is positioned directly over cornea. If it is not, close the eyelids, place index and middle fingers of one hand behind the lens, and gently but firmly massage lens back into place.	Correct position of lens allows easy removal from eye.
d. Place index finger on outer corner of client's eye and draw skin gently away from eye.	Maneuver tightens lids against eyeball.
e. Tell client to blink. Do not release pressure on lids until blink is completed.	Maneuver should cause lens to dislodge and pop out. Lid margins must clear top and bottom of lens until the blink.
f. If lens fails to pop out, gently retract eyelid beyond edges of lens. Press lower eyelid gently against lower edge of lens.	Pressure causes upper edge of lens to tip forward.
g. Allow both eyelids to close slightly and grasp lens as it rises from eye.	Maneuver causes lens to slide off easily.
h. Cup lens in your hand.	Protects lens from breakage.
i. Clean and rinse lens (see "Cleansing and Disinfecting Contact Lenses"). Place lens in proper storage case compartment: *R* for right lens and *L* for left lens. Center lens in storage case, convex side down.	Both lenses may not have the same prescription. Proper storage prevents cracking, tearing, or chipping.
j. Repeat Steps c through i for other lens. Secure cover over storage case.	Proper storage prevents damage to lens.
k. Dispose of towel and wash hands.	Reduces spread of infection and keeps client's environment neat.

Steps	Rationale
4. Cleansing and disinfecting lenses	

Cleansing and Disinfecting Contact Lenses

a. Wash hands.	Reduces transmission of micro-organisms.
b. Assemble supplies at bedside.	Provides easy access to supplies.
c. Place towel over work area.	Towel helps prevent lens breakage.
d. Open lens container carefully, taking care not to flip lens caps open suddenly.	Prevents lenses from being accidentally spilled or flipped out of case.
e. After removal of lens from eye, apply 1 to 2 drops of daily surfactant cleaner on the lens in palm of your hand (use cleanser recommended by lens manufacturer or eye care practitioner).	Removes tear components, including mucus, lipids, and proteins that collect on lens.
f. Rub lens gently but thoroughly on both sides for 20 to 30 seconds. Use index finger (soft lenses) or little finger or cotton-tipped applicator soaked with cleaner (rigid lenses) to clean inside lens. Be careful not to touch or scratch lens with fingernail.	It is easier to manipulate and clean lenses using fingertips. Cleans all surfaces for microorganisms.
g. Holding lens over emesis basin, rinse thoroughly with manufacturer-recommended rinsing solution (soft lenses) or cold tap water (rigid lenses).	Removes debris and cleaning agent from lens surface.

Steps	Rationale
h. Place lenses in storage case and fill with storage solution recommended by manufacturer or eye care practitioner.	Disinfects lenses, removes residue, enhances wettability of lenses, and prevents scratches from a dry case.

5. Lens Insertion

Inserting Soft Lenses

Steps	Rationale
a. Wash hands with mild, noncosmetic soap, rinse well, and dry with clean, lint-free towel or paper towel.	Lint or film left on hands from cosmetic or deodorant soaps can be transferred to lenses and irritate eye.
b. Place towel over client's chest.	Towel will catch dropped lens and avoid breakage, scratching, or tearing.
c. Remove right lens from storage case and rinse with recommended rinsing solution; inspect lens for foreign materials, tears, or other damage.	Removes disinfectant solution. Prevents irritation or damage to eye.
d. Check that lens is not inverted (inside out).	Soft lens is inverted if bowl has a lip; it is in proper position if curve is even from base to rim.
e. Using middle or index finger of opposite hand, retract upper lid until iris is exposed.	Soft lenses do not adhere as easily as hard lenses. Separating lids as much as possible allows room for lens to contact cornea without touching lids or lashes.
f. Use middle finger or the hand holding the lens to pull down lower lid.	
g. Tell client to look straight ahead and "through" the lens and finger, gently place lens directly on cornea, and release lens slowly.	Ensures secure fit and comfort.

Steps	Rationale
h. If lens is on sclera rather than cornea, tell client to slowly close eye and roll it towards the lens.	Maneuver centers soft lens over cornea.
i. Tell client to blink a few times.	Ensures lens is centered, free of trapped air, and comfortable.
j. Be sure lens is centered properly by asking client if vision is blurred.	Vision will blur if lens slips to side of cornea or into conjunctival sac.
k. Repeat Steps c through j for other eye.	
l. If client's vision is blurred: (1) Retract eyelids. (2) Locate position of lens. (3) Ask client to look in direction opposite of lens. With your index finger, apply pressure to lower eyelid margin and position lens over cornea. (4) Have client look slowly toward lens.	Technique repositions lens over center of cornea as client looks toward lens.
m. Assist client to comfortable position.	Promotes client's comfort.
n. Discard soiled supplies; discard solution in storage case; rinse case thoroughly and allow to air dry; wash hands.	Prevents infection.

Inserting Rigid Lenses

a. Wash hands thoroughly with mild, noncosmetic soap. Rinse well. Dry with clean, lint-free towel or paper towel.	Lint or film on hands from soaps containing perfumes, deodorants, or complexion creams can be transferred to lenses and cause eye irritation.

Steps	Rationale
b. Place towel over client's chest.	Towel will catch dropped lens and avoid breakage, scratching, or tearing.
c. Remove right lens from storage case. Attempt to lift lens straight up.	Sliding lens out of case can cause scratches on the surface.
d. Rinse with cold tap water.	Hot water causes lens to warp.
e. Wet lens on both sides using prescribed wetting solution.	Lubricates lens so that it slides easily over and adheres to cornea.
f. Place right lens concave side up on tip of index finger of dominant hand (Fig. 99).	Proper manipulation of lens ensures easy insertion. Inner surface of lens should be face up so that it is applied against cornea.

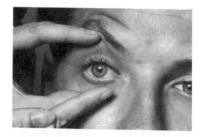

Fig. 99

g. Instruct client to look straight ahead while retracting both upper and lower eyelids; place lens gently over center of cornea.	Hard lens is rigid and can be placed as client looks straight ahead. Retraction of lids promotes easy insertion between lid margins.
h. Ask client to close eyes briefly and avoid blinking.	Helps to secure position of lens.

Steps	Rationale
i. Be sure lens is centered properly by asking client if vision is blurred.	If lens slips to side of cornea or into conjunctival sac, vision will blur.
j. Repeat Steps c through i for left eye.	
k. Assist client to comfortable position.	Promotes client's comfort.
l. Discard soiled supplies; discard solution in storage case; rinse case thoroughly and allow to air dry; wash hands.	Use of fresh solution daily prevents infection.
6. Record or report any signs or symptoms of visual alterations noted during procedure.	
7. Record on nursing care plan or Kardex times of lens insertion and removal if client is going to surgery or special procedure.	May indicate presence of eye injury or disease. In most institutions it is not necessary to record procedure unless it was ordered or client is going to surgery.

Nurse Alert

A critically ill client admitted to hospital should be assessed for the presence of contact lenses. If they are present but not detected, they can cause serious corneal injury. Suction cups are available in emergency rooms to lift a contact lens off the cornea.

Client Teaching

Clients who are relatively new wearers of contact lenses should be instructed in all aspects of lens care. Information to emphasize includes duration that lenses can safely remain inserted, cleaning methods, signs of corneal irritation, insertion techniques, and situations in which lenses should not be worn.

Pediatric Considerations

Parents or older children should learn all aspects of contact lens care.

Geriatric Considerations

Elderly clients who are able to wear contact lenses should be carefully assessed for their ability to insert and remove a lens. Any hand tremors or impairment in fine motor coordination or ability to grasp small objects may prevent them from performing self-care. If an older client suddenly becomes ill, a family member or friend should know how to remove contact lenses.

Care of
Hearing Aids

A hearing aid intensifies the sound reaching the tympanic membrane (eardrum). Each client requires a different level of sound amplification. The aid consists of an ear mold, a battery compartment, a microphone and amplifier, and a connecting tube. The "behind-the-ear" device is the most common type used (Fig. 100).

Care of a hearing aid includes proper cleaning, battery care, and storage. The nurse must also know the correct way to insert a hearing aid for a dependent client.

Potential Nursing Diagnoses

Client data derived during the assessment reveal defining characteristics to support the following nursing diagnoses in clients requiring this skill:

Sensory alteration

Knowledge deficit regarding care of a hearing aid

Equipment

Emesis basin
Mild soap and water
Pipe cleaner (optional)
Syringe needle (optional)
Soft towel
Washcloth
Storage case

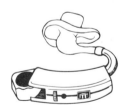

Fig. 100

Steps	Rationale
1. Wash hands.	Reduces transfer of microorganisms.

Steps	Rationale
2. Assemble supplies at bedside table or sink area.	Prevents delays in procedure.
3. Remove hearing aid from client's ear.	Eliminates unpleasant feedback squeal (harsh whistling sound), which can be caused by proximity of the aid to objects near wearer's body.
4. Determine if new battery is needed. ■ Close "battery door." ■ Turn volume slowly to high. ■ Cup hand over ear mold. ■ If no sound, replace battery and check again.	The desired effect is a high-pitched feedback sound, which indicates that the batteries are functional. Batteries usually need replacing after 1 week of daily wear.
5. Check that plastic connecting tube is not twisted or cracked.	Cracked or twisted tube prevents transmission of sound.
6. Check to see if ear mold is cracked or has rough edges.	Can cause irritation to external ear canal.
7. Check for accumulation of cerumen around ear mold and plugging of bore (opening) in mold.	Prevents clear sound reception and transmission.

Cleaning

1. Detach ear mold from hearing aid.	Moisture entering battery and transmitter will cause permanent damage.
2. Add warm water and soap to emesis basin. Soak ear mold for a few minutes. Be careful not to soak too long because cement holding ear mold to aid can become softened.	Removes cerumen that can accumulate on mold.
3. Wash client's ear canal with washcloth moistened in soap and water. Rinse and dry.	Removes cerumen and debris.

Steps	Rationale
4. If cerumen has built up in bore of ear mold, carefully clean hole with tip of syringe needle.	Wax will prevent normal sound transmission.
5. Rinse ear mold in clear water.	Soap may form residue that blocks opening in mold.
6. Allow mold to dry thoroughly after wiping with a soft towel.	Water droplets left in connecting tube could enter hearing aid and damage parts.
7. (Optional) Clean connecting tube carefully with pipe cleaner.	Removes moisture and debris, which can interfere with sound transmission and hearing aid function.
8. Reconnect ear mold to hearing aid.	Reassemble before inserting or storing hearing aid.

Storage

1. Open "battery door."	Ensures that there will be no contact, which would cause battery to run down.
2. Store hearing aid in storage case if client is about to do any of following: Bathe Walk in rain Use a hair dryer Sit in sun or under heat lamp Go to surgery or major diagnostic procedure Sleep Or is diaphoretic	Protects against damage and breakage.

Insertion

1. To reinsert hearing aid, first check battery and replace as needed.	Ensures proper sound amplification.
2. Turn aid off and turn volume control down.	Protects client from sudden exposure to sound.

Steps	Rationale
3. Place ear mold in external auditory meatus (ear canal). Be sure that ear bore in mold is first placed in ear canal. Shape of mold indicates which is correct ear. Slowly and with care, twist mold until it feels snug.	Proper fit ensures optimal sound transmission.
4. Gently bring connecting tube up and over ear toward back. Avoid kinking. Hearing aid fits around the upper ear.	Ensures correct function of hearing aid and maintains client comfort.
5. Adjust volume gradually to comfortable level for talking to client in regular voice at a distance of 1 to 1.25 meters (3 to 4 feet).	Gradual adjustment prevents exposing client to harsh squeal or feedback. Client should hear you comfortably.
6. Remove soiled equipment from bedside and dispose of used supplies. Wash your hands.	Maintains clean environment and reduces risk of infection.
7. If client is going to surgery or other special procedure, record removal and storage in nurse's notes.	Protects you from liability if aid is lost.

Client Teaching

Discuss with the client guidelines for hearing aid use and tips for care: avoiding exposure to excess heat or cold, not dropping the aid on a hard surface, changing the battery over a towel or bed, not exposing the aid to moisture, not applying hair spray while wearing the aid, and cleaning the battery to remove corrosion. The battery should be stored in a cool, dry place. Keep the contacts clean by removing residue with a pencil eraser. Remove the battery when the aid is being stored.

Pediatric Considerations

A hearing deficit in children can cause serious developmental problems, including speech impediments, poor recognition of verbal cues, delayed socialization, and impaired learning.

Geriatric Considerations

Isolation and social withdrawal are common among persons with a hearing deficit. Often the elderly client is sensitive about admitting that he cannot hear clearly. The nurse should use good communication techniques to help the person understand what is being said.

Brushing and Flossing Teeth of Dependent Clients

Brushing, flossing, and irrigation are necessary for proper cleansing of the teeth. Brushing removes food particles, loosens plaque, and stimulates gums. Flossing removes tartar that collects at the gum line. Irrigation removes dislodged food particles and excess toothpaste.

When the client is debilitated, the nurse must perform these skills for the client to ensure proper oral hygiene.

Potential Nursing Diagnoses

Client data derived during the assessment reveal defining characteristics to support the following nursing diagnoses in clients requiring this skill:

Altered oral mucous membranes
Pain
Knowledge deficit regarding oral hygiene care

Equipment

Toothbrush with straight handle and small soft bristles
Toothpaste or dentifrice
Dental floss
Glass with cool water
Mouthwash (optional)
Straw
Emesis basin
Face towel and paper towels
Disposable gloves

Steps	Rationale
1. Wash hands.	Reduces transmission of micro-organisms.
2. Place paper towels on over-bed table and arrange other equipment within easy reach.	Towels collect moisture and spills from emesis basin.
3. Pull curtain or close room door (optional if client is only brushing teeth).	Provides client privacy. When brushing is part of bathing and total hygiene, privacy is essential.
4. Raise bed to comfortable working position. Raise head of bed (if allowed) and lower side rail. Move client or help client move toward you. Side-lying position can be used.	Raising bed and positioning client prevent nurse from sustaining muscle strain. Semi-Fowler's position helps prevent client from choking or aspirating.
5. Place towel over client's chest.	Prevents soiling of gown and bed linen.
6. Position overbed table within easy reach and adjust height as needed.	Easy accessibility of supplies ensures smooth, safe procedure.
7. Apply gloves.	Prevents contact with microorganisms in saliva.
8. Apply toothpaste to brush, holding brush over emesis basin. Pour small amount of water over toothpaste.	Moisture aids in distribution of toothpaste over tooth surfaces.
9. Hold toothbrush bristles at 45-degree angle to gum line. Be sure tips of bristles rest against and penetrate under gum line. Brush inner and outer surfaces of upper and lower teeth by brushing from gum to crown of each tooth. Use short vibrating strokes and brush each tooth separately.	Angle allows brush to reach all tooth surfaces and to clean under gum line where plaque and tartar accumulate. Back-and-forth motion dislodges food particles caught between teeth and along chewing surfaces.

Steps	Rationale

Clean biting surfaces of teeth by holding top of bristles parallel with teeth and brushing gently back and forth (Fig. 101). Brush sides of teeth by moving bristles back and forth.

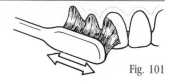

Fig. 101

10. Hold brush at 45-degree angle and lightly brush over surface and sides of tongue. Avoid initiating gag reflex.

Microorganisms collect and grow on tongue's surface. Gagging is uncomfortable and may cause aspiration of toothpaste.

11. Allow client to rinse mouth thoroughly by taking several sips of water, swishing across all tooth surfaces, and spitting into emesis basin.

Irrigation removes food particles.

12. Allow client to gargle or rinse mouth with mouthwash.

Mouthwash leaves pleasant taste in mouth.

13. Remove emesis basin and assist in wiping client's mouth.

Promotes sense of comfort.

14. Prepare for flossing by having client wash hands, if client is to floss independently.

Reduces transmission of microorganisms.

15. Prepare two pieces of dental floss approximately 25 cm (10 in) in length. Opinion differs over use of waxed vs unwaxed floss. Waxed floss frays less easily. Food particles adhere to unwaxed floss.

Need adequate length to grasp floss firmly and insert over surfaces of teeth.

Steps	Rationale
16. Wrap ends of floss around the third finger of each hand. Using thumb and index finger, stretch floss and insert between two upper teeth (Fig. 102). Move floss up and down in see-saw motion between teeth from under gum lines up to top of each tooth's crown. Be sure to clean outer surface of back molar. Make a figure C around the edge of the tooth being flossed. Work systematically along each set of teeth.	Proper insertion and movement of floss along tooth surfaces mechanically removes plaque and tartar.

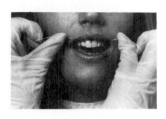

Fig. 102

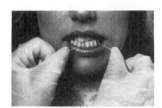

Fig. 103

17. Take a clean piece of floss and wrap around third finger of each hand. Using index fingers stretch floss and insert between two lower teeth (Fig. 103).	Frayed floss becomes caught between teeth and can be torn off. This can lead to gum inflammation and infection. Position of hands helps reach lower tooth surfaces.
18. Move floss up and down, between gum lines and crown of lower teeth one at a time.	Upward motion of floss removes plaque and tartar.

Steps	Rationale
19. Allow client to rinse mouth thoroughly with tepid water and spit into emesis basin. Assist in wiping client's mouth.	Irrigation removes plaque and tartar from oral cavity.
20. Assist client to comfortable position, remove bedside table, raise side rail, and lower bed to original position.	Provides client comfort and safety.
21. Wipe off overbed table, discard soiled linen and paper towels in appropriate containers, remove soiled gloves, and return equipment to proper place.	Reduces transmission of micro-organisms.
22. Remove gloves and wash hands.	
23. Record and report procedure in nurse's notes, mentioning specifically condition of oral cavity.	Documents response of client to hygiene measures.

Nurse Alert

All postoperative clients who receive general anesthesia are initially NPO after surgery and thus require frequent mouth care. Brushing is often contraindicated for these clients. Clients with sensitive gums or bleeding tendencies benefit from use of unflavored oral care sponges. A swab stick containing an aqueous solution of sorbitol, sodium, carboxymethylcellulose, and electrolytes may be used.

Client Teaching

The client may be weak and unable to assist in his own care. However, the nurse can still provide instructions and answer any questions. She should discuss guidelines in the prevention of tooth decay: reducing intake of carbohydrates between meals, brushing within 30 minutes of eating sweets, always rinsing the mouth thoroughly with water, brushing and flossing before bed-time, and using fluoridated water if available.

Pediatric Considerations

A child's toothbrush should be approximately 21 cm (6 inches) in length.

Geriatric Considerations

Elderly persons can have reduced gum vascularity, decreased periodontal tissue elasticity, and brittle, thin teeth. They also may have jaw bone atrophy. However, maintenance of regular dental hygiene should minimize periodontal disease.

Mouth Care for an Unconscious Client

The unconscious client poses special problems for the nurse with respect to mouth care. Many such clients have an absent or diminished gag reflex. Thus secretions tend to accumulate in the mouth, increasing the risk of aspiration. Critically ill clients often require an artificial airway and/or nasogastric tubes. These devices can cause considerable irritation to sensitive oral mucosal structures. Unconscious clients will require frequent mouth care to keep the mucosa well hydrated and intact.

Potential Nursing Diagnoses

Client data derived during the assessment reveal defining characteristics to support the following nursing diagnoses in clients requiring this skill:

  Altered oral mucous membranes
  High risk for injury
  High risk for infection

Equipment

Mouthwash or antiseptic solution
Toothettes or tongue blade wrapped in single layer of gauze
Padded tongue blade
Face towel
Emesis basin
Paper towels
Water glass with cool water
Petrolatum jelly
Suction catheter attached to suction

Steps	Rationale
1. Explain procedure to client.	Although unconscious, he may retain ability to hear explanation.
2. Wash your hands and don gloves.	Reduces transmission of microorganisms.
3. Place paper towels on overbed table and arrange equipment.	Provides easy access to equipment.
4. Pull curtain around bed or close door to room.	Provides privacy.
5. Raise bed to its highest horizontal level. Lower side rail.	Use of good body mechanics prevents injury to both you and client.
6. Position client on side near you. Make sure that his head is turned toward mattress.	Protects client from aspirating secretions.
7. Place towel under client's face and emesis basin under his chin.	Prevents soiling of bed linen.
8. Carefully retract client's upper and lower teeth with tongue blade by inserting blade, quickly but gently, between the back molars. Insert when client is relaxed, if possible.	Prevents client from biting down on nurse's padded fingers. Provides access to oral cavity.

Steps	Rationale
9. Clean client's mouth using toothettes or tongue blade moistened with mouthwash or water. Suction as needed during cleansing. Clean chewing and inner surfaces first. Swab roof of mouth and inside cheeks and lips. Swab tongue but avoid causing gag reflex if present. Moisten a clean applicator with water and swab mouth to rinse. Repeat as needed.	Swabbing stimulates gums and helps remove large food particles when brushing is impossible. Water or mouthwash provides lubricant for dry mucosa. Rinsing helps remove secretions and food particles. Suctioning minimizes risk of aspiration in clients with reduced gag reflex.
10. Apply petrolatum jelly to client's lips.	Prevents lips from drying and cracking.
11. Explain to client that you have completed procedure.	Hearing and responsive capability are often still intact in unconscious clients.
12. Remove gloves and dispose in proper receptacle.	Prevents transmission of microorganisms.
13. Reposition client comfortably, raise side rail, and return bed to its original position.	Maintains client's comfort and safety.
14. Clean equipment and return it to proper place. Dispose of soiled linen in proper receptacle.	Prevents spread of infection.
15. Wash your hands.	Reduces transmission of microorganisms.
16. Record and report procedure in nurse's notes, mentioning pertinent observations (e.g., presence of bleeding gums, dry mucosa, or crusts on tongue).	Accurate documentation should be timely and descriptive.

Nurse Alert

To ensure that any secretions in the client's pharynx are not aspirated, it may be helpful to have a second nurse assist with suctioning. Avoid the use of lemon glycerine swabs, which can
cause drying of the mucosa and loss of tooth enamel.

Chemotherapy, radiation, and nasogastric tube intubation can
cause stomatitis. Clients should rinse their mouths before and after each meal with a solution containing 0.5 to 1 teaspoon of salt
to 1 pint of water (Wilson, 1986).

Geriatric Considerations

With aging there is reduced vascularity of the gums. In elderly
persons the teeth may be brittle, drier, and darker in color. If
dental hygiene is not maintained, inflammation and swelling of
periodontal tissues can easily occur.

ELIMINATION

Female Urinary

Catheterization

Indwelling and Straight

Catheterization of the bladder involves the introduction of a rubber or plastic tube through the urethra into the bladder. The catheter allows a continuous flow of urine in clients unable to control micturition or in those with obstruction to urinary outflow. In female clients the urethra is close to the anus, therefore the risk of infection is always great and thorough cleaning of the perineum before catheter insertion is vital. Frequent perineal care must be provided thereafter.

Potential Nursing Diagnoses

Client data derived during the assessment reveal defining characteristics to support the following nursing diagnoses in clients requiring this skill:

    Urinary retention
    Pain

Equipment

Sterile catheterization tray
    Sterile gloves
    Clean gloves
    Sterile drapes, one fenestrated
    Lubricant
    Antiseptic cleansing solution
    Cotton balls or gauze sponges
    Forceps
    Straight or indwelling catheter
    Prefilled syringe with solution to inflate balloon for indwelling catheter

   Receptacle or basin (usually bottom of tray)
   Specimen container
Flashlight or gooseneck lamp
Sterile drainage tubing and collection bag
Tape, rubber band, and safety pin
Bath blanket
Waterproof pad
Trash bag
Basin with warm water and soap
Bath towel

Steps	Rationale
1. Explain procedure to the client.	Minimizes client's anxiety and promotes cooperation.
2. Raise bed to appropriate height.	Promotes use of proper body mechanics.
3. Close cubicle or room curtains.	Reduces client's embarrassment and aids in relaxation during procedure.
4. Wash hands.	Reduces transmission of micro-organisms.
5. Stand at left side of bed if you are right-handed (at the right if left-handed). Clear bedside table and arrange equipment.	Successful catheter insertion requires that you assume a comfortable position with all equipment easily accessible.
6. Raise side rail on opposite side of bed. Place waterproof pad under client.	Promotes client's safety. Pad prevents soiling of bed linen.
7. Assist client to a dorsal recumbent position (supine with knees flexed). Ask client to relax thighs so as to promote external rotation. If client cannot abduct her leg at hip joint (e.g., arthritic joints), position in side-lying (Sims') position with upper leg flexed at knee and hip.	Provides good access to perineal structures.

Steps	Rationale
8. Drape client with bath blanket. Place blanket diamond fashion over client: one corner over each foot, and last corner over perineum.	Unnecessary exposure of body parts is avoided, and client's comfort is maintained.
9. Don disposable gloves and wash perineal area with soap and water as needed, and dry.	Presence of microorganisms near urethral meatus is reduced.
10. Remove gloves and wash hands.	Reduces transmission of microorganisms.
11. If inserting indwelling catheter, open drainage system. Place drainage bag over edge of bottom bed frame. Bring drainage tube up between side rail and mattress.	Once catheter is inserted, you must immediately connect drainage system. Easy access prevents possible contamination. System is positioned to promote gravity drainage.
12. Position lamp to illuminate perineal area. (When using a flashlight, have another nurse hold it.)	Permits accurate identification and good visualization of urethral meatus.
13. Open catheterization kit according to directions, keeping bottom of container sterile.	Transmission of microorganisms from table or work area to sterile supplies is prevented.
14. Don sterile gloves.	Allows you to handle sterile supplies.
15. Pick up solid sterile drape by one corner and allow it to unfold. Be sure that it does not touch a contaminated surface.	Sterility of drape to be used as work surface is maintained.

Steps	Rationale
16. Allow top edge of drape to form a cuff over both your hands. Place drape down on bed between client's thighs. Slip cuffed edge just under client's buttocks, taking care not to touch a contaminated surface with your gloves.	Outer surface of drape covering hands remains sterile. Sterile drape against sterile gloves is sterile.
17. Pick up fenestrated (the drape with the hole) sterile drape and allow it to unfold as in Step 15. Apply drape over client's perineum, exposing labia and being careful not to touch a contaminated surface.	Fenestrated drape provides a clean work area near catheter insertion site.
18. Place sterile tray and its contents on sterile drape between client's thighs.	Easy access to supplies during catheter insertion is provided.
19. Open packet containing antiseptic cleaning solution and pour contents over sterile cotton balls or gauze. (Be sure not to pour solution in receptacle that is to receive urine.)	All equipment is prepared before catheter is handled to maintain aseptic technique during procedure.
20. Open urine specimen container, keeping top sterile.	Prepared to receive specimen.
21. Apply lubricant to bottom 2.5 to 5 cm (1 to 2 inches) of catheter tip.	Lubricant allows easy insertion of catheter tip through urethral meatus.
22. With your nondominant hand, carefully retract labia to fully expose urethral meatus. Maintain your nondominant hand in this position throughout remainder of procedure (Fig. 104).	Full visualization of meatus is provided. Full retraction prevents contamination of meatus during cleansing. Closure of labia during cleansing requires that procedure be repeated.

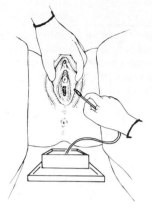

Fig. 104

Steps	Rationale
23. With your dominant hand, pick up a cotton ball with forceps and clean perineal area, wiping front to back from clitoris toward anus. Use a new clean cotton ball for each wipe: along near labial fold, and along far labial fold, and directly over meatus.	Cleaning reduces number of microorganisms at urethral meatus. Using single cotton ball for each wipe prevents transfer of microorganisms. Preparation moves from area of least contamination to area of most contamination. Your dominant hand remains sterile.
24. With your dominant hand, pick up catheter approximately 7.5 to 10 cm (3 to 4 inches) from the tip. Place the end of catheter in the urine tray receptacle.	Collection of urine prevents soiling of client's bed linen and allows accurate measurement of urinary output. Holding catheter near tip allows easier manipulation during insertion into meatus.
25. Ask client to bear down as if to void and slowly insert catheter through meatus.	Relaxation of external sphincter aids in insertion of the catheter.

Steps	Rationale
26. Advance catheter approximately 5 to 7.5 cm (2 to 3 inches) in adult, 2.5 cm (1 inch) in child, or until urine flows out the catheter end. When urine appears, advance catheter another 5 cm (1 inch).	Female urethra is short. Appearance of urine indicates that catheter tip is in bladder or lower urethra. Further advancement of catheter ensures bladder placement.
27. Release labia and hold catheter securely with your nondominant hand.	Bladder or sphincter contraction may cause accidental expulsion of catheter.
28. Collect urine specimen as needed: ■ Fill specimen cup or jar to desired level (20 to 30 ml) by holding end of catheter in your nondominant hand over cup. With your dominant hand, pinch catheter to stop urine flow temporarily. Release catheter to allow remaining urine in bladder to drain into collection tray. Cover specimen cup and set it aside for labeling.	
29. Allow bladder to empty fully (usually 750 to 1000 ml), unless institutional policy restricts maximal volume of urine to drain with each catheterization.	Retained urine may serve as reservoir for growth of microorganisms. (In obstetric clients, caution must be taken to avoid hypotension resulting from sudden release of pressure against pelvic floor blood vessels.)
30. Withdraw straight, single-use catheter slowly but smoothly until removed.	Discomfort to client is minimized.
31. With indwelling catheter:	

Steps	Rationale
▪ While holding with thumb and little finger of your nondominant hand at meatus, take end of catheter and place it between first two fingers of that hand.	Catheter should be anchored while syringe is manipulated.
▪ With your free dominant hand, attach syringe to injection port at end of catheter.	Port connects to lumen leading to inflatable balloon.
▪ Slowly inject total amount of solution. If client complains of sudden pain, aspirate back and advance catheter farther.	Balloon within bladder is inflated. If malpositioned in urethra, it will cause pain during inflation.
▪ After inflating balloon fully, release catheter with your nondominant hand and pull gently to feel resistance.	Inflation of balloon anchors catheter tip in place above bladder outlet (Fig. 105).

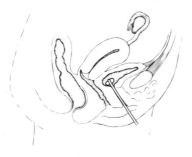

Fig. 105

32. Attach end of catheter to collecting tube of the drainage system.	Closed system for urine drainage is established.

Steps	Rationale
33. Tape catheter to client's inner thigh with a strip of nonallergenic tape. (Velcro catheter strips are also available.) Allow for slack so movement of thigh does not create tension on catheter.	Anchoring of catheter minimizes trauma to urethra and meatus during client movement. Nonallergenic tape prevents skin breakdown.
34. Be sure that no obstructions or kinks are in tubing. Place excess coil of tubing on bed and fasten it to bottom bedsheet with a clip from drainage set or with rubber band and safety pin.	Patent tubing allows free drainage of urine by gravity and prevents backflow of urine into bladder.
35. Remove gloves and dispose of equipment, drapes, and urine in proper receptacles.	Transmission of microorganisms is prevented.
36. Assist client to a comfortable position. Wash and dry perineal area as needed.	Client comfort and security are maintained.
37. Instruct client on ways to position herself in bed with catheter: side-lying facing drainage system—catheter and tubing on bed unobstructed; supine—catheter and tubing draped over thigh; side-lying facing away from system—catheter and tubing extending between legs.	Urine should drain freely without obstruction. Placing catheter under extremities can result in obstruction caused by compression of the tubing from client's weight. Catheter should not be placed over the upper thigh when the client is on one side facing away from the system; this forces urine to drain uphill.
38. Caution client against pulling on catheter.	
39. Wash your hands.	Reduces transfer of microorganisms.

Steps	Rationale
40. Record results of procedure in nurse's notes, including size of catheter, amount and character of urine, and client's tolerance.	Documents client's response and results of therapy.

Nurse Alert

If the catheter is mistakenly introduced into the client's vagina, leave it in place. Open a new sterile catheter and place it in the urethra (which is immediately anterior to the vagina). Then remove the misplaced catheter.

If catheter is definitely in bladder and no urine is produced, absence of urine should be reported to physician immediately.

Women who have just had a baby or who have had gynecologic surgery and clients who have just undergone bladder surgery are at risk for bladder distention.

Client Teaching

Instruct the client to keep the continuous drainage bag below the level of her bladder. This reduces the risk of urinary tract infections from backflow from the collection bag into the bladder. If the client is to be discharged with intermittent straight catheterization or with an indwelling (Foley) catheter, instruct her or a responsible person in catheter care, catheter insertion, and catheter removal.

Pediatric Considerations

Catheterization is most often used when urethral obstruction or anuria resulting from renal failure is believed to be the cause of the child's failure to void. Most female infants and children accommodate an 8- or 10-gauge French catheter. Special care must be exercised to restrain and reassure the child during the procedure.

Geriatric Considerations

Foley catheters should be avoided if at all possible in an older client who is incontinent. The nurse must modify the client's fluid intake patterns and must adjust toileting procedures to accommodate a routine that will maintain proper fluid balance, independence in toileting, and integrity of the perineal skin.

Male Urinary

Catheterization

Indwelling and Straight

Catheterization of the bladder involves introduction of a rubber or plastic tube through the urethra and into the bladder. It is used for the following purposes: immediate relief of bladder distention, management of an incompetent bladder, obtaining a sterile urine specimen, and assessment of residual urine after voiding. Introduction of a catheter into a male client may be difficult if the prostate gland is enlarged. The nurse must not force a catheter through the urethra. Doing so might cause tissue injury.

Potential Nursing Diagnoses

Client data derived during the assessment reveal defining characteristics to support the following nursing diagnoses in clients requiring this skill:

Urinary retention

Pain

Equipment

Sterile catheterization tray

Sterile gloves

Clean gloves

Sterile drapes, one fenestrated

Lubricant

Antiseptic cleansing solution

Cotton balls or gauze sponges

Forceps

Straight or indwelling catheter

Prefilled syringe with solution to inflate balloon for indwelling catheter

Receptacle or basin (usually bottom of tray)
    Specimen container
Flashlight or gooseneck lamp
Sterile drainage tubing and collection bag
Tape, rubber band, and safety pin
Bath blanket
Waterproof pad
Trash bag
Basin with warm water and soap
Bath towel

Steps	Rationale
1. Explain procedure to the client.	Minimizes client anxiety and promotes cooperation.
2. Raise bed to appropriate height.	Promotes use of proper body mechanics.
3. Close cubicle or room curtains.	Reduces client embarrassment and aids in relaxation during procedure.
4. Wash hands.	Reduces transmission of micro-organisms.
5. Stand at left side of bed if right-handed (at left side if left-handed). Clear bedside table and arrange equipment.	Successful catheter insertion requires that you assume a comfortable position with all equipment easily accessible.
6. Raise side rail on opposite side of bed. Assist client to a supine position with thighs slightly abducted.	Promotes client safety. Prevents tensing of abdominal and pelvic muscles.
7. Drape client's upper trunk with bath blanket and cover lower extremities with bedsheets, exposing only genitalia.	Unnecessary exposure of body parts is prevented, and client comfort is maintained.
8. Place bath towel under genitalia.	Prevents soiling of bed linen.

Steps	Rationale
9. Don gloves and wash perineum with soap and water as needed. In uncircumcised males, be sure to retract foreskin to clean urethral meatus. (Do *not* allow soap to get into meatus.)	Presence of microorganisms near urethral meatus is reduced.
10. Remove gloves and wash hands.	Prevents transmission of bacteria from your hands to meatus.
11. If inserting an indwelling catheter, open drainage system. Place drainage bag over edge of bottom bed frame. Bring drainage tube up between side rail and mattress.	Once catheter is inserted, drainage system is immediately connected. Easy access prevents possible contamination. System is positioned to promote gravity drainage.
12. Open catheterization kit according to directions, keeping bottom of container sterile.	Transmission of microorganisms from table or work area to sterile supplies is prevented.
13. Don sterile gloves.	Maintains asepsis throughout procedure.
14. Apply sterile drapes. Pick up solid sterile drape by corner and allow it to unfold. Be sure that drape does not touch a contaminated surface. Apply drape over client's thighs just below penis. Pick up fenestrated sterile drape, allow it to unfold, and drape it over penis with fenestrated slit resting over penis.	Sterility of drape as work surface is maintained.
15. Place sterile tray and its contents on drape alongside client's thigh or on top of thighs.	Easy access to supplies during catheter insertion is provided.

Steps	Rationale
16. Obtain cotton balls or gauze with antiseptic solution. Open urine specimen container, keeping top sterile.	Prepares container for specimen.
17. Apply lubricant to bottom 12.5 to 17.5 cm (5 to 7 inches) of catheter tip.	Lubricant allows easy insertion of catheter tip through urethral meatus.
18. With your nondominant hand, retract foreskin of uncircumcised male. Grasp penis at shaft just below glans. Retract urethral meatus between thumb and forefinger. Maintain nondominant hand in this position throughout procedure.	Firm grasp minimizes chance that erection will occur (if an erection develops, discontinue procedure). Accidental release of foreskin or dropping of penis during cleaning requires process to be repeated.
19. With dominant hand, pick up a cotton ball with forceps and clean penis. Move it in a circular motion from meatus down to base of glans. Repeat cleaning two more times using a clean cotton ball each time.	Reduces number of microorganisms at meatus and moves from least contaminated to most contaminated area. Dominant hand remains sterile.
20. Pick up catheter with gloved dominant hand approximately 7.5 to 10 cm (3 to 4 inches) from catheter tip. Hold end of the catheter loosely coiled in the palm of your dominant hand (optional: grasp catheter with forceps).	Holding catheter near tip allows easier manipulation during insertion into meatus and prevents distal end from striking a contaminated surface.
21. Lift penis to a position perpendicular to client's body and apply light traction (Fig. 106).	Straightens urethral canal to ease catheter insertion.

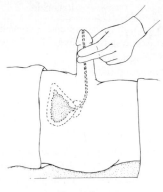

Fig. 106

Steps	Rationale
22. Ask client to bear down as if to void and slowly insert catheter through meatus.	Relaxation of external sphincter aids in insertion of catheter.
23. Advance catheter 17.5 to 22 cm (7 to 9 inches) in an adult and 5 to 7.5 cm (2 to 3 inches) in a young child, or until urine flows out catheter end. If resistance is felt, withdraw catheter; do not force it through urethra. When urine appears, advance catheter another 5 cm (2 inches).	The adult male urethra is long. Appearance of urine indicates catheter tip is in bladder or urethra. Resistance to catheter passage may be caused by urethral strictures or enlarged prostate. Further advancement of catheter ensures proper placement.
24. Lower penis and hold catheter securely in nondominant hand. Place end of catheter in urine tray receptacle.	Catheter may be accidentally expelled by bladder or urethral contraction. Collection of urine prevents soiling and provides output measurement.

Steps	Rationale
25. Collect urine specimen according to Step 26 in female catheterization procedure (see Skill 8-1). If an indwelling catheter is ordered, inflate balloon and check for proper anchoring as in Step 31 of Skill 8-1.	Ensures that tip will remain in place above bladder outlet (Fig. 107).

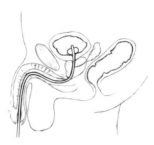

Fig. 107

26. Allow bladder to empty fully, unless institutional policy restricts maximal volume of urine to drain with each catheterization.	Retained urine serves as reservoir for growth of microorganisms. (Precaution may prevent hypotension resulting from sudden release of pressure against pelvic floor blood vessels under bladder.)
27. Replace foreskin over glans. With straight, single-use catheters, withdraw slowly but smoothly until removed.	Minimizes discomfort during removal. Tightening of foreskin around shaft of penis can cause localized edema and discomfort.
28. Attach end of catheter to collecting tube of drainage system.	Establishes closed system for urine drainage.

Steps	Rationale
29. Tape catheter to top of client's thigh or lower abdomen (with penis directed toward client's chest). Use strip of nonallergenic tape. Provide slack so movement does not create tension on catheter (Fig 108).	Anchoring of catheter minimizes trauma to urethra and meatus. Taping to abdomen minimizes irritation at angle of penis and scrotum. Nonallergenic tape prevents skin breakdown.

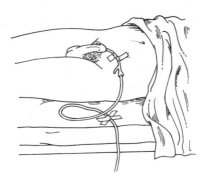

Fig. 108

30. Be sure that there are no obstructions or kinks in tubing. Place excess coil of tubing on bed and fasten it to bottom bedsheet with a clip to drainage set or with a rubber band and safety pin (Fig. 109).	Patent tubing allows free drainage of urine by gravity and prevents backflow of urine into bladder.
31. Remove gloves and dispose of all equipment.	Prevents transmission of microorganisms.
32. Assist client to a comfortable position and wash and dry perineal areas as needed.	Promotes client comfort.

Steps	Rationale

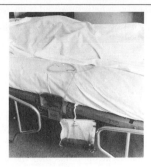

Fig. 109

33. Instruct client on proper positioning and the importance of not pulling on catheter (see Steps 32 and 34 of Skill 8-1). | Ensures unobstructed drainage through a closed system.

34. Wash your hands. | Reduces transmission of microorganisms.

35. Record in nurse's notes results of procedure, including size of catheter, amount of urine drained, character of urine, and client's tolerance. | Documents client's response and results of therapy.

Nurse Alert

Do not force the catheter if resistance is met. In older men, prostatic hypertrophy may partially obstruct the urethra and prevent easy passage of the catheter. If resistance is met, notify the client's physician.

Client Teaching

Instruct the client to keep the continuous drainage bag below the level of his bladder. This reduces the risk of urinary tract infections resulting from backflow from the collection bag into the bladder. If the client is to be discharged with intermittent straight catheterization or with an indwelling Foley catheter, instruct him or his family on catheter care, insertion, and removal.

Pediatric Considerations

Male infants may not be able to accommodate the 8- or 10-gauge French catheters. In such instances a smaller soft plastic feeding tube may be used. Caution is necessary in catheterizing young males to avoid trauma that might result in sterility from damage to the ductal and glandular openings into the urethra.

Geriatric Considerations

Foley catheters should be avoided whenever possible in older adult clients who are incontinent. The nurse must modify the client's fluid intake patterns and schedule toileting procedures so that a routine for bladder elimination will be developed that maintains proper fluid balance, independence in toileting, and skin integrity.

Applying a Condom Catheter

A condom catheter is an external urinary drainage device that is convenient to use and safe for draining urine in male clients. It is a soft, pliable rubber sheath that slips over the penis, and it is suitable for incontinent or comatose clients who still have complete and spontaneous bladder emptying. This catheter may be preferred over an indwelling (Foley) type because drainage is maintained with less risk of infection.

Potential Nursing Diagnoses

Client data derived during the assessment reveal defining characteristics to support the following nursing diagnoses in clients requiring this skill:

Incontinence, total
High risk for or actual impaired skin integrity
Self-care deficit, toileting

Equipment

Rubber condom sheath
Strip of elastic or Velcro adhesive
Urinary collection bag with drainage tubing
Basin with warm water and soap
Towel and washcloth
Bath blanket
Disposable gloves
Scissors

Steps	Rationale
1. Wash hands.	Reduces transmission of micro-organisms.

Steps	Rationale
2. Close door or bedside curtain.	Provides privacy.
3. Explain procedure to client.	Reduces client anxiety and improves cooperation.
4. Don disposable gloves.	Reduces transmission of microorganisms.
5. Assist client to a supine position. Place bath blanket over his upper trunk and cover his lower extremities with bedsheets so only the genitalia are exposed.	Supine position promotes comfort, and draping prevents unnecessary exposure of body parts.
6. Clean the genitalia with soap and water. Dry thoroughly.	Secretions that may irritate client's skin are removed. Rubber sheath rolls onto dry skin more easily.
7. Prepare urinary drainage bag by attaching it to bed frame. Bring drainage tubing up through side rails onto bed.	Easy access to equipment during connection of condom catheter is provided.
8. With nondominant hand grasp client's penis firmly along shaft. With dominant hand, hold condom sheath at tip of penis and smoothly roll sheath up onto penile shaft.	Firm grasp reduces chances that erection will occur. Condom should fit smoothly to prevent sites of constriction.
9. Allow 2.5 to 5 cm (1 to 2 inches) of space between glans penis and end of condom catheter (Fig. 110).	Avoids excess pressure on glans penis.
10. Encircle penile shaft with strip of Velcro or elastic adhesive. Strip should touch only condom sheath. Apply snugly but not tightly.	Adhesive strip anchors condom in place. Snug fit prevents constriction of blood flow.

Steps   Rationale

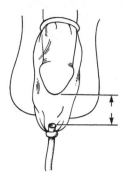

Fig. 110

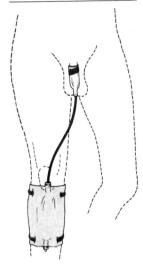

Fig. 111

11. Connect drainage tubing to end of condom catheter (Fig 111).	Prevents soiling of bed linen and provides for collection of all voided urine.
12. Place excess coil of tubing on bed and secure to bottom bedsheet.	Patent tubing promotes free drainage of urine.
13. Reposition client in a safe comfortable position.	Promotes client comfort.
14. Dispose of soiled equipment, remove gloves, and wash hands.	Reduces transmission of microorganisms.
15. Record when condom catheter was applied and presence of urine in drainage bag.	Documents procedure. Also notes that client is able to empty his bladder and that urine is contained in drainage bag.

Nurse Alert

Adhesive tape should never be used to secure a condom catheter. It can cause constriction and reduction of blood flow to the penis. Velcro or elastic adhesive expands with changes in size of the penis and does not reduce blood flow.

Remove condom catheter for 30 minutes every 24 hours for perineal skin care. Inspect glans every 4 hours to determine that circulation to penis is adequate.

Client Teaching

Occasionally the client will return home and wear a condom catheter intermittently or throughout the day. Instruct him and his family in perineal care, catheter application, and use of the optional leg bag.

Pediatric Considerations

Pediatric urinary collection bags are applied to the male infant or child when exact urinary output is required. The adolescent male may be catheterized only if there is no other method of obtaining exact urinary output.

Geriatric Considerations

Older men may require more frequent bladder emptying and should be offered the urinal or taken to the bathroom more frequently rather than subjected to condom catheter application.

Continuous Ambulatory Peritoneal Dialysis

Peritoneal dialysis is a type of dialysis in which the peritoneal membrane is used to promote the removal of fluid, electrolytes, and toxins from the client's blood. A form of peritoneal dialysis is continuous ambulatory peritoneal dialysis (CAPD). CAPD is a type of therapy that has made home dialysis feasible for the client with end-stage renal disease (ESRD). During this type of dialysis, a permanent peritoneal catheter is surgically implanted into the peritoneal cavity and the principles of osmosis and diffusion remove fluid, excess electrolytes, and toxins from the client's blood (Perras et al, 1983). CAPD has the same three phases as routine peritoneal dialysis except the time cycle changes. The dwell time ranges from 4 to 8 hours. During this time an empty plastic bag and drainage tubing are folded and concealed under the client's clothes. After the dwell time, the client drains the abdominal cavity, which is followed by a period of reinstilling fresh dialysate into the peritoneal cavity. CAPD requires changes in the dialysate ranging from three to five times a day. One major advantage of CAPD is that it allows clients to be out of the hospital, maintain their systems at home, and continue with daily activities. This method is not appropriate for all clients with ESRD and requires thorough education from nursing and routine follow-up in an outpatient renal clinic (Lane et al, 1982; Perras et al, 1983).

Potential Nursing Diagnoses

Client data derived during the assessment reveal defining characteristic to support the following nursing diagnoses in clients requiring this skill:

Fluid volume excess
High risk for infection
Urinary elimination, altered

Equipment

Collect the following equipment for PD catheter site care:
Sterile gloves
Occlusive dressing materials
Hydrogen peroxide
Providone solution
Providone ointment
Mask
IV pole
Y-connector tubing (some CAPD clients may not need this tubing)
Sterile drainage bag

Steps	Rationale
1. Obtain client's weight.	Provides baseline information about weight attributed to fluid retention. A daily weight gain of 1 kg is equivalent to 1 liter of fluid.
2. Obtain vital signs.	Fluid volume changes associated with peritoneal dialysis increase the client's risk for hemodynamic blood pressure changes. This is especially true for clients having in-hospital peritoneal dialysis.
3. Measure abdominal girth. ■ Mark midpoint of the client's abdomen. Maintain this mark as a reference for future abdominal girth measurements.	Provides baseline data regarding the amount of fluid in the client's peritoneal cavity.
4. Inspect catheter site for: Erythema Tenderness Drainage	Indicates possible infection at catheter entry site. Increases client's risk for peritonitis (Breckenridge et al, 1982).
5. Measure client's body temperature.	Provides baseline data regarding client's febrile status.

Steps	Rationale
6. Review hospital or dialysis unit's procedure for CAPD.	There may be institutional variations regarding ordering of supplies; fill, dwell, and drain times; catheter care; and discharge teaching plans.
7. Review physician's orders. ■ CAPD orders usually include three to four exchanges with a specific dialysate volume and composition as well as a specific dwell time, which can range from 4 to 8 hours.	PD and CAPD require specific orders, which are individualized to the client's fluid needs and disease process.
8. Obtain laboratory data as ordered. ■ CAPD orders can vary, depending on individual client needs.	Documents client's fluid and electrolyte status and changes that occur from CAPD.
9. Ordered dialysate should be at room temperature. ■ Dialysate is warmed by placing solution bag on a warming pad, not into a warming solution.	Dialysate that is too cold results in intolerance, cramps, or hypothermia. Plastic dialysate bags are permeable. Immersing them in warm water when the protective wrapper is removed risks the introduction of bacteria from the nonsterile water. In addition, the osmotic concentration of the dialysate can change (Strangio, 1988).
10. Have a Deane prosthesis or PD button at the bedside.	Button is aseptically applied to the PD site at the end of the treatment. The button maintains patency of the insertion site for another treatment.
11. Explain procedure to the client.	Assists in reducing anxiety and promoting cooperation.

Initiating the Dialysis Exchanges

Steps	Rationale
1. Don mask and gloves, and wash hands. Instruct client to don mask.	Reduces transmission of micro-organisms.
2. Place client in semi- or high Fowler's position.	Instilling fluid into the perito-neal cavity decreases diaphrag-matic excursion. These positions promote optimal lung expansion.
3. Make sure all clamps on the inflow and outflow tub-ings are in the "off" posi-tions.	Prevents accidental instillation of air or dialysate into client's peritoneal cavity. Also prevents unscheduled removal of dialy-sate from the cavity before completion of ordered dwell time.
4. Add any medications as listed in the physician's order.	Medications can include: ■ Heparin, which reduces accumulation of fibrin around the catheter tip. ■ Local anesthetic, which aids in reducing back or abdominal pain related only to the infusion of the dialysate and no other causes (Birdsall, 1988). ■ Prophylactic antibiotics, which reduce risk of peritonitis.

Steps	Rationale
5. Attach two warmed dialysate bags to inflow tubing and attach to IV pole (Fig. 112). Note that these bags are punctured exactly as are IV solution bags (see Unit 13).	Attachment of two dialysate bags promotes timely, organized follow-up exchanges. Standard peritoneal dialysis usually includes 24 exchanges. CAPD clients are instructed to hang only one bag because these clients have three to seven exchanges daily.
6. Prime inflow tubing by removing protective cap and maintaining sterility of the cap. Hold tubing over basin or sink, open inflow clamp, and allow fluid to run through the tubing until all air has been removed.	Maintaining sterility of the cap allows safe, sterile reapplication of cap on inflow tubing. Prevents air from entering the peritoneal cavity.

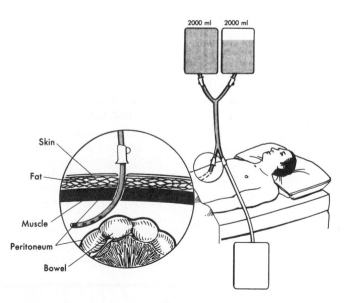

Fig. 112

Steps	Rationale
7. Open the clamp on dialysate bag. Infuse solution over prescribed time. Time usually includes 2 liters over 15 minutes.	Permits instillation of dialysate into the peritoneal cavity.
8. Clamp inflow tubing for prescribed dwell time.	Clamping prevents air from entering the peritoneal cavity.
■ CAPD dwell time ranges from 3 to 5 hours. The CAPD client folds the tubing and infusion bag on the abdomen, which is concealed by clothing. The CAPD client uses the same bag and tubing for the drain cycle.	This dwell time permits the peritoneal membrane to exchange fluid, electrolytes, and toxins from the client's blood.
9. Unclamp outflow tubing and drain; the time usually ordered for this is 20 minutes.	Permits drainage of dialysate and wastes from abdominal cavity. During the first two to three exchanges it is not uncommon for dialysate to remain in the cavity. However, this excess should drain with later exchanges.
10. Clamp outflow tubing.	Prevents untimed drain during subsequent exchange.
11. Empty and measure fluid in drainage bag.	Provides assessment of fluid balance of the dialysate solution. If a greater volume of fluid was infused than the amount drained, then the balance is a negative number. For example: 2000 ml of dialysate was infused and 1800 ml drained; then the balance is negative 200 ml (-200 ml).

Steps	Rationale
12. When the exchange is complete either:	
■ Cover catheter with a sterile cap.	Catheter remains in place if future PD is anticipated.
■ Remove catheter and insert Deane button into catheter insertion site. This can be a medical procedure or designated to nurses in specialty units.	Maintains patency of catheter insertion site.
13. Inspect catheter dressing. If dressing is reapplied, use transparent occlusive dressing.	Dressing remains intact and dry, which reduces the risk of infection.
14. Remove mask and gloves, wash hands, and dispose of contaminated supplies according to agency policy.	Reduces transmission of microorganisms and blood-borne pathogens.
15. Document client's pre-PD and post-PD weight, abdominal girth, and dialysis fluid balance.	Notes the presence or absence of retained fluid in abdominal cavity.
■ Document client's vital signs before, during, and after dialysis.	Notes client's hemodynamic response.
■ Document temperature and status of catheter site.	Notes presence or absence of local or systemic infection.
■ Record color of drainage.	Notes any abnormalities in drainage color.
■ Record status of the catheter dressing or if new dressing was applied.	Provides a record of the status of the dressing's condition and most recent dressing change.

Nurse Alert

Stop dialysis and notify physician for change in vital signs, respiratory distress, bright red bleeding, fecal contents in the drainage, or scrotal swelling. These findings can indicate intolerance to the procedure, distention of the peritoneal cavity, perforation of the organ or vessel, perforation of bowel, or catheter displacement, respectively.

Clients on CAPD may experience weight gain caused by dextrose absorption. The glucose in the dialysate may provide a third or more of daily caloric intake (Ulrich, 1989). A potassium-free dialysate is usually employed in peritoneal dialysis because the peritoneal membrane clears potassium slowly. However, if a client is receiving digoxin, especially during the initial dialysis period, potassium should be added. The amount varies, but is usually 3 to 4 mEq/L (Levine et al, 1983).

Complaints of cramps can indicate that the dialysate is too cold or being infused too rapidly. In addition, cramps can indicate the presence of an electrolyte imbalance.

Teaching Considerations

Clients who receive CAPD require meticulous teaching. These clients must be taught principles of surgical asepsis as well as the specific steps of their therapy. Before initiating CAPD, a specific teaching plan is individualized for the client. The implementation of the teaching plan is usually done by dialysis nurses and is based on national or regional teaching protocols.

Pediatric Considerations

Because small children are at risk for fluid and electrolyte imbalances, this therapy may not be selected. When it is used, it is selected for the adolescent in end-stage renal disease.

Geriatric Considerations

In the presence of other chronic diseases, the older adult may not be a candidate for this therapy. When it is selected, the nurse should do a detailed assessment of the client's learning needs and ability as well as the client's ability to implement the procedure in the home setting.

SKILL 8-5

Continuous Bladder
Irrigation

Continuous bladder irrigation is performed to maintain patency of
the urethral catheter. This irrigation is maintained by way of a
closed irrigating system. The closed system ensures sterility of
the irrigant and the irrigation system. Continuous bladder irrigation is commonly used in clients after genitourinary surgery.
Such clients are at risk for small blood clots and mucus frag-
ments that can occlude the urinary catheter.

Potential Nursing Diagnoses

Client data derived during the assessment reveal defining characteristics to support the following nursing diagnoses in clients requiring this skill:
  High risk for infection
  Pain

Equipment

Sterile irrigating solution (as ordered by physician)
Irrigation tubing with clamp (with or without Y-connector)
IV pole
Antiseptic swab
Metric container
Y-connector
Bath blanket (optional)
Clean gloves

Steps	Rationale
1. Explain procedure to client.	Reduces anxiety and promotes cooperation.
2. Close curtains or room door.	Provides privacy.

Steps	Rationale
3. Don gloves and wash hands.	Reduces transmission of micro-organisms.
4. Arrange client in a comfort-able position that does not occlude inflow or outflow tubing.	Maintains client comfort. Prevents accidental occlusion of drainage tubing and subsequent bladder distention.
5. Assess lower abdomen for signs of bladder distention.	Detects whether catheter or urinary drainage system is malfunctioning, blocking urinary drainage.
6. Using aseptic technique, insert tip of sterile irrigation tubing into bag containing irrigation solution.	Reduces transmission of micro-organisms.
7. Close clamp on tubing and hang bag of solution on IV pole.	Prevents loss of irrigating solution.
8. Open clamp and allow solution to flow through tubing, keeping end of tubing sterile; close clamp.	Removes air from tubing.
9. Wipe off irrigation port of triple-lumen catheter or attach sterile Y-connector to double-lumen catheter, then connect to irrigation tubing (Fig. 113).	The third catheter lumen or Y-connector provides means for irrigating solution to enter bladder. System must remain sterile.
10. Be sure drainage bag and tubing are securely connected to drainage port of triple-Y-connector to double lumen catheter.	Ensures that urine and irrigating solution will drain from bladder.

Steps   Rationale

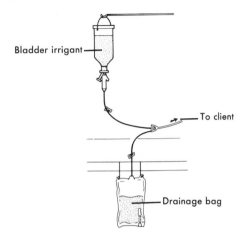

Fig. 113

11. For intermittent flow, clamp tubing on drainage system, open clamp on irrigation tubing, and allow prescribed amount of fluid to enter bladder (100 ml is normal for adults). Close irrigation tubing clamp, then open drainage tubing clamp.

Fluid instills through catheter into bladder, flushing system. Fluid drains out after irrigation is complete.

12. For continuous irrigation, calculate drip rate and adjust clamp on irrigation tubing accordingly; be sure clamp on drainage tubing is open and check volume of drainage in drainage bag.

Ensures continuous, even irrigation of catheter system. Prevents accumulation of solution in bladder, which may cause bladder distention and possible injury.

13. Dispose of contaminated supplies, remove gloves, and wash hands.

Reduces spread of microorganisms.

Steps	Rationale
14. Record amount of solution used as irrigant, amount returned as drainage, and consistency of drainage in nurses' notes and intake and output (I & O) sheet. Report catheter occlusion, sudden bleeding, infection, or increased pain to physician.	Documents procedure and client's tolerance of it.

Nurse Alert

If the irrigant is too cold, bladder spasms can result, causing the client increased pain. If blood and blood clots are present, the nurse may need to seek an order to increase the rate of flow. The purpose of this intervention is to maintain catheter patency. Blood clots have the potential to occlude the catheter.

Teaching Considerations

Clients need to be instructed to observe the urine drainage for signs of blood or mucus, changes in color, or changes in consistency. In addition, clients are instructed to report increased frequency, duration, or intensity of bladder spasms and/or pain.

Unless contraindicated, clients should be instructed to maintain an oral intake of at least 2 liters per day. This dilutes urine and increases urine flow.

Geriatric Considerations

Continuous bladder irrigations are commonly ordered following prostate surgery. The majority of males needing this surgery are older adults.

Teaching
Self-Catheterization

Self-catheterization enables the client who no longer has voluntary bladder control to independently maintain urinary continence. Self-catheterization can be taught to clients with paraplegia, hemiplegia, or other illnesses that limit voluntary bladder control. When self-catheterization is included in the care plan, the nurse must also teach a family member or significant other how to perform the procedure. It is necessary for another person to know the technique in case the client becomes incapacitated and is unable to empty the bladder.

Self-catheterization is an important component of a client's rehabilitation and return to maximal level of functioning. Therefore instruction is integrated into the rehabilitation program at an early stage and not merely tacked onto the end of the hospital stay.

Self-catheterization is taught to clients requiring intermittent straight catheterization and those with indwelling Foley catheters. However, the greater proportion of clients using this technique require intermittent catheterization.

Potential Nursing Diagnoses

Client data derived during the assessment reveal defining characteristics to support the following nursing diagnoses in clients requiring this skill:

Knowledge deficit of self-catheterization

Equipment

Assemble equipment required for Skill 8-1 or 8-2

Steps	Rationale
1. Assess status of client to determine: (1) Learning needs. What does client need to know about self-catheterization? (2) Readiness to learn. Does client want to learn to perform this skill? What does client already know about procedure? (3) Ability to learn. Consider developmental stage, cognitive status, physical attributes. (4) Learning environment. Choose setting where nurse can help client to focus on learning task.	Aids in developing appropriate teaching strategy and selecting proper environment for teaching sessions. It is important to include client and family member in this process.
2. Develop individualized goals for the client	Based on identified learner needs.
a. Client will perform self-catheterization.	Objectives relate to psychomotor, cognitive, and affective domain, are stated in behavioral terms, and serve as bases to measure learning. Nurse should collaborate with client when developing objectives.
b. Client will be able to correctly identify urethral meatus.	
c. Client will be able to discuss the importance of handwashing before beginning the procedure, and of aseptic technique.	
d. Client will be able to correctly identify equipment and supplies used for procedure.	
e. Client will be able to position self correctly.	
f. Client will be able to cleanse perineal area correctly before catheter insertion.	
g. Client will be able to state how far catheter should be inserted.	

Steps	Rationale

h. Client will be able to demonstrate caring for equipment after it is used.

3. Carry out individualized plan, allowing client to return demonstrations each time:

a. Reduction of microorganisms:
  ■ Teach theory and importance of hand washing. Demonstrate how to wash hands thoroughly (medical asepsis).
  ■ Explain and demonstrate opening catheterization package and manipulation of supplies. (Read directions on label.)
  ■ Explain and demonstrate technique for handling catheter.
  ■ Explain and demonstrate preparation of urethral meatus.

Starting with simple concepts and working toward more complex ones facilitates learning. Return demonstration actively involves client in performing procedure on self, or client may need to start with model and work up to performing procedure on self with nurse's supervision.

b. Insertion of catheter into bladder:
  ■ Explain suitable position for client to assume (sitting on a bed with legs bent and knees apart or sitting on a toilet).

Practicing psychomotor skills after cognitive learning allows client to apply and practice principles learned.

Steps	Rationale

- Explain and demonstrate insertion of catheter: how to separate labia or hold penis, cleansing urethra, and distance to insert catheter. Explain normal sensations client will feel.

c. Care of equipment:

- Discuss and demonstrate principles of aseptic technique.

Proper care of equipment ensures maintenance of aseptic technique.

4. Have client independently demonstrate entire procedure.

Feedback on independent demonstration of psychomotor skill is means of evaluating ability.

5. Document teaching content and learner's progress in client's record.

Documents client's learning for other health care workers.

Nurse Alert

- Positioning may depend on physical ability. Paraplegics frequently assume sitting position.
- Clients with spinal cord injuries may be unable to perceive pain associated with urinary tract infections.
- Client with hearing problem may respond best to visual material.
- Female client may need mirror to visualize perineal area.
- Video tape demonstrations can be used as long as teacher is available for feedback or discussion. Include family member's participation if appropriate. Implement individualized plan with step-by-step skill progression. Client gradually performs independent self-catheterization.
- Disposable supplies are preferred. If it is necessary to reuse catheters, client should learn boiling technique. (Boil rubber catheter 20 minutes and wrap in clean cloth.)
- Clients should be instructed to switch from clean to sterile catheter technique when signs of urinary tract infection occur.
- Teach family members catheterization technique.

Administering an
Enema

An enema is the instillation of a solution into the rectum and sigmoid colon. It is administered to promote defecation by stimulating peristalsis. Medications are occasionally given by enema to exert a local effect on the rectal mucosa. A cleansing enema can be used to soften feces that have become impacted or to empty the rectum and lower colon for diagnostic or surgical procedures.

Potential Nursing Diagnoses

Client data derived during the assessment reveal defining characteristics to support the following nursing diagnoses in clients requiring this skill:

> Constipation
> Self-care deficit, toileting
> Pain

Equipment
Administration Via Rectal Tube With Container

Enema container
Ordered volume of warmed solution (with soap, salt, or other additives):
> Adult: 700 to 1000 ml, 40.5° to 43° C (105° to 109° F)
> Child: 37° C (98.6° F)
>> Infant: 150 to 250 ml
>> Toddler: 250 to 350 ml
>> School age: 300 to 500 ml
>> Adolescent: 500 to 700 ml
Rectal tube with rounded tip
> Adult: No. 22- 30-gauge French (Fr)
> Child: No. 12- 18-gauge Fr

Tubing to connect rectal tube to container
Regulating clamp on tubing
Bath thermometer to measure solution's temperature
Water-soluble lubricant
Waterproof pad
Bath blanket
Toilet paper
Bedpan or commode
Wash basin, washcloth and towel, and soap
Disposable gloves

Administration Via Prepackaged Disposable Container

Prepackaged bottle with rectal tip
Disposable gloves
Water-soluble lubricant
Waterproof pad
Bath blanket
Toilet paper
Bedpan or commode
Wash basin, washcloth and towel, and soap

Steps	Rationale
Rectal Tube with Container	
1. Explain procedure to client.	Reduces client anxiety and promotes cooperation during procedure.
2. Close room or cubicle curtains.	Provides client privacy.
3. Assist client into a left side-lying (Sims') position with right knee flexed. Children may also be placed in dorsal recumbent position. (Position clients with poor sphincter control on bedpan.)	Allows enema solution to flow downward by gravity along natural curve of sigmoid colon and rectum, thus improving retention of solution. (Clients with poor sphincter control will not be able to retain all enema solution.)
4. Place waterproof pad under client's hips and buttocks.	Prevents soiling of bed linen.

Steps	Rationale
5. Drape client's trunk and lower extremities with bath blanket, leaving only anal area exposed.	Prevents unnecessary exposure of body parts and reduces client embarrassment.
6. Assemble enema container—connecting tubing, clamp, and rectal tube. Size of rectal tube should be 10- to 12-gauge French for infant or child and 22-26-gauge French for adult.	Rectal tubing should be small enough to fit diameter of client's anus but large enough to prevent leakage around tube.
7. Close regulating clamp.	Prevents initial loss of solution as it is added to container.
8. Add warmed solution to container. Warm the water as it flows from faucet. Place saline container in basin of hot water before adding saline to enema container. Check temperature of solution with bath thermometer or by pouring small amount of solution over your inner wrist.	Hot water can burn intestinal mucosa. Cold water can cause abdominal cramping and is difficult to retain.
9. Raise container, release clamp, and allow solution to flow enough to fill tubing. Reclamp tubing.	Removes air from tubing. Prevent loss of solution.
10. Place bedpan near bedside unit.	To be easily accessible if client is unable to retain enema.
11. Wash hands and don gloves.	Reduces transmission of infection.
12. Lubricate 3 to 4 inches of tip of rectal tube with lubricating jelly.	Allows smooth insertion of tube without risk of irritation or trauma to rectal mucosa.

Steps	Rationale
13. Gently separate buttocks and locate anus. Instruct client to relax by breathing out slowly through his mouth.	Breathing out promotes relaxation of external anal sphincter.
14. Insert tip of rectal tube slowly by pointing it in direction of client's umbilicus. Length of insertion varies: 7.5 to 10 cm (3 to 4 inches) for adult; 5 to 7.5 cm (2 to 3 inches) for child; 2.5 to 3.25 cm (1 to 1.5 inches) for infant. Withdraw tube immediately if it meets obstruction.	Careful insertion prevents trauma to rectal mucosa from accidental lodging of tube against wall. Insertion beyond proper limit can cause bowel perforation.
15. Continue to hold tubing until end of fluid instillation.	Bowel contraction can cause expulsion of rectal tube.
16. Open regulating clamp and allow solution to enter slowly, with container at client's hip level.	Rapid infusion can stimulate evacuation prematurely, before sufficient volume is infused.
17. Raise height of container slowly to appropriate level above anus (30 to 45 cm or 12 to 18 inches for high enema, 30 cm or 12 inches for low enema, and 7.5 cm or 3 inches for infant). Infusion time varies with volume of solution administered (e.g., 1 liter in 10 minutes).	Allows for continuous slow infusion. Raising container too high causes rapid infusion and possible painful distention of colon.
18. Lower the container or clamp tubing if client complains of cramping or if fluid escapes from anus around tube.	Temporary cessation of infusion prevents cramping. Cramping may prevent client from retaining all fluid.

Steps	Rationale
19. Clamp tubing after all solution is infused.	Prevents entrance of air into rectum.
20. Place layers of toilet tissue around tube at anus and gently withdraw tube.	Provides for client's comfort and cleanliness.
21. Explain to client that feeling of distention is normal. Ask him to retain solution as long as possible while lying quietly in bed. (For an infant or young child, gently hold buttocks together for a few minutes.)	Solution distends bowel. Length of retention varies with type of enema and client's ability to contract anal sphincter. Longer retention promotes more effective stimulation of peristalsis and defecation. (Infants and young children have poor sphincter control.)
22. Discard enema container and tubing in proper receptacle or rinse out thoroughly with warm water and soap if container is to be reused.	Controls transmission and growth of microorganisms.
23. Remove gloves by pulling them inside out and discard in proper receptacle.	Prevents microorganism transmission.
24. Assist client to bathroom or help position him on bedpan.	Normal squatting position promotes defecation.
25. Observe character of feces and solution (caution client against flushing toilet before inspection).	When enemas are ordered "until clear," it is essential to observe the contents of solution passed.
26. Assist client as needed to wash anal area with warm water and soap.	Fecal contents can irritate skin. Hygiene promotes client's comfort.
27. Wash your hands and record results of enema in nurse's notes.	Prompt recording improves documentation of treatment results.

Steps	Rationale

Prepackaged Disposable Container

1. Follow Steps 1 through 5 for "Rectal Tube with Container".

2. Place bedpan near bedside unit.

   To be easily accessible if client unable to retain enema.

3. Wash your hands.

   Reduces transmission of infection.

4. Don disposable gloves.

   Prevents transmission of organisms from feces.

5. Remove plastic cap from rectal tip. Although tip is already lubricated, more jelly can be applied as needed.

   Lubrication provides for smooth insertion of rectal tube without causing rectal irritation or trauma.

6. Gently separate buttocks and locate anus. Instruct client to relax by breathing out slowly through his mouth.

   Breathing out promotes relaxation of external anal sphincter.

7. Insert tip of bottle gently into rectum. Advance it 7.5 to 10 cm (3 to 4 inches) in adult (Fig. 114). (Children and infants usually do not receive prepackaged hypertonic enemas.)

   Gentle insertion prevents trauma to rectal mucosa.

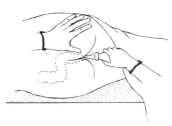

Fig. 114

Steps	Rationale
8. Squeeze bottle until all solution has entered rectum and colon. (Most bottles contain approximately 250 ml.)	Hypertonic solutions require only small volumes to stimulate defecation.
9. Follow Steps 20 through 27 for "Rectal Tube with Container".	

Nurse Alert

If a client has an order for enemas "until clear," the nurse should not give more than three without verifying with the physician the need for more. Repeated enema administration can result in serious fluid and electrolyte imbalances.

Client Teaching

Clients should be instructed not to rely on enemas to maintain bowel regularity. Repeated use of enemas destroys defecation reflexes and leads to further alterations in bowel elimination.

Pediatric Considerations

The procedure for giving an enema to an infant or a child does not differ essentially from that for giving one to an adult. However, because of lack of motor control in the rectum, infants and small children may be unable to retain the instilled fluid. Plain tap water is rarely used in children because, being hypotonic, it can cause rapid fluid shifts and fluid overload. The Fleet enema is not advised for children because of the harsh action of its ingredients, which may produce severe diarrhea (leading to metabolic acidosis).

Geriatric Considerations

A frail elderly client may be more susceptible than would be a young adult client to fluid and electrolyte imbalances resulting from enema administration. Caution should be used when administering repeated cleansing enemas. In addition, the nurse should frequently monitor fluid and electrolyte status.

Removing Stool Digitally

Digital stool removal involves the introduction of the nurse's fingers into the client's rectum to break up a fecal mass and remove it in sections. This procedure is used when the fecal mass is too large to be passed voluntarily and enema administration is unsuccessful. Elderly or immobilized clients who are unable to ambulate regularly and who fail to maintain a balanced diet or fluid intake are susceptible to fecal impaction.

Potential Nursing Diagnoses

Client data derived during the assessment reveal defining characteristics to support the following nursing diagnoses in clients requiring this skill:

Constipation
Diarrhea
Pain

Equipment

Water-soluble lubricant
Gloves
Bedpan
Waterproof pad
Bath blanket
Wash basin, washcloth and towel, and soap.

Steps	Rationale
1. Measure client's pulse rate.	Serves as baseline for determining changes during procedure.

Steps	Rationale
2. Explain procedure to client, noting that manipulation of the rectum can cause discomfort.	Explanation reduces client anxiety. Cooperation is necessary to minimize risk of injury.
3. Assist client to a side-lying position with knees flexed.	Provides access to rectum.
4. Drape client's trunk and lower extremities with bath blanket.	Prevents unnecessary exposure of body parts.
5. Place waterproof pad under client's buttocks.	Prevents soiling of bed linen.
6. Place bedpan next to client.	To be receptacle for stool.
7. Wash hands and don disposable gloves.	Prevents transmission of microorganisms.
8. Lubricate your gloved index finger with ample amount of lubricating jelly.	Permits smooth insertion of finger into rectum.
9. Insert your finger into client's rectum and advance it slowly along rectal wall toward umbilicus.	Allows you to reach impacted stool high in rectum.
10. Gently loosen fecal mass by massaging around it. Work finger into hardened core.	Loosening mass allows you to penetrate it with less discomfort to client.
11. Work stool downward toward anus. Remove small sections of feces at a time.	Prevents need to force finger up into rectum and minimizes trauma to mucosa.
12. Periodically assess client's pulse and look for signs of fatigue. Stop procedure if client's pulse rate drops or rhythm changes.	Vagal stimulation slows heart rate. Procedure may exhaust client.
13. Continue to clear rectum of feces and allow client to rest at intervals.	Rest improves client's tolerance of procedure.

Steps	Rationale
14. After disimpaction, use washcloth and towel to wash buttocks and anal area.	Promotes client's sense of comfort and cleanliness.
15. Remove bedpan and dispose of feces. Remove gloves by turning them inside out and discard in proper receptacle.	Prevents transmission of microorganisms.
16. Assist client to toilet or a clean bedpan.	Disimpaction may stimulate defecation reflex.
17. Wash your hands and record in nurse's notes results of disimpaction. Describe fecal characteristics. (Procedure may be followed by enemas or cathartics.)	Prompt recording improves accuracy of documentation.

Nurse Alert

Excessive rectal manipulation can cause irritation to the mucosa, bleeding, and stimulation of the vagus nerve. When there is vagal stimulation, a reflexive slowing of the heart rate occurs and can cause dangerous dysrhythmias in some clients.

Client Teaching

Clients and their families should be instructed on how to avoid fecal impactions—by modifying their diets to include more fruits and vegetables, by increasing their fluid intake (if not contraindicated), and by altering sedentary activity patterns.

Pediatric Considerations

Digital removal of stool is rarely needed in children. If it does become necessary, it should be preceded by a careful explanation to both the parent and the child. Preventive measures are more common and include stool softeners, diet changes, and adequate hydration.

Geriatric Considerations

In the older adult population, constipation tends to be more of a problem than in younger persons, and along with it the more frequent use of laxatives and/or enemas. In addition, a higher percentage of elderly clients have chronic cardiovascular disease, which puts these persons at greater risk of dysrhythmias induced by vagal stimulation during digital stool removal.

CARE OF THE SURGICAL CLIENT

Demonstrating Postoperative Exercises

The manner in which the nurse prepares a client for surgery can have a positive influence on his recovery. With well-planned instruction a client can learn how to cough and deep breathe regularly, ambulate and resume activities of daily living early after surgery, and participate in the recovery process to attain a sense of well-being. A few simple maneuvers—diaphragmatic breathing, coughing, turning, and leg exercises—serve to prevent respiratory and circulatory complications that otherwise might develop in a client who stays inactive postoperatively. The exercises are important for any client undergoing general anesthesia.

Structured preoperative teaching can influence postoperative factors such as:

1. Ventilatory function—improved ability to cough and deep breathe.
2. Physical functional capacity—improved ability to ambulate and resume activities earlier.
3. Sense of well-being—decreased anxiety.
4. Length of hospital stay—reduced length of stay.

When the nurse plans postoperative exercises it is important to know the client's risks of complications. Chronic smoking, a history of respiratory disease, and a painful surgical incision all can contribute to impairing a client's ventilatory capacity. Likewise, a history of peripheral vascular disease or forced immobilization from an applied cast or traction can increase the risk of poor tissue perfusion. By helping clients learn how to participate actively in postoperative recovery, the nurse provides an effective and preventive plan of care.

Potential Nursing Diagnoses

Client data derived during the assessment reveal defining characteristics to support the following nursing diagnoses in clients requiring this skill:

Airway clearance, ineffective
Pain
Mobility, impaired physical

Equipment

Pillow (optional)
Incentive spirometer

Steps	Rationale

Diaphragmatic Breathing

Demonstrate the following steps
to client:

1. Sit or stand upright, placing your hands palm down along lower borders of your anterior rib cage (Fig. 115).	Upright position facilitates diaphragmatic excursion. This placement of hands allows individual to feel movement of chest and abdomen as diaphragm descends and lungs expand.

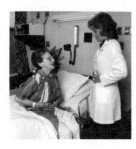

Fig. 115

2. Take slow deep breath, inhaling through your nose.	Discourages panting or hyperventilation. Breathing through nose warms, humidifies, and filters air.

Steps	Rationale
3. Give attention to normal downward movement of your diaphragm during inspiration. Abdominal organs descend, and thorax expands slowly.	Your explanation focuses on normal ventilatory movements so the client can anticipate how diaphragmatic breathing feels.
4. Avoid using your chest and shoulders while inhaling.	Use of auxiliary chest and shoulder muscles increases energy expenditure during breathing.
5. After holding your breath to a count of 3, slowly exhale through your mouth.	Allows gradual expulsion of all air.
6. Repeat exercise three to five times.	Establishes slow, rhythmic breathing pattern.
7. Have client practice exercise.	Reinforces learning.

Incentive Spirometry

Instruct client to:

1. Wash hands.	Reduces transmission of microorganisms.
2. Assume semi-Fowler's or high-Fowler's position.	Promotes optimal lung expansion during respiratory maneuver.
3. Place mouthpiece in mouth so that lips completely cover mouth piece (Fig. 116).	Demonstration is a reliable technique for documentation of psychomotor skill.

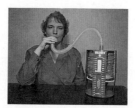

Fig. 116

Steps	Rationale
4. Client inhales slowly to maintain a constant flow through the mouthpiece. When maximal inspiration is reached, client holds breath for 2 to 3 seconds and then exhales slowly. Number of breaths should not exceed 10 to 12 per minute (Dettenmeier, 1992).	Maintains maximal inspiration and reduces risk of progressive collapse of individual alveoli. Slow breath prevents or minimizes pain from sudden pressure changes in chest (Dettenmeier, 1992).
5. Client breathes normally for a short period.	Prevents hyperventilation and fatigue.
6. Client repeats maneuver. Instruct client on importance of performing incentive spirometry every 2 hours while awake during the postoperative period.	Demonstrates correct use of spirometer. Frequent postoperative use of spirometer promotes lung expansion and reduces risk of pulmonary complications.
7. Wash hands.	Reduces transmission of microorganisms.

Controlled Coughing

Demonstrate the following steps to client:

1. Assume an upright position in bed or on side of bed.	Facilitates diaphragmatic movement and enhances expansion of lungs.
2. Take two or three slow diaphragmatic breaths.	Expands lungs fully to move air behind mucus in airways.
3. Inhale deeply, hold your breath to count of 3, and cough once and then again.	Two successive coughs help remove mucus more effectively and completely than one forceful cough.
4. Do not merely clear your throat.	Clearing of throat does not remove mucus from deep inside airways.

Steps	Rationale
5. If surgical incision is to be in chest or abdominal area, place one hand over the incisional area and other hand on top of first. During inhalation and coughing, press gently against that area to splint incision. (A pillow over incision is optional.) (Fig. 117.)	Surgical incision results in cutting of muscles and tissues. Breathing and coughing place strain on a suture line and cause discomfort. Splinting minimizes incisional pulling. Hands provide firm support to incision.

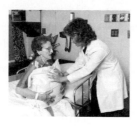

Fig. 117

6. Have client practice coughing with splinting.	You are trying to emphasize value of deep coughing with splinting to effectively expectorate mucus with minimal discomfort.
7. Instruct client on importance of performing controlled cough every 2 hours while awake during the postoperative period.	Promotes lung expansion and reduces risk of pulmonary complications.

Turning

NOTE: This is for turning client to his left side.

1. Instruct client to assume a supine position on right half of bed. (Side rails should be up on both sides.)	You cannot demonstrate exercise in client's bed for obvious reasons of asepsis. Positioning begins toward right side of bed so turning to left will not cause client to roll toward bed's edge.

Steps	Rationale
2. Place client's left hand over incisional area for splinting.	Supports incisional area to minimize pulling of suture line during turning.
3. Have client keep his left leg straight and flex right knee up and over left leg.	Straight left leg stabilizes client's position. Flexed right leg shifts weight for easier turning.
4. Grasping side rail on left side of bed with his right hand, client pulls toward left and rolls onto his left side.	Minimizes effort needed to turn.
5. Instruct client on importance of turning every 2 hours while awake during the postoperative period.	Promotes lung expansion and reduces risk of pulmonary complications. Reduces risk of vascular complications.

Leg Exercises

NOTE: If client's surgery involves one or both extremities, a surgeon's order is required before exercises can be performed postoperatively. Legs unaffected by surgery can be safely exercised unless a client has preexisting alterations.

1. Place client supine in bed. Demonstrate leg exercises by putting him through passive range of motion.	Provides for normal anatomic position of lower extremities.
2. Instruct client to rotate each ankle in a complete circle by pretending to draw circles with his big toe (Fig. 118).	Maintains joint mobility and promotes venous return.
3. Alternate dorsiflexion and plantar flexion of the feet. Client will feel his calf muscles first contract and then relax.	Stretches and contracts gastrocnemius muscles.
4. Have client flex and extend his knees (Fig. 119).	

Steps   Rationale

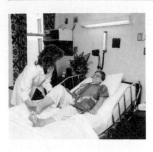

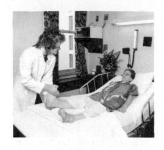

Fig. 118   Fig. 119

5. Keeping his legs straight,   Promotes contraction and relax-
   client then alternately raises   ation of quadriceps muscles.
   each leg from surface of bed
   and lets it drop gently.

6. Instruct client to do leg exer-   Reduces risk of vascular com-
   cises every 2 hours while   plications.
   awake.

All preoperative exercises:

1. Observe client's ability to   Demonstration enables the nurse
   perform all exercises inde-   to monitor that client is doing
   pendently.   the exercises correctly, or if
                                         exercises are done incorrectly,
                                         to develop interventions to cor-
                                         rect errors.

2. Record teaching and client's   Documents client teaching and
   return demonstrations of   provides information for instruc-
   postoperative exercises.   tional follow-up.

Nurse Alert

Know whether a client will be allowed to do active exercising of
his extremities postoperatively. Some vascular procedures, such
as repair of the femoral-popliteal artery, prohibit active exercising until the vascular graft has healed. Likewise, certain procedures may contraindicate turning.

Client Teaching

The nurse must demonstrate each exercise carefully and then have the client practice doing it under supervision. Eventually the client should be able to perform the exercises independently. During a routine postoperative day it is hoped that he will become able to initiate exercises on his own.

Pediatric Considerations

Children usually are at lower risk of postoperative complications because they tend to resume activity quickly. However, seriously ill children may require guidance and support. Parents can be helpful in demonstrating and reinforcing exercises.

Geriatric Considerations

Elderly persons usually are at greater risk of postoperative complications because of the aging process. They often have increased calcium and cholesterol deposits in small arteries, and vessel walls thicken. These changes predispose to clot formation. The elderly person's rib cage also tends to stiffen and diaphragmatic movement declines, reducing lung expansion. It often takes longer for an elderly client to become oriented following surgery because of neurologic and sensory changes. Thus active participation in exercises may be lessened.

Surgical Skin
Preparation

Before any surgical procedure the skin is prepared so as to minimize the number of resident microorganisms that could enter a surgical wound. Skin preparation routinely requires thorough cleaning with scrubs and/or showers. Hair clipping or shaving may also be performed to remove body hair that harbors microorganisms and obstructs the view of the surgical field. An area of skin larger than the actual surgical site is always prepared to ensure that the surgical site is as clean as possible.

The Centers for Disease Control (CDC) recommends avoiding hair removal or, if necessary, shaving only immediately before the operation (Garner, 1985). Hair removal can injure the skin, especially if a razor is used. Minor nicks or cuts in the skin are prime sites for bacterial growth. The longer the period between the shave and surgery, the greater is the potential for bacterial growth.

Potential Nursing Diagnoses

Client data derived during the assessment reveal defining characteristics to support the following nursing diagnoses in clients requiring this skill:

Infection, high risk for

Equipment

Electric clippers
Scissors
Towel
Cotton balls, applicators, and antiseptic solution (optional)
Portable lamp
Bath blanket

Steps	Rationale
1. Inspect general condition of skin.	If lesions, irritations, or signs of skin infection are present, shaving should not be done. These conditions increase chances for postoperative wound infections.
2. Review physician's order for area to be clipped. (Review institution's operating room manual as needed.)	Extent of area for hair removal depends upon site of incision, nature of surgery, and physician's preference. Area is always larger than actual incision to ensure wide perimeter with minimal bacteria.
3. Explain procedure and rationale for removal of hair over large surface area.	Promotes cooperation and minimizes anxiety because client may think incision will be as large as clipped site.
4. Wash hands.	Reduces transmission of infection.
5. Close room doors or bedside curtains.	Provides client privacy.
6. Raise bed to high position.	Avoids need to bend over for long periods.
7. Position client comfortably with surgical site accessible.	Hair removal and skin preparation can take several minutes. Nurse should have easy access to hard-to-reach areas.
8. Lightly dry area to be clipped with towel.	Removes moisture, which interferes with clean cut of clippers.
9. Hold clippers in dominant hand, about 1 cm above skin, and cut hair in direction it grows. Clip small area at time.	Prevents pulling on hair and abrasion of skin.
10. Arrange drapes as necessary.	Prevents unnecessary exposure of body parts.
11. Lightly brush off cut hair with towel.	Removes contaminated hair and promotes client's comfort. Improves visibility of area being clipped.

Steps	Rationale
12. When clipped area is over body crevices (e.g., umbilicus or groin), clean crevices with cotton-tipped applicators or cotton ball dipped in antiseptic solution, then dry.	Removes secretions, dirt, and any remaining hair clippings, which harbor microorganisms.
13. Tell client that procedure is completed.	Relieves client's anxiety.
14. Clean and dispose of equipment according to policy and dispose of gloves.	Proper disposal of soiled equipment prevents spread of infection and reduces risk of injury.
15. Inspect condition of skin after completion of hair removal.	Determines if there is remaining hair or if skin was cut.
16. Record procedure, area clipped or shaved, and condition of skin before and after in nurse's notes.	Documents procedure performed and condition of skin before surgery.

Nurse Alert

Use extra caution if the client has a preexisting bleeding tendency such as leukemia, aplastic anemia, or hemophilia, or has been receiving anticoagulant therapy. If a client has a bleeding tendency or is on anticoagulant therapy, dry shaving may be ordered.

Client Teaching

Explain the purpose of shaving and its importance to the client's welfare. The client should understand that it is necessary to shave a larger surface area than the immediate surgical site. He may fear that the surgical incision will be as large as the shaved area.

Pediatric Considerations

A shave will sometimes be deferred because the amount of body hair on a young child is limited. An adolescent has more body hair and may need to be shaved.

Geriatric Considerations

The elderly client's skin can be thin and fragile. Use caution when shaving to avoid cuts.

NUTRITION

Insertion, Placement, and Anchoring of Nasogastric Tubes

Large-bore and small-bore

Insertion of a nasogastric tube involves placing a pliable plastic tube through the client's nasopharynx into the stomach. The tube has a hollow lumen that allows both the removal of gastric secretions from and the introduction of solutions into the stomach.

Potential Nursing Diagnoses

Client data derived during assessment reveal defining characteristics to support the following nursing diagnoses in clients requiring this skill:

Nutrition, altered: less than body requirements

Equipment

Large-bore tube placement
  NG tube (14-18 French)
  Water-soluble lubricant
  60-ml catheter tip syringe
  Stethoscope
  Hypoallergenic tape and tincture of benzoin
  pH indicator strip
  Glass of water and straw
  Emesis basin
  Tongue blade
  Towel
  Clean gloves

Facial tissue
Normal saline solution
Small-bore tube placement
    NG tube (8-12 French)
    30-ml or larger Luer-Lok or tip syringe
    Stethoscope
    Hypoallergenic tape and tincture of benzoin
    pH indicator strip
    Glass of water and straw
    Emesis basin
    Towel
    Guide wire or stylet
    Facial tissues
    Clean gloves

Steps	Rationale
Tube Insertion	
1. Explain the procedure fully to client, as well as purpose of nasogastric decompression.	Procedure is easier to complete with client's full cooperation.
2. Wash hands.	Reduces transfer of microorganisms.
3. Assemble all equipment at bedside.	Organized procedure can be performed in a timely fashion, limiting client's discomfort.
4. Assist client to high Fowler position with pillows behind head and shoulders.	Promotes client's ability to swallow.
5. Place bath towel over client's chest. Keep facial tissues within client's reach.	Prevents soiling of client's gown. Insertion of tube through nasal passages may cause tearing.
6. Stand on right side of bed if you are right-handed (or on left side if left-handed).	Allows easier manipulating of tubing.
7. Instruct client to relax and breathe normally while occluding one naris. Then	Tube passes more easily through naris that is more patent.

Steps	Rationale

repeat procedure for other naris. Select one with greater air flow.

8. Determine length of tube to be inserted and mark with tape.

   a. Traditional method (Fig. 120): Measure distance from tip of nose to ear- lobe to xiphoid process to sternum. — Approximates depth of NG tube insertion.

   b. Hanson method: First mark 50-cm point on tube; then do traditional measurement. Tube in- sertion should be to midway point between 50 cm (25 inches) and traditional mark.

9. Cut a 10-cm (4-in) piece of tape.

10. Prepare nasogastric tube for intubation:

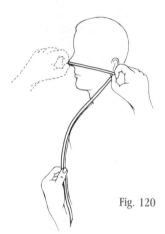

Fig. 120

Large-Bore Intubation

   a. Plastic tubes should not be iced. — Tubes will become stiff and inflexible, causing trauma to mucous membranes.

   b. Close off the end of the tube by attaching a sy- ringe. — Protects nurse from spread of microorganisms through contact with GI contents.

   c. Lubricate nasogastric tube 10 to 20 cm. — Lubrication decreases friction between nasal mucous mem- brane and tube.

Small-Bore Intubation

   a. Plastic tubes should not be iced. — Tubes will become stiff and inflexible, causing trauma to mucous membranes.

Steps	Rationale
b. Inject 10 ml of water from 30-ml or larger Luer-Lok tip syringe into the tube.	Aids in guide wire or stylet insertion.
c. Insert guide wire or stylet into tube, making certain it is securely positioned against weighted tip and that both Luer-Lok connections are snugly fitted together.	Promotes smooth passage of tube into GI tract. Improperly positioned stylet can induce serious trauma.
d. Dip weighted tip of tube into glass of water.	Activates lubricant to facilitate passage of tube into naris to GI tract.
11. Wash hands and don clean gloves.	Reduces spread of microorganisms. Protects nurse from transmission of microorganisms from gastric contents.
12. Alert client that insertion is to begin. Insert tube gently through nostril to back of throat (posterior nasopharynx). May cause client to gag. Aim back and down toward ear.	Natural contours facilitate passage of tube into gastrointestinal tract.
13. Flex client's head toward chest after tube has passed through nasopharynx. Allow client to relax a moment.	Closes off glottis and reduces risk of tube entering trachea. Allows client to "catch breath" and remain calm.
14. Encourage client to swallow by giving small sips of water or ice chips when possible. Advance tube as client swallows. Rotate tube 180 degrees while inserting.	Swallowing facilitates passage of tube past oropharynx. Rotating tube decreases friction.

Steps	Rationale
15. Emphasize need to mouth breathe and swallow during procedure.	Helps facilitate passage of tube and alleviates client's fears during procedure.
16. Advance tube each time client swallows until desired length has been passed.	Reduces discomfort and trauma to client.
17. Do not force tube. When resistance is met or client starts to gag, choke, or become cyanotic, stop advancing tube and pull tube back. Check for position of tube in back of throat with tongue blade.	Tube may be coiled, kinked, in oropharynx, or entering trachea.

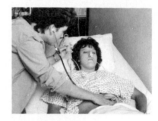

Fig. 121

18. Check placement of tube.	Proper position is essential before initiating feedings.
a. Attach a syringe to end of nasogastric tube. Place diaphragm of stethoscope over upper left quadrant of client's abdomen just below costal margin. Inject 10 to 20 ml of air while auscultating abdomen. (Fig. 121).	Air entering stomach creates "whooshing" sound and confirms tube placement. Absence of sound indicates tip of tube is still in esophagus. However, the nurse must know this is not always the most reliable method.
b. Aspirate gently to obtain gastric contents and measure pH.	Gastric pH ranges 1 to 4. If tip is not in stomach, contents cannot be aspirated.
c. If tube is not in stomach, advance another 2.5 to 5 cm (1 to 2 inches) and again check position.	Tube must be in stomach to provide adequate decompression.

Steps	Rationale
19. Apply tincture of benzoin on tip of client's nose and tube. Allow to dry.	Helps tape adhere better.
20. Secure tube with tape and avoid pressure on naris.	Prevents trauma to nasal mucosa and permits client mobility.
a. Cut 10 cm (4 inches) long piece of tape. Split one end lengthwise 5 cm (2 inches). Place other end of tape over bridge of patient's nose. Wrap 1.3 cm (½ inch) strips around tube as it exits nose (Fig. 122).	Prevents tissue necrosis to naris. Secures tape to nares.

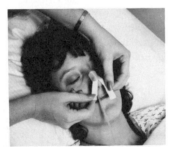

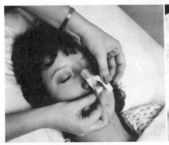 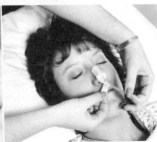

Fig. 122

Steps	Rationale
b. Fasten end of nasogastric tube to client's gown by looping rubber band around tube in slip knot and pinning to gown.	Reduces traction on the naris if tube moves. Provides slack to take if client moves.
21. Obtain x-ray of abdomen (tube must be radiopaque).	Determines placement of tube.
SMALL-BORE ONLY	
a. Position client on right side when possible until radiologic confirmation of correct placement has been verified.	Allow tube to pass small intestine (duodenum or jejunum).
b. Leave stylet in place until correct position is ensured by x-ray. Never attempt to reinsert partially or fully removed stylet while feeding tube is in place.	Guide wire or stylet may perforate GI tract, especially esophagus or nearby tissue and seriously injure the client.
22. Administer oral hygiene frequently. Cleanse tubing at nostril.	Promotes client comfort and integrity of oral mucous membranes.
23. Remain and talk with client.	Decreases anxiety after tube insertion.
24. Remove gloves, dispose of equipment, and wash hands.	Reduces transmission of microorganisms.
25. Record type of tube placed and client's tolerance to the procedure.	Documents the exact procedure.

Nurse Alert

Nasogastric tube placement can only be confirmed accurately by x-ray visualization and must be reassessed after the client's position changes or if severe coughing or vomiting develops. Verification determines that the tube is not displaced into the airway.

Client Teaching

Pre-procedure instruction in relaxation and deep breathing exercises can help reduce client anxiety and promote cooperation during tube insertion.

Pediatric Considerations

Nasogastric tubes may be placed in infants or small children through either the mouth or the nares. The size of the tube varies with the size of the child and the viscosity of any solution being introduced (infants: 5 to 8 Fr; children: 10 to 14 Fr). Measurement is from the tip of the nose to the earlobe and then to the tip of the xiphoid process.

Geriatric Considerations

With aging there is a reduction in the amount of secretions produced by the stomach and intestinal tract.

Nasogastric Tube Feedings

Initiating and maintaining nutrition

Enteral feeding is preferred over parenteral nutrition because it improves utilization of nutrients, is safer for clients, and is less expensive. Not all clients are able to be fed enterally, but if the GI system is able to digest and absorb nutrients, it should be used. Indications for nasogastric tube feedings include clients who cannot eat, clients who will not eat, and clients who cannot maintain adequate oral nutrition (e.g., clients with cancer, sepsis, trauma, or clients who are comatose).

Potential Nursing Diagnoses

Client data derived during the assessment reveal defining characteristics to support the following nursing diagnoses in clients requiring this skill:

Pain
Nutrition, altered: less than body requirements
Diarrhea
Gas exchange, impaired

Equipment

Disposable gavage bag and tubing
60-ml catheter tip syringe (large-bore NG tube)
30 ml or larger Luer-Lok or tip syringe (small-bore NG tube)
Stethoscope
Ph indicator strips
Prescribed tube feeding formula
Infusion pump (use pump designed for tube feedings)
Disposable gloves

Steps	Rationale
1. Wash hands and don gloves.	Reduces transmission of micro-organisms.
2. Auscultate for bowel sounds.	Bowel sounds indicate presence of peristalsis and ability of the GI tract to digest nutrients. When bowel sounds are absent, hold feeding and notify physician.
3. Verify physician's order for formula, rate, route, and frequency.	Tube feedings must be ordered by physician.
4. Prepare bag and tubing to administer formula:	
a. Connect tubing and bag.	Tubing must be free of contamination to prevent bacterial growth.
b. Fill bag and tubing with formula.	Placement of formula through tubing prevents excess air from entering gastrointestinal tract.
5. Explain procedure to client.	Reduces anxiety and increases cooperation.
6. Position client in high-Fowler's position or elevate head of bed 30 degrees.	Reduces risk of aspiration.
7. Verify placement of NG tube (see Skill 10-1, Step 18).	Reduces risk of aspiration of gastric contents into the respiratory tract.
8. Initiate feeding:	
a. Bolus or intermittent method	
■ Pinch proximal end of the feeding tube.	Prevents air from entering client's stomach.
■ Attach syringe to end of tube and elevate to 18 inches above the client's head.	Gradual emptying of tube feeding by gravity from syringe or gavage bag reduces risk of diarrhea induced by bolus tube feedings.
■ Fill syringe with formula. Allow syringe to empty gradually,	

Steps	Rationale

refilling until pre-
scribed amount has
been delivered to the
client.

- If gavage bag is used,
  attach bag to the end
  of the feeding tube
  and raise bag 18
  inches above client's
  head. Fill bag with
  prescribed amount of
  formula, then allow
  bag to empty gradu-
  ally over 30 min.

b. Continuous drip method
   (Fig. 123)
   - Hang gavage bag to
     IV pole.

Continuous feeding method is
designed to deliver prescribed
hourly rate of feeding. This
method reduces risk of diarrhea.
Clients who receive continuous
drip feedings should have resid-
uals checked every 4 hours.

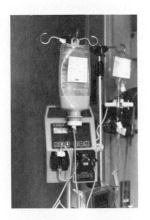

Fig. 123

- Connect end of bag to
  the proximal end of
  the feeding tube.
- Connect infusion
  pump and set rate.

Steps	Rationale
9. When tube feedings are not being administered, clamp the proximal end of the feeding tube.	Prevents air from entering stomach between feedings.
10. Administer water via feeding tube as ordered with or between feedings.	Provides client with source of water to help maintain fluid and electrolyte balance.
11. Rinse bag and tubing with warm water after all bolus feedings.	Rinsing bag and tube with warm water clears old tube feedings and prevents bacterial growth.
12. Advance tube feeding (see box on page 366).	Tube feedings should be advanced gradually to prevent diarrhea and gastric intolerance of formula.
13. Client remains in high-Fowler's position or with head of bed elevated 30 degrees or more for 30 minutes after tube feeding. With continual feedings client should be in one of these positions throughout feeding.	Position uses gravity to assist in keeping formula in the GI tract. These positions reduce the client's risk of aspiration.
14. Record amount and type of feeding, verification of tube placement, patency of tube, client's response to feeding, and any adverse effects.	Documents status of tube feeding and client's response.

Nurse Alert

Some tube feedings are ordered over a 24-hour period, whereas others are ordered at intermittent periods. The physician determines the client's status and nutritional requirements when writing the nutritional orders. NG formulas should be hung for only 8 to 12 hours at room temperature.

Advance Tube Feeding

Bolus
1. Advance concentration before increasing volume.
2. After client has tolerated desired concentration of feeding, advance volume over 24- to 48-hour period until maximum nutrient requirements are reached.
3. Aspirate before each feeding.
   a. Volume: 150 ml or more. Notify physician and withhold feeding. Check residual in 2 hours (if volume 150 ml or more again notify the physician so that client can be evaluated for delayed gastric emptying).
   b. Volume: less than 150 ml. Give tube feeding as ordered.

Continuous Feeding
1. Advance concentration, then volume.
2. Initial infusion rate is usually 50 ml/hr.
3. After determining tolerance, advance in increments of 25 ml/hr daily until the necessary volume is reached or an infusion rate of 125 ml/hr.

Teaching Considerations

Teach the client and caregiver to keep tubing clamped between feedings and to give feedings with client in sitting position. If tolerated, client should remain upright for 30 minutes after feedings.

Pediatric Considerations

Intermittent feeding is preferred in infants because of possible perforation of stomach, nasal airway obstruction, ulceration, and irritation to mucous membrane.

Geriatric Considerations

Older adults may require a slower advance in tube feeding formula. The slower rate of formula advancement may assist in reducing the risk of diarrhea as a complication of NG tube feedings in this population.

Irrigating a
Nasogastric Tube
Large-bore

An NG tube is irrigated to maintain patency. If the distal tip of the tube rests against the stomach wall or if the tube becomes occluded with secretions, it must be irrigated. Obstruction of the tube can result in abdominal distention and possible vomiting. NG tube irrigations are routinely ordered when intermittent gastric suction is ordered.

Potential Nursing Diagnoses

Client data derived during the assessment reveal defining characteristics to support the following nursing diagnoses in clients requiring this skill:

Pain
Skin integrity, impaired

Equipment

Disposable gloves
Soft or small bulb syringe or GU syringe
Normal saline, 30 ml
Emesis basin or irrigation tray
Towel
Facial tissues

Steps	Rationale
1. Wash hands and don gloves.	Reduces transmission of micro-organisms.
2. Verify tube placement.	Prevents accidental entrance of irrigating solution into lungs.

Steps	Rationale
a. Attach a syringe to end of NG tube. Place diaphragm of stethoscope over upper left quadrant of client's abdomen just below costal margin. Inject 10 to 20 ml of air while auscultating abdomen (see Skill 10-1, Fig. 119).	Air entering stomach creates "whooshing" sound and confirms tube placement. Absence of sound indicates tip of tube is still in esophagus.
b. Aspirate gently to obtain gastric contents and measure pH.	Gastric pH ranges 1 to 4. If tip is not in stomach, contents cannot be aspirated.
c. If tube is not in stomach, advance another 2.5 to 5 cm (1 to 2 inches) and check position again.	Tube must be in stomach to provide adequate decompression.
3. Draw up 30 ml of normal saline into bulb syringe.	Isotonic solution maintains osmotic pressure and minimizes loss of electrolytes from stomach.
4. Kink or clamp off tube proximal to connection site of drainage or suction apparatus. Disconnect suction tube and lay end on towel.	Prevents backflow of secretions and soiling of client's gown and bed linen.
5. Insert tip of irrigating syringe into end of NG tube. Release clamp or kink in tube. Holding syringe with tip toward floor, inject saline slowly but evenly. (Do not force.)	Position of syringe prevents introduction of air into tubing. Air can cause distention. Fluid introduced under pressure can cause trauma.
6. If resistance occurs, check for kinks in tubing. Turn client on his side. Repeated resistance should be reported to physician.	Buildup of secretions will cause abdominal distention.

Steps	Rationale
7. After instilling saline, immediately aspirate to withdraw fluid. Measure volume returned.	Stomach should remain empty. Fluid in stomach is measured as intake.
8. Reconnect nasogastric tube to drainage or suction. (If flow does not return, irrigation may be repeated.)	Reestablishes means of collecting drainage.
9. Record irrigation procedure in nurse's notes. Mention specifically amount of normal saline instilled, amount and type of drainage returned, and client's tolerance.	Documents performance of procedure.

Nurse Alert

If an NG tube continues to drain improperly after irrigation, the nurse must reposition it by advancing or withdrawing it slightly. Changes in the client's position or severe coughing or vomiting require reassessment of tube placement.

Client Teaching

Instruct the client to notify nursing personnel if the NG tube becomes displaced or he feels nauseated. Nausea may be associated with abdominal distention caused by improper draining of the tube. Irrigation of the tube may improve drainage and relieve the nausea.

Pediatric Considerations

Children are vulnerable to fluid and electrolyte imbalances associated with NG suctioning. Therefore a meticulously accurate record of drainage and irrigating solution is essential. For irrigation an electrolyte solution is used to prevent further body depletion.

Geriatric Considerations

The older adult is vulnerable to fluid and electrolyte imbalances associated with NG suctioning. Therefore accurate recording of drainage and irrigating solution is essential.

Clients with an NG tube are NPO. An elderly person's oral mucosa can become dry and inflamed without thorough hygiene. Thus it is essential to keep the mucosa well hydrated during NG suctioning.

Discontinuing a
Nasogastric Tube

Large-bore and small-bore

Discontinuing an NG tube is done when the client no longer needs gastric decompression, feeding, or lavage. Discontinuing the NG tube requires a physician's order.

Potential Nursing Diagnoses

Client data derived during the assessment reveal defining characteristics to support the following nursing diagnoses in clients requiring this skill:

Pain

Skin integrity, impaired

Equipment

Disposable gloves

Facial tissue

Towel

Emesis basin

Toothbrush or sponge applicators for mouth care

Steps	Rationale
1. Wash hands and don gloves.	Reduces transfer of microorganisms.
2. Place towel under client's chin.	Prevents contamination of bed or gown from gastric secretions.
3. Turn off suction and disconnect NG tube from drainage bag. Remove tape from bridge of nose and remove pin from gown.	Tube should be free of connection when removed.

Steps	Rationale
4. Explain procedure to client, reassuring him that removal is less distressing than insertion.	Minimizes client's anxiety.
5. Hand client a facial tissue. Instruct him to take a deep breath and hold.	Airway may be temporarily obstructed during removal of tube. NOTE: Some clients may experience paroxysms of coughing during procedure.
6. Pull tube steadily and smoothly as client is holding his breath. (Do not pull too slowly or too rapidly.)	Reduces trauma to mucosa and minimizes client discomfort.
7. Dispose of tube and drainage equipment and wash hands.	Reduces transfer of microorganisms.
8. Clean client's nares and provide mouth care.	Promotes comfort. Nares often become excoriated.
9. Record procedure in nurse's notes. Mention specifically tube removal, final volume of secretions collected in drainage system, and client's response.	Timely recording accurately documents procedure.

Nurse Alert

After discontinuing an NG tube the nurse should observe the client for abdominal distention, nausea, or vomiting. Any of these signs or symptoms could indicate the need for reinserting the tube.

DRESSINGS,
BINDERS,
BANDAGES, AND
APPLICATION OF HOT
AND COLD THERAPY

Changing a
Dry Dressing

A dry dressing protects wounds with minimal drainage against microorganism contamination. The dressing can simply be a gauze pad that does not adhere to wound tissues and causes very little irritation. Or it can be a Telfa pad that likewise does not adhere to the incision or wound opening but allows drainage through the nonadherent surface to the softened gauze beneath.

As long as an incision or wound remains open, the application of a dry dressing requires sterile technique.

Potential Nursing Diagnoses

Client data derived during assessment reveal defining characteristics to support the following nursing diagnoses in clients requiring this skill:

Skin integrity, impaired
Pain
Infection, high risk for

Equipment

Sterile dressing set or individual supplies of following:
Sterile gloves
Dressing set (scissors and forceps)
Gauze dressings and pads
Basin for antiseptic or cleaning solution
Antiseptic ointment (if ordered)
Cleaning solution prescribed by physician
Sterile normal saline or water
Disposable gloves
Tape, ties, or bandage as needed
Waterproof bag for disposal
Extra gauze dressings and Surgipads or ABD pads.

Bath blanket
Adhesive remover (optional)
Measurement device (optional)

Steps	Rationale
1. Explain procedure to client by describing steps of wound care.	Relieves client anxiety and promotes understanding of healing process.
2. Assemble all necessary supplies at bedside table (do not yet open supplies).	Prevents chances of break in sterile technique by accidental omission of needed supplies.
3. Take disposable bag and make cuff at top. Place bag within reach of your work area.	Prevents accidental contamination of top of outer bag surface. Do not reach across sterile field to dispose of soiled dressing.
4. Close room or cubicle curtains or arrange partition around bed. Close any open windows.	Provides client privacy and reduces air currents that may transmit microorganisms.
5. Assist client to comfortable position and drape him with bath blanket to expose only wound site. Instruct client not to touch wound area or sterile supplies.	Sudden movement by client during dressing change can cause contamination of wound or supplies. Draping provides access to wound and minimizes unnecessary exposure.
6. Wash hands thoroughly.	Removes microorganisms resident on skin surface and reduces transmission of pathogens to exposed tissues.
7. Don clean disposable gloves and remove tape, ties, or bandage.	Gloves prevent transmission of infectious organisms from soiled dressings to your hands.
8. Remove tape by loosening end and pulling gently, parallel to skin and toward dressing. (If adhesive remains on skin, it may be removed with acetone.)	Reduces tension against suture line or wound edges.

Steps	Rationale
9. With your gloved hand or forceps, lift dressings off, keeping soiled undersurface away from client's sight. NOTE: If drains are present, remove only one dressing at a time.	Appearance of drainage may upset client emotionally. Cautious removal of dressings prevents accidental withdrawal of drain.
10. If dressing sticks to wound, loosen it by applying sterile saline or water.	Prevents disruption of epidermal surface.
11. Observe character and amount of drainage on dressings.	Provides estimate of drainage lost and assessment of wound's condition.
12. Dispose of soiled dressings in trash bag, avoiding contamination of bag's outer surface. Remove disposable gloves by pulling them inside out. Dispose of them properly.	Procedures reduce transmission of microorganisms to other persons.
13. Open sterile dressing tray or individually wrapped sterile supplies. Place on bedside table or at client's side on bed. Dressings, scissors, and forceps should remain in sterile tray or can be placed on open sterile drape used as a sterile field. Open bottle or packet of antiseptic solution and pour it into sterile basin or over sterile gauze (Fig. 124).	Sterile dressings and supplies remain sterile while on or within a sterile surface. Preparation of all supplies prevents break in technique during actual dressing change.

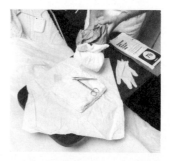

Fig. 124

Steps	Rationale
14. If sterile drape or gauze packages become wet from antiseptic solution, repeat preparation of supplies.	Fluids move through material by capillary action. Microorganisms travel from unsterile environment on table top or bed linen through dressing package to dressing itself.
15. Don sterile gloves (Fig. 125).	Allows you to handle sterile dressings, instruments, and solutions without contaminating them.

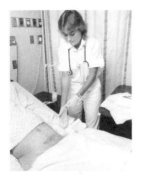

Fig. 125

Steps	Rationale
16. Inspect wound. Note its condition, placement of drain, integrity of suture or skin closure, and character of drainage. (Palpate wound, if necessary, with portion of nondominant hand that will not touch sterile supplies; Fig. 126).	Determines state of wound healing. (Contact with skin surface or drainage contaminates glove.)

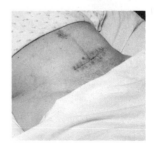

Fig. 126

Steps	Rationale
17. Clean wound with prescribed antiseptic solution or normal saline. Grasp gauze moistened in solution with forceps. Use separate gauze for each cleaning stroke. Clean from least contaminated to most contaminated area. Move in progressive strokes away from incision or wound edges.	Use of forceps prevents contamination of gloved fingers. Direction of cleaning strokes prevents introduction of organisms into wound.
18. Use fresh gauze to dry wound or incision line. Swab in same manner as described in Step 17.	Reduces moisture at wound site, which eventually could harbor microorganisms.
19. Apply antiseptic ointment (if ordered), using same technique as for cleaning. Do not apply over drainage site.	Application directly to dressing or drainage site can occlude drainage.
20. Apply dry sterile dressings to incision or wound site. ■ Apply dressings one at a time (Fig. 127).	Prevents application of large bulky dressings that may impair client's movement, and ensures proper coverage of entire wound.

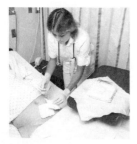

Fig. 127

Steps	Rationale
■ Apply loose woven gauze (4 × 4) or Telfa as contact layer.	Promotes proper absorption of drainage.
■ If a drain is present, take scissors and cut 4 × 4 gauze square to fit around it.	Dressing around drain secures its placement and absorbs drainage.
■ Apply second layer of gauze as an absorbent layer.	Protects wound from entrance of microorganisms.
■ Apply thicker woven Surgipad or ABD pad. (Blue line down middle of pad marks outside surface.) (Fig. 128).	

Fig. 128

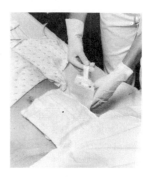

21. Use tape over dressing or secure with Montgomery ties, bandage, or binder (Fig. 129).	Provides support to wound and ensures complete coverage with minimized exposure to microorganisms.

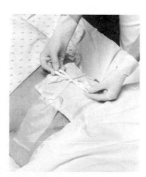

Fig. 129

Steps	Rationale
22. Remove gloves and dispose of them properly in container.	Reduces transmission of microorganisms.
23. Dispose of all supplies and help client return to comfortable position.	Clean environment enhances client comfort.
24. Wash hands.	Reduces microorganism transmission.
25. Record in nurse's notes observations of wound, dressing, and drainage. Document dressing change, including statement of client's response.	Accurate timely documentation notifies personnel of any changes in wound condition and status of client.

Nurse Alert

When removing or positioning the dressing, take care not to dislodge or pull on a drain. If the wound is dry and intact, healing may be optimized by exposing it to air. Contact the physician for an order to discontinue wound dressing.

Protective eyewear should be worn when there is a risk of ocular contamination, such as splash from wound.

Client Teaching

Clients often go home with a simple dry dressing in place. They, or their family, must be instructed in handwashing techniques, wound cleaning, and proper disposal of soiled dressings. It is not necessary to use sterile technique.

Pediatric Considerations

When a dressing is absolutely necessary in an infant or young child, the nurse should incorporate diversional activities into her care plan so the chances of the child's displacing the dressing will be minimized.

Geriatric Considerations

An elderly client's skin is normally inelastic and thin. Use special care, therefore, when removing tape.

Changing a

Wet-to-Dry

Dressing

A wet-to-dry dressing is the treatment of choice for wounds requiring debridement. The wet portion of the dressing effectively cleans an infected and necrotic wound. The moist gauze directly absorbs all exudate and wound debris. The dry outer layer helps pull moisture from the wound into the dressing by capillary action.

Potential Nursing Diagnoses

Client data derived during the assessment reveal defining characteristics to support the following nursing diagnoses in clients requiring this skill:

    Infection, high risk for
    Skin integrity, impaired
    Pain
    Self-esteem disturbance related to wound drainage

Equipment

A sterile dressing set or individual supplies of following:
    Sterile gloves
    Sterile scissors and forceps
    Sterile drape (optional)
    Gauze dressings and fine-mesh 4 × 4 gauze pads
    Basin for antiseptic or cleaning solution
    Antiseptic ointment (optional)
Cleaning solution prescribed by physician
Normal saline or water
Disposable gloves

Tape, ties, or bandage as needed
Waterproof bag for disposal
Extra gauze dressings and Surgipads or ABD pads
Bath blanket
Acetone (optional)
Waterproof pad

Steps	Rationale
1. Explain procedure to client by describing steps of wound care.	Relieves client's anxiety and promotes understanding of healing process.
2. Assemble all necessary supplies at bedside table (do not yet open supplies).	Prevents chances of break in sterile technique by accidental omission of a needed supply.
3. Take disposable bag and make cuff at top. Place bag within reach of your work area.	Cuff prevents accidental contamination of top of outer bag surface. You should not reach across sterile field to dispose of soiled dressing.
4. Close room or cubicle curtains or arrange partition around bed. Close any open windows.	Provides client privacy and reduces air currents that may transmit microorganisms.
5. Assist client to comfortable position and drape him with bath blanket to expose only wound site. Instruct client not to touch wound area or sterile supplies.	Sudden movement by client during dressing change can cause contamination of wound or supplies. Draping provides access to wound and minimizes unnecessary exposure.
6. Wash hands thoroughly.	Removes microorganisms resident on skin surface and reduces transmission of pathogens to exposed tissues.
7. Place waterproof pad under client.	Prevents soiling of bed linen.
8. Don clean disposable gloves and remove tape, ties, or bandage.	Gloves prevent transmission of infectious organisms from soiled dressings to your hands.

Steps	Rationale
9. Remove tape by loosening end and pulling gently, parallel to skin and toward dressing. (If adhesive remains on skin, it may be removed with acetone.)	Reduces tension against suture line or wound edges.
10. With gloved hand or forceps, lift dressings off, keeping soiled undersurface away from client's sight. NOTE: If drains are present, remove only a layer at a time.	Appearance of drainage may upset client emotionally. Cautious removal of dressings prevents accidental withdrawal of drain.
11. If dressing adheres to underlying tissues, do not moisten it. Gently free the dressing from dried exudate. Warn client about pulling and possible discomfort.	Wet-to-dry dressing is designed to clean contaminated or infected wounds by debridement of necrotic tissue and exudate.
12. Observe character and amount of drainage on dressing.	Provides estimate of drainage lost and assessment of wound condition.
13. Dispose of soiled dressings in appropriate container, avoiding contamination of outer surface of container. Remove disposable gloves by pulling them inside out. Dispose of them properly.	Reduces transmission of microorganisms to other persons.
14. Prepare sterile dressing supplies. Pour the prescribed solution into a sterile basin and add fine-mesh gauze.	Contact layer of gauze must be totally moistened to increase dressing's absorptive abilities.
15. Don sterile gloves.	Allows you to handle sterile dressings, instruments, and solutions without contaminating them with microorganisms.

Steps	Rationale
16. Inspect wound. Note its condition, placement of drain, integrity of sutures or skin closure, and character of drainage. (Palpate wound, if necessary, with portion of your nondominant hand that will not be touching sterile supplies.)	Determines state of wound healing. (Contact with skin surface or drainage contaminates glove.)
17. Clean wound with prescribed antiseptic solution or normal saline. Grasp gauze moistened in solution with forceps. Use separate gauze square for each cleaning stroke. Clean from least contaminated to most contaminated area. Move in progressive strokes away from incision line or wound edges.	Use of forceps prevents contamination of your gloved fingers. Direction of cleaning prevents introduction of organisms into wound.
18. Apply moist fine-mesh gauze directly on wound surface. If wound is deep, gently pack it by first picking up end of gauze with forceps. Gradually feed gauze into wound so all surfaces of wound are in contact with moist gauze (Figs. 130 and 131).	Moist gauze absorbs drainage and adheres to debris. Pack gauze so it is evenly distributed within wound bed.
19. Apply dry sterile gauze (4 × 4) over wet gauze.	Dry layer serves as absorbent layer to pull moisture from wound surface.
20. Cover with gauze, Surgipad, or ABD pad.	Gauze or pad protects wound from entrance of microorganisms.

Dressings, Binders, and Bandages

Steps   Rationale

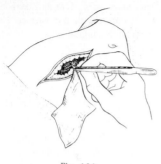
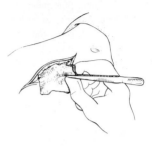

Fig. 130   Fig. 131

21. Apply tape over dressing or   Provides support to wound and
    secure with Montgomery   ensures complete coverage of
    ties, bandage, or binder.   wound to minimize exposure to
                                       microorganisms.

22. Assist client to comfortable   Enhances client's sense of well-
    position.   being.

23. Wash hands.   Reduces transmission of micro-
                                       organisms.

24. Record in nurse's notes   Accurate and timely documenta-
    observations of wound,   tion notifies personnel of any
    dressing, drainage, and cli-   changes in wound condition and
    ent's response.   status of client.

Nurse Alert

Removal of the old dressing and reapplication of a new wet-to-
dry dressing may cause the client pain. The nurse should administer an analgesic and time the dressing change to coincide with
the drug's peak effect.

Protective eyewear should be worn when there is a risk for
ocular contamination, such as splash from wound.

Client Teaching

A client is not usually discharged home while a wet-to-dry dressing is still required. He can be taught wound care in anticipation of use of a dry dressing at home.

Pediatric Considerations

It may be necessary to reinforce a wet-to-dry dressing with a gauze roll to prevent its accidental removal by an active toddler. Whenever possible, reinforce the dressing rather than restrain the child.

Geriatric Considerations

An elderly client's skin is normally thin and inelastic. Use special care, therefore, when removing tape.

Wound Irrigation

The purpose of wound irrigation is to remove exudate and debris from slow-healing wounds. It requires sterile technique and is particularly useful for open deep wounds, when access to all wound surfaces is limited. Wound irrigation can deliver heat to an affected area to promote healing or facilitate the application of local medications.

Potential Nursing Diagnoses

Client data derived during the assessment reveal defining characteristics to support the following nursing diagnoses in clients requiring this skill:

Skin integrity, impaired
Infection, high risk for
Pain

Equipment

Sterile basin
Irrigating solution (200 to 500 ml as ordered) warmed to body temperature (32° to 37° C or 90° to 98.6° F)
Sterile irrigating syringe (sterile red rubber catheter as an attachment for deep wounds with small openings)
Clean basin to receive solution
Sterile dressing tray and supplies for dressing change
Waterproof pad
Lubricating jelly and tongue blade (optional)

Steps	Rationale
1. Explain procedure to client. Describe sensations to be felt during irrigation.	Client's anxiety will be reduced through awareness of what procedure involves and sensations to be expected.
2. Assemble supplies at bedside.	Prevents break in procedure.
3. Position client so irrigating solution will flow from upper end of wound into basin held below wound (Fig. 132).	Fluid flows by gravity from least to most contaminated area.

Fig. 132

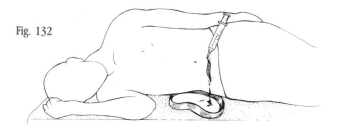

4. Place waterproof pad under client.	Prevents soiling of bed linen.
5. Wash hands.	Reduces microorganism transmission.
6. Don clean disposable gloves and remove tape, ties, or bandage.	Gloves prevent transmission of infectious organisms from soiled dressings to your hands.
7. Remove tape by loosening end and pulling gently, parallel with skin and toward dressing. (If adhesive remains on the skin, it may be removed with acetone.)	Reduces tension against suture line or wound edges.

Steps	Rationale
8. With your gloved hand or forceps, lift dressings off, keeping soiled undersurface away from client's sight. Remove one dressing layer at a time.	Appearance of drainage may upset client emotionally. Cautious removal of dressings prevents accidental withdrawal of drain.
9. If dressing sticks to wound, loosen it by applying sterile saline or water.	Prevents disruption of epidermal surface.
10. Observe character and amount of drainage on dressings.	Provides estimate of drainage lost and assessment of wound's condition.
11. Dispose of soiled dressings in proper receptacle, avoiding contamination of receptacle's outer surface. Remove disposable gloves by pulling them inside out. Dispose of them properly.	Reduces transmission of microorganisms to other persons.
12. Prepare sterile supplies. Open basin and pour in solution (volume varies depending on size of wound and extent of drainage). Open syringe. Prepare dressing tray. Don sterile gloves.	Prevents introduction of microorganisms into wound.
13. Place clean basin against client's skin below incision or wound site.	Collects contaminated irrigating solution.
14. Draw up some solution into syringe. While holding syringe tip just above top of wound, irrigate slowly but continuously with enough force to flush away drainage and debris. Avoid sudden spurts or splashing of fluid. Irrigate pockets in wound.	Irrigation mechanically removes drainage and debris. Pockets or depressions in wound bed can easily trap debris.

Steps	Rationale
15. Continue irrigating until solution draining into basin is clear.	Ensures that all debris has been removed.
16. With sterile gauze, dry off wound edges. Clean from least contaminated to most contaminated area. Move in progressive strokes away from incision line or wound edges.	Removes excess moisture, which can serve as medium for microorganism growth or as irritant to skin.
17. Apply sterile dressing.	Sterile dressing prevents infection and promotes wound healing.
18. Assist client to comfortable position.	Promotes client comfort.
19. Dispose of equipment and wash hands.	Controls transfer of microorganisms.
20. Record in nurse's notes volume and type of solution, character of drainage, appearance of wound, and client's response.	Timely recording provides accurate documentation of therapy and progress of wound healing.

Nurse Alert

If drains are present, remove only one layer of dressing at a time so accidental withdrawal of a drain does not occur. Do not forcibly introduce irrigant into a wound pocket that is not visible. You could damage tissue.

Protective eyewear should be worn when there is a risk for ocular contamination, such as a splash from a wound.

Client Teaching

The client is not usually discharged home when irrigations are still necessary. However, instruct him regarding the procedure for wound irrigations so he can monitor the progress of his healing. In addition, early instruction helps him and his family prepare for discharge and any necessary home care.

Pediatric Considerations

If a child is unable to remain still during the procedure, it may be helpful for another nurse or the parent to use diversional activities such as reading, singing, or storytelling. Cautious use of restraints may be necessary.

Ear Irrigation

Irrigation of the auditory canal is performed to remove cerumen or a foreign object or to apply heat. The irrigating solution should be sterile to prevent transmission of microorganisms in the event of tympanic membrane rupture. The solution must be at room temperature so it does not cause nausea or vertigo (severe dizziness). At home the client or family can be instructed in proper cleaning of the ear to reduce the need for further irrigation.

Potential Nursing Diagnoses

Client data derived during the assessment reveal defining characteristics to support the following nursing diagnoses in clients requiring this skill:

Injury, high risk for

Sensory/perceptual alteration: auditory

Pain

Equipment

Prescribed irrigating solution; volume depends on purpose: 200 to 500 ml at 37° C (98.6° F)

Sterile basin for solution

Soft or small bulb syringe

Curved emesis basin

Moisture-proof towel or pad

Cotton-tip applicators

Bath thermometer

Cotton balls

Steps	Rationale
1. Wash hands.	Reduces transmission of micro-organisms.
2. Explain steps of procedure and warn client about sensations that might be experienced.	Relieves client's anxiety.
3. Assist client to either a side-lying or a sitting position with head tilted toward affected ear. Position emesis basin under ear. (Client may help hold basin.)	Irrigating solution will flow from auditory canal into basin.
4. Place towel over client's shoulder just under ear and emesis basin.	Prevents soiling of gown and bed linen.
5. Inspect auditory canal for any accumulation of cerumen or debris. Remove with cotton applicator and solution.	Prevents reentry of debris into canal during irrigation.
6. Check irrigating solution for proper temperature. Fill bulb syringe with appropriate volume.	Solution at body temperature minimizes onset of dizziness and discomfort.
7. Straighten auditory canal for introduction of solution. In infants, pull auricle (or pinna) down and back. In adults, pull auricle up and back.	Facilitates entrance and flow of irrigating solution.
8. With tip of syringe just above canal, irrigate gently by creating steady flow of solution against roof of canal.	Occlusion of canal with syringe causes pressure against tympanic membrane during irrigation. Solution drains safely out of canal while loosening debris.
9. Continue irrigation until all debris has been removed or all solution has been used.	Purpose of irrigation may be to clean canal, instill antiseptics, or provide local heat.

Steps	Rationale
10. Assess client for onset of dizziness or nausea. Onset of symptoms may require temporary cessation of procedure.	Irritation of semicircular canals may cause dizziness and nausea.
11. Dry off auricle and apply cotton ball to auditory meatus.	Drying promotes client's comfort. Cotton ball collects excess drainage.
12. Position client on side of affected ear for 10 minutes.	Remaining solution in auditory canal will drain out.
13. Remove equipment and wash hands.	Controls transfer of microorganisms.
14. Return to client to assess character and amount of drainage and determine his level of comfort.	Enables you to evaluate client's tolerance of procedure.
15. Record in nurse's notes client's response to irrigation and note type, temperature, and volume of solution used and character of drainage.	Timely recording provides accurate documentation of client's response to procedure.
16. Return to client after 10 minutes to remove cotton ball and reassess drainage. Client may resume normal level of activity.	Increase in drainage or onset of pain may indicate injury to tympanic membrane.

Nurse Alert

Although the external auditory canal is not sterile, you should use sterile drops and solutions in case the tympanic membrane (eardrum) is ruptured. Entrance of nonsterile solutions into the middle ear could result in infection. Never occlude the external auditory canal with the syringe. Forceful delivery of solution can damage the tympanic membrane.

Client Teaching

Family members as well as the client should be instructed not to
force medication into an occluded auditory canal. Instilling medication or solution under pressure can injure the eardrum.

Pediatric Considerations

The auditory canal of infants and young children is straightened
by grasping the pinna and pulling it gently downward and backward. Failure to straighten the canal properly may prevent medic-
inal solutions from reaching the deeper external ear structures.

Geriatric Considerations

The skin lining the auditory canal of an elderly person often becomes dry, flaky, and irritated. It is thus very important to be
gentle when performing irrigations or cleanings of the ear in
older clients.

Eye Irrigation

Eye irrigation is performed to relieve local inflammation of the conjunctiva, apply antiseptic solution, or flush out exudate or caustic or irritating solutions. It is a procedure commonly used in emergency situations when a foreign object or some other substance has entered the eye.

Potential Nursing Diagnoses

Client data derived during the assessment reveal defining characteristics to support the following nursing diagnoses in clients requiring this skill:

Sensory/perceptual alteration: visual

Pain

Anxiety

Equipment

Prescribed irrigating solution; volume varies: 30 to 180 ml at 37° C (98.6° F) (For chemical flushing: tap water in volume to provide continuous irrigation over 15 minutes.)

Sterile basin for solution

Curved emesis basin

Waterproof pad or towel

Cotton balls

Soft bulb syringe or eye dropper

Disposable gloves (optional)

Steps	Rationale
1. Explain procedure fully to client. Explain that he will be allowed to close eye periodically and that no object will touch eye.	Relieves client's anxiety and improves his ability to cooperate.
2. Assist client to lying position on side of affected eye. Turn his head toward affected eye.	Irrigating solution will flow from inner to outer canthus and into collecting basin.
3. Wash your hands.	Reduces number of microorganisms on skin surface.
4. Don disposable gloves (if client's eye is infected).	Prevents exposure of your hands to pathogens.
5. Place waterproof pad under client's face.	Prevents soiling of bed linen.
6. With cotton ball moistened in prescribed solution (or normal saline), gently clean lid margins and eyelashes. Clean from inner to outer canthus.	Minimizes transfer of debris from lids or lashes into eye during irrigation. Cleaning motion prevents entrance of drainage into nasolacrimal duct.
7. Place curved emesis basin just below client's cheek on side of affected eye.	Basin collects irrigating solution.
8. Fill irrigating syringe or eye dropper. Gently retract lower and upper eyelids (conjunctival sacs) by applying pressure to lower bony orbit and bony prominence beneath eyebrow. Do not apply pressure over eye.	Retraction minimizes blinking and exposes upper and lower conjunctival membranes for irrigation. Pressure on internal eye structures could cause permanent injury.
9. Hold irrigating syringe or dropper approximately 2.5 cm (1 inch) above inner canthus.	If dropper or syringe touches eye, there is risk of injury. Dropper or syringe becomes contaminated.

Steps	Rationale
10. Ask client to look up. Gently irrigate by directing solution into lower conjunctival sac toward outer canthus. Use only enough force to remove secretions gently.	Flushing of conjunctival sac prevents exposure of sensitive cornea to solution. Fluid flows away from nasolacrimal duct, minimizing absorption of contaminated solution.
11. Allow client to close his eye periodically, particularly if burning or excess blinking occurs. Encourage his cooperation.	Lid closure moves secretions from upper to lower conjunctival sac. Also promotes client's ability to relax during procedure.
12. Continue irrigation until all solution is used or secretions have been cleaned. (Remember: a 15-minute irrigation is needed to flush chemicals.)	Serves to clean exudate, relieve inflammation, or flush caustic solution.
13. Dry eyelids and facial area with sterile cotton ball. Client may resume normal position.	Removes excess solution and provides for client's comfort.
14. Remove equipment and wash hands.	Reduces transfer of microorganisms.
15. Record in nurse's notes client's response to irrigation (burning, itching, pain) as well as volume and type of solution used, character of drainage, and appearance of conjunctiva.	Timely recording provides accurate documentation of client's response to procedure.

Nurse Alert

Be sure that a client's contact lenses are removed before beginning any irrigation. When caustic chemicals enter the eye, it is necessary to flush the eye continuously for at least 15 minutes. Continuous flushing prevents burning of the sensitive cornea. Do not apply pressure directly on the eye during irrigation. This could injure the eye.

Client Teaching

Clients can be taught to administer eye irrigations at home. However, they may need to use an eye cup, which should be practiced before it is attempted alone.

Pediatric Considerations

Young children are at risk of getting objects in their eyes accidentally during the normal course of play. The parent should act quickly because a child's natural response is to begin rubbing his eye. It may be necessary to restrain a young child so the eye can be properly and thoroughly irrigated. The easiest technique is to have the child stand over a sink as the parent flushes the eye with tap water.

Geriatric Considerations

An elderly client may have reduced coordination of the hand or fingers and require assistance from an available family member or friend in administering the irrigation. If a client lives alone, he should try to perform the irrigation himself. Any delay could result in burns to the cornea.

Applying Binders

Abdominal, perineal T, and breast binders

Binders provide support to large incisions. These incisions are vulnerable to tension or stress as the client moves or coughs. An abdominal binder is a rectangular piece of cotton or elasticized material that has long extensions on each side to surround the abdomen (Fig. 133).

Perineal binders are designed for both male and female clients (Fig. 134). The male binder (also called a double T-binder) has two tails, which secure perineal or rectal dressings. The female binder (also called a T-binder) has one tail, which secures perineal or rectal dressings.

A properly secured binder provides support and comfort so the client can resume normal activities.

Potential Nursing Diagnoses

Client data derived during assessment reveal defining characteristics to support the following nursing diagnoses in clients requiring this skill:

Pain
Skin integrity, impaired
Mobility, impaired physical

Equipment

Binder: abdominal or perineal
Clean gloves

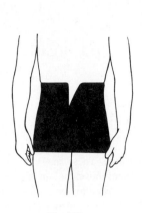

Fig. 133

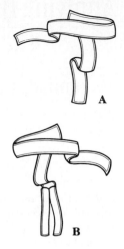

Fig. 134

Steps	Rationale
1. Wash hands and don gloves.	Reduces transmission of micro-organisms.
2. Explain to client that binder serves to support abdominal incision and provides comfort.	Reduces client's anxiety.
3. Instruct client to roll onto one side while supporting abdominal incision and dressing firmly with hands.	Reduces pain.

4. Apply binder.
  a. Abdominal
    ■ Place binder (fan folded) under client in same manner as when applying sheet for an occupied bed.
	Allows client to roll over binder to ease positioning and centering.

Steps	Rationale
■ Have client roll to opposite side. Unfold binder beneath him.	
■ Position client supine over center of binder. Bottom edge of binder should be just above symphysis pubis, and top edge below costal margins.	Ensures that adequate pressure will be applied over wound. Also prevents interference with chest expansion.
■ Close the binder: *Straight*: Pull left end of binder toward center of client's abdomen. While keeping tension on left end, pull right end over left. Secure by smoothing Velcro edges together.	Firm, even application provides optimal wound support and comfort.
b. Perineal	
■ Provide perineal hygiene.	Ensures application of binder to clean skin.
■ Apply new perineal or rectal dressings according to physician's order.	Dressings to the perineal or rectal areas require frequent dressing changes, which assist in reducing the number of bacteria near the wound site.
■ Secure binder *Female:* Secure waist band. Bring vertical strip over perineal dressing and continue up and under center front, until vertical band can be secured to the waist band with safety pins.	Provides support to perineal muscles and organs.

Steps	Rationale
Male: Secure waist band. Bring remaining vertical strips over dressing with each tail supporting one side of scrotum and proceeding upward on either side of penis. Continue until vertical tails can be secured to the waist band with safety pins.	

c. Breast

Steps	Rationale
■ Assist client in placing arms through binder's armholes.	
■ Assist client to supine position in bed.	Supine positioning facilitates normal anatomic alignment of breasts, facilitates healing, and comfort.
■ Pad area under breasts if necessary.	Reduces risk of skin irritation and breakdown.
■ Using Velcro closure tabs or horizontally placed safety pins secure binder at nipple level first. Continue closure process above and then below nipple line until entire binder is closed.	Horizontal placement of pins may reduce risk of uneven pressure or localized irritation.
■ Make appropriate adjustments, including individualizing fit of shoulder straps and pinning waistline darts to reduce binder size.	Maintains better support of client's breasts.
5. Assess client's comfort and ability to deep breathe and cough. Readjust as necessary.	Binders should exert pressure over abdomen but should not impair chest expansion. Perineal binders support perineal structures.

Steps	Rationale
6. Wash hands.	Reduces transmission of micro-organisms.
7. Record in nurse's notes application and client's tolerance.	Prompt documentation improves accuracy of record.

Nurse Alert

An abdominal binder should apply support to the abdominal structures but should never be so tight as to cause pain or impede deep breathing or coughing.

Client Teaching

Explanation of the procedure promotes client cooperation. In addition, teaching the client about why the binder is necessary can improve his mobility and his deep breathing and coughing.

Geriatric Considerations

As a result of the aging process, an elderly person normally has reduced chest expansion and a diminished vital capacity. A binder should not restrict his ability to ventilate fully.

Applying Hot
Compresses

A hot moist compress is effective for improving circulation, relieving edema, and promoting the consolidation and drainage of pus. Because the compress is applied to an open wound, it must be sterile.

Potential Nursing Diagnoses

Client data derived during the assessment reveal defining characteristics to support the following nursing diagnoses in clients requiring this skill:

Infection, high risk for
Pain
Mobility, impaired physical

Equipment

Prescribed solution warmed to proper temperature (approximately 43° to 46° C [110° to 115° F])
Sterile gauze dressings
Sterile container for solution
Commercially prepared compresses (optional)
Sterile gloves
Petrolatum jelly
Sterile cotton swabs
Waterproof pad
Tape or ties
Dry bath towel
Water-flow or heating pad (optional)
Disposable gloves
Bath thermometer

Steps	Rationale
1. Explain procedure to client, including sensations that will be felt (e.g., feeling of warmth and wetness). Explain precautions to prevent burning.	Improves client cooperation and lessens anxiety.
2. Assist client to comfortable position in proper body alignment.	Compress will remain in place for several minutes. Limited mobility in uncomfortable position can cause muscular stress.
3. Place waterproof pad under area to be treated.	Prevents soiling of bed linen.
4. Expose body part to be covered with compress. Drape rest of body with bath blanket.	Prevents unnecessary cooling and exposure of body part.
5. Wash hands.	Reduces transmission of infection.
6. Assemble equipment. Pour warmed solution in sterile container. (If using a portable heating source, keep solution warm. Commercially prepared compresses may remain under infrared lamp until just before use.) Open sterile packages and drop gauze into container to become immersed in solution. Turn electrical heating pad to correct temperature.	Compresses must retain warmth for therapeutic benefit.
7. Don disposable gloves. Remove any dressings covering wound. Dispose of gloves and dressings in proper receptacle.	Proper disposal prevents spread of microorganisms.

Steps	Rationale
8. Assess condition of wound and surrounding skin.	Provides baseline for determining skin changes after compress application.
9. Don sterile gloves.	Sterile touching sterile remains sterile.
10. Apply petrolatum jelly with a cotton swab to skin surrounding wound. Do not place jelly on areas of broken skin.	Protects skin from possible burns and maceration (softening).
11. Pick up one layer of immersed gauze and wring out any excess water.	Excess moisture macerates skin and increases risk of burns and infection.
12. Apply gauze lightly to open wound. Watch client's response and ask if he feels discomfort. In a few seconds, lift edge of gauze to assess skin for redness.	Skin is most sensitive to sudden change in temperature. Redness indicates a burn.
13. If client tolerates hot compress, pack gauze snugly against wound. Be sure that all wound surfaces are covered.	Packing of compress prevents rapid cooling from underlying air currents.
14. Wrap moist compress with dry bath towel. If necessary, pin or tie in place.	Insulates compress to prevent heat loss.
15. Change the hot compress every 5 minutes.	Prevents cooling, thus maintaining therapeutic benefit of compress.
16. (Optional) Apply waterflow or waterproof heating pad over towel. Keep it in place for desired duration of application (usually 20 to 30 minutes).	Provides constant temperature to compress.

Steps	Rationale
17. Ask client periodically if there is any discomfort or burning sensation.	Continued exposure to heat can cause burning of skin.
18. Remove pad, towel, and compress. Assess wound and condition of surrounding skin.	Continued exposure to moisture will macerate skin.
19. Replace sterile dressing.	Prevents entrance of microorganisms into wound site.
20. Dispose of equipment and wash hands.	
21. Record in nurse's notes type of application, solution, temperature of solution, duration of application, and condition of skin before and after procedure.	Accurate documentation protects you legally and provides information on the treatment.

Nurse Alert

The nurse must use caution to avoid burning the client's skin. Because moisture conducts heat, the temperature setting on any device applied to a moist compress need not be as high as if the device is used for a dry application.

Client Teaching

Clients may frequently use compresses or heating devices in the home. Instruct them on ways to avoid burns: always time applications carefully to avoid overexposure; do not adjust the temperature of a heating pad to a high setting; do not lie directly on a heating device but instead wrap it in a towel and apply it onto the skin.

Pediatric Considerations

When applying a hot moist compress to a child, determine the need to restrain him so he does not contaminate the wound. If possible, you may use this time to cuddle and read to the child so as not to dislodge the compress.

Geriatric Considerations

Elderly persons frequently suffer a loss of or reduction in temperature sensation because of aging or chronic disease. Therefore, watch the client's skin condition carefully during heat application.

Using Hypothermia/ Hyperthermia Blankets

Clients can have high, prolonged fevers from infectious neurologic diseases and side effects from anesthesia. One such measure for fever control is a hypothermia (cooling) blanket. Hypothermia blankets are fluid-filled rubberized blankets that circulate cooled solution (usually distilled water) through the blanket. When the client lies on the device, the cooling blanket helps to reduce the client's body temperature.

Conversely, a client whose body temperature is abnormally low because of extreme exposure to cold or as a result of hypothermia from neurologic or cardiac surgery requires a hyperthermia (warming) blanket to assist the body to return to near-normal temperature. In the case of hyperthermia, or rewarming, therapy a warmed solution is circulated through the blanket to help return the client's body temperature to normal.

Potential Nursing Diagnoses

Client data derived during the assessment reveal defining characteristics to support the following nursing diagnoses in clients requiring this skill:

Hyperthermia
Hypothermia

Equipment

Hypothermia/hyperthermia blanket with control panel and rectal probe
Sheet or thin bath blanket
Distilled water to fill the units if necessary
Gloves
Rectal thermometer

Steps	Rationale
1. Obtain client's vital signs, neurologic/mental status, and peripheral circulation.	Established baseline data to use for comparison during the therapy.
2. Verify that client's body temperature cannot be returned to normal by other less intensive measures.	Hypothermia/hyperthermia blankets are not without risk and should only be used when other measures are not effective.
3. Assess client's skin: ears, hands, fingers, heels, sacrum, and other bony prominences before therapy.	These areas are more exposed to the hypothermia/hyperthermia blanket and consequently are at greater risk for injury. Baseline data enable the nurse to quickly determine if injury to the skin is a result of the therapy.
4. Verify physician's order and double check that client's current body temperature requires a hypothermia/hyperthermia blanket.	Institution of therapy requires a physician's order.
5. Explain procedure to client.	Increases cooperation and reduces anxiety.
6. Prepare client: a. Prepare the blanket according to agency policy and manufacturer's instructions.	Agencies have specific policies as to who should maintain the equipment in functioning order. Each type of blanket varies from one manufacturer to another. Manufacturer's instructions are located on the machine. Read before using.
7. Wash hands and don gloves.	Reduces transmission of microorganisms.
8. Place the blanket on the client's mattress and precool or prewarm the blanket. Set the pad temperature to the desired level.	Prepares the blanket for the prescribed therapy.

Steps	Rationale
9. Observe that the cool/warm light is on.	Verifies that the blanket is correctly set to assist in reducing (cool) or increasing (warm) the client's body temperature.
10. Verify that the pad temperature limits are set at the desired safety ranges.	Safety ranges prevent excessive cooling/warming. The blanket automatically shuts off when the preset body temperature is achieved.
11. Place sheet or thin bath blanket over the blanket.	Protects the client's skin from direct contact with blanket, and in so doing reduces the risk of injury to the skin.
12. Lubricate rectal probe and insert into client's rectum.	When using hypothermia/hyperthermia blankets it is imperative that the nurse have continuous access to the client's core internal (rectal) temperature.
13. Place client on the blanket. Hypothermia: wrap client's hands and feet in towels.	Reduces the risk of frostbite to the body's distal areas.
14. Properly position client on blanket so that client's body surface is directly on the blanket, while at the same time ensuring that the client is protected from pressure ulcer development or impaired body alignment.	Client has an increased risk of pressure ulcer development because of the skin moisture created by the blanket and client's body temperature.
15. Double-check the fluid thermometer on the control panel of the blanket.	Verifies that pad temperature is maintained at desired level.
16. Remove gloves and wash hands.	Reduces transmission of microorganisms.

Steps	Rationale
17. Monitor the client's temperature and vital signs every 15 minutes during the first hour, every 30 minutes during the second hour, and every hour of therapy thereafter.	Provides continuous evaluation of response of client's body temperature to therapy during initial and continual therapy.
18. Assess the automatic temperature control every 4 hours by taking client's rectal temperature with a glass thermometer.	Verifies accuracy of rectal probe and automatic temperature control device.
19. Determine client's level of comfort.	Therapy has the potential of causing discomfort. Prompt assessment reduces risk for severe injuries.
20. Record baseline data: vital signs, neurologic/mental status, status of peripheral circulation, skin integrity, when therapy was initiated, temperature control setting, and the client's response to therapy.	Documents client's status prior to instituting therapy, care provided, and client's response to therapy.

Nurse Alert

If the client experiences a rapid change in body temperature, the blanket must be turned off, and the therapy may need to be adjusted. Should the client's core temperature remain unchanged, the nurse should check to determine that the system is set up and functioning correctly. Other sites on the client's body, such as the groin, axilla, or neck, may be used to check the temperature. If the client begins to shiver, the hypothermia (cooling) blanket should also be turned off. The physician may order the blanket be warmed a few degrees, and the client's temperature should be monitored carefully.

The material of the hyperthermia/hypothermia blanket itself can cause the client's skin to become moist, thus increasing the risk of skin breakdown.

Teaching Considerations

Clients and their families need to be instructed not to move the client off the blanket.

OXYGENATION

Postural

Drainage

Postural drainage is the gravitational clearance of airway secretions from specific bronchial segments. It is achieved by assuming one or more of 10 different body positions. Each position drains a specific section of the tracheobronchial tree—the upper, middle, or lower lung field—into the trachea. Coughing or suctioning can then remove secretions from the trachea. The figures and list that follow show the bronchial area and the corresponding body posture for its drainage.

Potential Nursing Diagnoses

Client data derived during the assessment reveal defining characteristics to support the following nursing diagnoses in clients requiring this skill:

Airway clearance ineffective
Breathing pattern, ineffective
Gas exchange, impaired
Infection, high risk for

Equipment

Pillows—two to three extra
Slant or tilt board (if drainage to be performed in home)
Facial tissues
Glass of water
Clear jar

Positions for Postural Drainage
Left and Right Upper Lobe Anterior Apical Bronchi

Have client sit in chair, leaning back against pillow (Figs. 135 and 136).

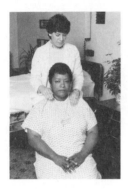

Fig. 135

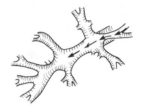

Fig. 136

Left and Right Upper Lobe Posterior Apical Bronchi

Have client sit in chair, leaning forward on pillow or table (Figs. 137 and 138).

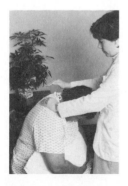

Fig. 137

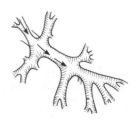

Fig. 138

Right and Left Anterior Upper Lobe Bronchi

Have client lie flat on back with small pillow under knees (Figs. 139 and 140).

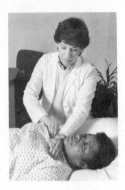

Fig. 139

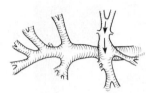

Fig. 140

Left Upper Lobe Lingual Bronchus

Have client lie on right side with arm over head in Trendelenburg position, with foot of bed raised 30 cm (12 inches). Place pillow behind back, and roll client one-fourth turn onto pillow (Figs. 141 and 142).

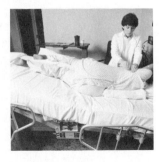

Fig. 141

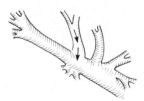

Fig. 142

Right Middle Lobe Bronchus

Have client lie on left side and raise foot of bed 30 cm (12 inches). Place pillow behind back and roll client one fourth turn onto pillow (Figs. 143 and 144).

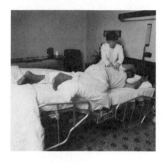

Fig. 143

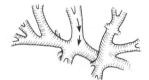

Fig. 144

Left and Right Anterior Lower Lobe Bronchi

Have client lie on back in Trendelenburg position, with foot of bed elevated 45 to 50 cm (18 to 20 inches). Have knees bent on pillow (Figs. 145 and 146).

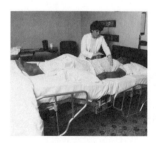

Fig. 145

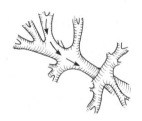

Fig. 146

Right Lower Lobe Lateral Bronchus

Have client lie on left side in Trendelenburg position with foot of
bed raised 45 to 50 cm (18 to 20 inches) (Figs. 147 and 148).

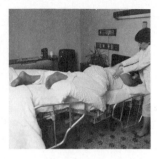

Fig. 147

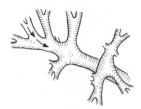

Fig. 148

Left Lower Lobe Lateral Bronchus

Have client lie on right side in Trendelenburg position with foot
of bed raised 45 to 50 cm (18 to 20 inches) (Figs. 149 and 150).

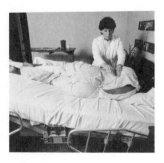

Fig. 149

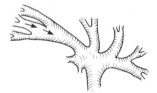

Fig. 150

Right and Left Lower Lobe Superior Bronchi

Have client lie flat on stomach with pillow under stomach (Figs. 151 and 152).

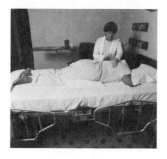

Fig. 151

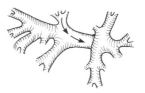

Fig. 152

Left and Right Posterior Basal Bronchi

Have client lie on stomach in Trendelenburg position with foot of bed elevated 45 to 50 cm (18 to 20 inches) (Figs. 153 and 154).

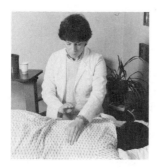

Fig. 153

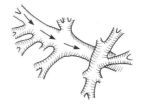

Fig. 154

Steps	Rationale
1. Wash hands.	Reduces transmission of micro-organisms.
2. Select congested areas to be drained based on assessment of all lung fields, clinical data, and chest x-ray views.	To be effective, treatment must be individualized to treat specific areas involved.
3. Place client in position to drain congested areas. (First area selected may vary from client to client.) Help client assume position as needed. Teach client correct posture and arm and leg positioning. Place pillows for support and comfort.	Specific positions are selected to drain each area involved. (See Figs. 135 through 154 for positioning.)
4. Have client maintain posture for 10 to 15 minutes.	In adults, draining each area takes time. In children, 3 to 5 minutes is sufficient.
5. During 10 to 15 minutes of drainage in this posture, perform chest percussion, vibration, and/or rib shaking over area being drained.	Provides mechanical forces that aid in mobilization of airway secretions.
6. After drainage in first posture, have client sit up and cough. Save expectorated secretions in clear container. If client cannot cough, suctioning should be performed.	Any secretions mobilized into central airways should be removed by cough and/or suctioning before client is placed in next drainage position. Coughing is most effective when client is sitting up and leaning forward.
7. Have client rest briefly if necessary.	Short rest periods between postures can prevent fatigue and help client to tolerate therapy better.

Steps	Rationale
8. Have client take sips of water.	Keeping mouth moist aids in expectoration of secretions.
9. Repeat Steps 3 to 8 until all congested areas selected have been drained. Each treatment should not exceed 30 to 60 minutes.	Postural drainage is used only to drain areas involved and is based on individual assessment.
10. Repeat chest assessment of all lung fields.	Allows you to assess need for further drainage or changes in drainage program.
11. Wash your hands.	Reduces transmission of micro-organisms.

Nurse Alert

Bronchospasm can be induced in some clients receiving postural drainage. It is caused by mobilization of secretions into the large central airways, which increases the work of breathing. To counteract the risk of bronchospasm, the nurse may ask the physician to start the client on bronchodilator therapy 20 minutes before postural drainage.

Client Teaching

The client and family should be taught how to assume postures at home. Some postures may need to be modified to meet individual needs. For example, the side-lying Trendelenburg position to drain the lateral lower lobes may have to be done with the client lying flat on his side or in a side-lying semi-Fowler position if he is very short of breath (dyspneic).

Pediatric Considerations

It is unrealistic to expect a child to cooperate fully in assuming all positions used for postural drainage. The nurse should set four to six positions as priority. More than six will frequently exceed the child's limit of tolerance.

Geriatric Considerations

Clients on antihypertensive medication may not be able to tolerate the postural changes required. The nurse must then modify
the procedure to meet the client's tolerance and still clear his airways.

Oropharyngeal and Nasopharyngeal Suctioning

Oropharyngeal or nasopharyngeal suctioning is used when the client is able to cough effectively but is unable to clear secretions by expectorating or swallowing. It is frequently used after the client has coughed. Oropharyngeal and nasopharyngeal suction may also be appropriate in less responsive or comatose clients who require removal of oral secretions.

Potential Nursing Diagnoses

Client data derived during the assessment reveal defining characteristics to support the following nursing diagnoses in client requiring this skill:

Infection, high risk for
Airway clearance, ineffective

Equipment

Portable or wall suction unit with connecting tubing and Y-connector if needed
Sterile catheter (12 or 16 French) (see box)
Sterile water or normal saline
Sterile gloves
Water-soluble lubricant
Drape or towel to protect linen and client's bedclothes
Goggles

Steps	Rationale
1. Prepare equipment at bedside.	Allows smooth performance of procedure without interruption.
2. Wash hands and don goggles.	Reduces transmission of microorganisms.

Suction Catheter of Appropriate Size

Newborn	6-8 Fr
Infant to 6 mo	6-8 Fr
18 mo	8-10 Fr
24 mo	10 Fr
2-4 years	10-12 Fr
4-7 years	12 Fr
7-10 years	12-14 Fr
10-12 years	14 Fr
Adults	12-16 Fr

Steps	Rationale
3. Explain to client how procedure will help clear airway and relieve some of his breathing problems. Explain that coughing, sneezing, or gagging is normal.	
4. Properly position client:	
■ If conscious with a functional gag reflex—Place him in semi-Fowler position with head turned to one side for oral suctioning. Place him in semi-Fowler position with neck hyperextended for nasal suctioning.	Gag reflex helps prevent aspiration of gastrointestinal contents. Positioning head to one side or hyperextending neck promotes smooth insertion of catheter into oropharynx or nasopharynx respectively.
■ If unconscious—Place him in lateral position facing you for oral or nasal suctioning.	Prevents client's tongue from obstructing airway, promotes drainage of pulmonary secretions, and prevents aspiration of gastrointestinal contents.
5. Place towel on pillow or under client's chin.	Soiling of bed linen or bed clothes from secretions is prevented. Towel can be discarded, reducing spread of bacteria.

Steps	Rationale
6. Select proper suction pressure and the type of suction unit. For wall suction units this is 120 to 150 mm Hg in adults, 100 to 120 mm Hg in children, or 60 to 100 mm Hg in infants (see box).	Ensures safe negative pressure according to client's age. Excessive negative pressure can precipitate injury to mucosa.

Vacuum Regulator

Vacuum Settings—Wall	
Infants	60-100 mm Hg
Children	100-120 mm Hg
Adults	120-150 mm Hg

Vacuum Setting—Portable	
Infants	3-5 inches Hg
Children	5-10 inches Hg
Adults	7-15 inches Hg

Steps	Rationale
7. Pour sterile water or saline into sterile container.	Needed to lubricate catheter to decrease friction and promote smooth passage.
8. Put sterile glove on your dominant hand.	Maintains asepsis as catheter is passed into client's mouth or nose.
9. Using your gloved hand, attach catheter to suction machine.	Sterility is maintained.
10. Approximate the distance between client's earlobe and tip of nose and place thumb and forefinger of gloved hand at that point.	This distance ensures that suction catheter will remain in pharyngeal region. Insertion of catheter past this point places catheter in trachea.

Steps	Rationale
11. Moisten catheter tip with sterile solution. Apply suction with tip in solution.	Moistening catheter tip reduces friction and eases insertion. Applying suction while catheter is in sterile solution ensures that suction equipment is functioning before catheter is inserted.
12. Suction ■ Oropharyngeal—Gently insert catheter into one side of client's mouth and guide it to oropharynx. Do not apply suction during insertion.	Stimulation of gag reflex is reduced.
■ Nasopharyngeal—Gently insert catheter into one naris. Guide it medially along floor of nasal cavity. Do not force catheter. If one naris is not patent, try other. Do not apply suction during insertion.	Catheter avoids nasal turbinates and enters more easily into nasopharynx. Risk of trauma to oral and nasal mucosa during catheter insertion is reduced.
13. Occlude suction port with your thumb. Gently rotate catheter as you withdraw it. Entire procedure should not take longer than 15 seconds.	Occlusion of suction port activates suction pressure. Suctioning is intermittently done as catheter is withdrawn. Rotation removes secretions from all surfaces of airway and prevents trauma from suction pressure on one area of airway. NOTE: Suctioning also removes air. Client's oxygen supply can be severely reduced if procedure lasts longer than 15 seconds.
14. Flush catheter with sterile solution by placing it in solution and applying suction.	Removes secretions from catheter and lubricates it for next suctioning.

Steps	Rationale
15. If client is not in respiratory distress, allow him to rest for 20 to 30 seconds before reinserting catheter.	Allows client opportunity to increase his oxygen intake.
16. If client is able, ask him to deep breathe and cough between suctions.	Promotes mobilization of secretions to upper airway, where they can be removed with catheter. If client is able to cough productively, further suctioning may not be needed so long as his airways are clear to auscultation.
17. If resuctioning is needed, repeat Steps 11 through 13.	
18. Suction secretions in mouth or under tongue after suctioning oropharynx or nasopharynx.	Sterile asepsis is maintained. Mouth should be suctioned only after sterile areas have been thoroughly suctioned.
19. Discard catheter by wrapping it around your gloved hand and pulling glove off around catheter.	Spread of bacteria from suction catheter is reduced.
20. Prepare equipment for next suctioning.	Ready access to suction equipment is provided, especially if the client is experiencing respiratory distress.
21. Record in nurse's notes amount, consistency, color, and odor of secretions, as well as client's response to procedure.	Documents that procedure was completed.

Nurse Alert

If the client is unable to cough or has an artificial airway, orotracheal or nasotracheal suctioning is necessary.

Client Teaching

Clients who have undergone head and neck surgery (such as laryngectomy or neck dissection) often learn to self-administer oral suctioning while in the hospital. This can give them a sense of independence.

Pediatric Considerations

Children require smaller-diameter suction catheters. The newborn to 18-month-old child requires a 6 to 8 French, the 18-to-24-month old an 8 to 10 French, and the older child a 10 to 14 French.

Geriatric Considerations

Elderly clients with underlying cardiac or pulmonary disease may be able to tolerate only a 10-second period of suctioning. These clients are at greater risk of hypoxia-induced cardiac dysrhythmias.

Nasotracheal

Suctioning

Nasotracheal suctioning involves the insertion of a small rubber tube into the client's naris and down to the trachea. The purpose of this procedure is to remove secretions from the client's airway and to stimulate the client to cough deeply. Secretions that are not removed from the airways increase the client's risk for infection and/or respiratory failure.

Potential Nursing Diagnoses

Client data derived during the assessment reveal defining characteristics to support the following nursing diagnoses in clients requiring this skill:

Infection, high risk for
Gas exchange, impaired
Airway clearance, ineffective

Equipment

Portable or wall suction unit with connecting tubing and Y-connector if needed
Sterile catheter (12 or 16 French)*
Sterile water or normal saline
Sterile cup*
Sterile gloves*
Water-soluble lubricant
Drape or towel to protect linen and client's bedclothes
Goggles

*These materials are usually supplied in disposable suction kits.

Steps	Rationale
1. Explain procedure to client.	Reduces anxiety and promotes cooperation.
2. Place client in semi- or high-Fowler's position.	Position promotes maximum lung expansion.
3. Wash hands.	Reduces transmission of micro-organisms.
4. Don goggles.	Protects the nurse from risk of transmission of blood-borne pathogens via droplet transmission.
5. If using suction kit: a. Open package. If sterile drape is available, place it across client's chest or use a towel.	Reduces transmission of micro-organisms.
b. Open suction catheter package. Do not allow suction catheter to touch any surface other than inside of its package.	Prepares catheter and reduces transmission of microorganisms. Maintains medical asepsis.
c. Unwrap or open sterile basin and place on bed-side table. Be careful not to touch inside of basin. Fill with about 100 ml sterile normal saline.	Saline is used to clean tubing after each suction pass.
6. Open lubricant. Squeeze onto open sterile catheter package without touching package.	Prepares lubricant while maintaining sterility. Water-soluble lubricant is used to avoid lipoid aspiration pneumonia.
7. Apply sterile glove to each hand or apply nonsterile glove to nondominant hand and sterile glove to dominant hand.	Reduces transmission of micro-organisms and allows nurse to maintain sterility of suction catheter.

Steps	Rationale
8. Pick up suction catheter with dominant hand without touching nonsterile surfaces. Pick up connecting tubing with nondominant hand. Secure catheter to tubing (Fig. 155).	Maintains catheter sterility. Connects catheter to suction.

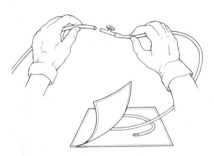

Fig. 155

9. Check that equipment is functioning properly by suctioning small amount of normal saline from basin.	Ensures equipment function. Lubricates internal catheter and tubing.
10. Coat distal 6 to 8 cm of catheter with water-soluble lubricant.	Lubricates catheter for easier insertion.
11. Remove oxygen delivery device, if applicable, with nondominant hand. Without applying suction, gently but quickly insert catheter with dominant thumb and fore-finger into naris using slight downward slant or through mouth when client breathes in. Do not force through naris (Fig. 156).	

Steps	Rationale

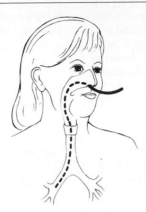

Fig. 156

a. Tracheal suctioning: in adults, insert catheter 20 to 24 cm; in older children, 14 to 20 cm; and in young children and infants, 8 to 14 cm.   If resistance is felt after insertion of catheter for recommended distance, nurse has probably hit carina. Pull catheter back 1 cm before applying suction.

b. Positioning: in some instances turning client's head to right helps nurse suction left mainstem bronchus; turning head to left helps nurse suction right mainstem bronchus.

Application of suction pressure while introducing catheter into trachea increases risk of damage to mucosa, as well as increased risk of hypoxia because of removal of inhaled oxygen present in airways. Epiglottis is open on inspiration and facilitates insertion into trachea. Client should cough. If client gags or becomes nauseated, catheter is most likely in esophagus.

Steps	Rationale
12. Apply intermittent suction for up to 10 seconds by placing and releasing non-dominant thumb over vent of catheter and slowly withdraw catheter while rotating it back and forth between dominant thumb and forefinger. Encourage client to cough. Replace oxygen device, if applicable.	Intermittent suction and rotation of catheter prevents injury to mucosa. If catheter "grabs" mucosa, remove thumb to release suction. Suctioning for longer than 10 seconds can cause cardiopulmonary compromise.
13. Rinse catheter and connecting tubing with normal saline until cleared.	Removes secretions from catheter.
14. Repeat Steps 10 through 12 as needed to clear pharynx or trachea of secretions. Allow adequate time between suction passes for ventilation.	Repeated passes with the suction catheter clear the airway of excessive secretions and promote oxygenation.
15. Monitor client's cardiopulmonary status between suction passes. Ask client to breathe deeply and cough.	Observe for alterations in cardiopulmonary status. Suctioning can induce hypoxia, dysrhythmias, and bronchospasm. Deep breathing reventilates and reoxygenates alveoli.
16. When pharynx and trachea are sufficiently cleared of secretions, perform oral pharyngeal suctioning to clear mouth of secretions.	Removes upper-airway secretions.
17. When suctioning is completed, roll catheter around fingers of dominant hand. Pull glove off inside out so that catheter remains coiled in glove. Pull off other glove in same way. Discard in appropriate receptacle. Turn off suction device.	Reduces transmission of microorganisms.

Steps	Rationale
18. Remove towel, place in laundry.	Reduces transmission of micro-organisms.
19. Reposition client.	Promotes comfort.
20. If indicated, readjust oxygen to original level.	Prevents absorption atelectasis and oxygen toxicity.
21. Discard remainder of normal saline into appropriate receptacle. If basin is disposable, discard into appropriate receptacle. If basin is reusable, rinse it out and place it in soiled utility room.	Reduces transmission of micro-organisms.
22. Wash hands.	Reduces transmission of micro-organisms.
23. Place unopened suction kit on suction machine or at head of bed.	Provides immediate access to suction catheter.
24. Chart in nurse's notes respiratory assessments before and after suctioning; size of suction catheter used; duration of suctioning period; route(s) used to suction; secretions obtained; odor, amount, color, consistency of secretions; frequency of suctioning; client's tolerance of procedure; and amount of negative suction pressure used.	Documents cardiopulmonary status, nursing care, expected and unexpected outcomes, and provides baseline for future assessment.

Nurse Alert

Clients with a history of deviated septum or facial trauma may require placement of nasal airway before nasal tracheal suctioning is attempted. Frequent nasotracheal suctioning may result in trauma to the nasal mucosa and bloody returns from the suction catheter.

Client Teaching

Clients who have undergone head and neck surgery (such as laryngectomy or neck dissection) often learn to self-administer oral suctioning while in the hospital. This can give them a sense of independence.

Pediatric Considerations

Children require smaller-diameter suction catheters. The newborn to 18-month-old child requires a 6 to 8 French, the 18-to-24-month old an 8 to 10 French, and the older child a 10 to 14 French.

Geriatric Considerations

Elderly clients with underlying cardiac or pulmonary disease may be able to tolerate only a 10-second period of suctioning. These clients are at greater risk of hypoxia-induced cardiac dysrhythmias.

Tracheal Suctioning

Tracheal suctioning involves the insertion of a suction catheter into the client's artificial tracheal airway. Tracheal suctioning maintains airway patency, facilitates removal of airway secretions, and stimulates a deep cough. In the acute health care environment tracheal suctioning is a sterile process. In the home setting the client may be instructed to use a clean suction technique as long as there are no signs of infection.

Potential Nursing Diagnoses

Client data derived during the assessment reveal defining characteristics to support the following nursing diagnoses in clients requiring this skill:

Infection, high risk for

Gas exchange, impaired

Airway clearance, ineffective

Equipment

Bedside table

Suction catheter of appropriate size (see box)

Water-soluble lubricant

2 sterile gloves or 1 sterile and 1 nonsterile glove

Sterile basin

Approximately 100 ml sterile normal saline

Clean towel or sterile drape from kit

Portable or wall suction apparatus

6 ft of connecting tubing

Sterile suction kit can be used, if available (be sure all listed items not in kit are assembled)

Goggles

Suction Catheter of Appropriate Size

Newborn	6-8 Fr
Infant to 6 mo	6-8 Fr
18 mo	8-10 Fr
24 mo	10 Fr
2-4 years	10-12 Fr
4-7 years	12 Fr
7-10 years	12-14 Fr
10-12 years	14 Fr
Adults	12-16 Fr

Steps	Rationale
1. Prepare client:	
a. Explain procedure and client's participation.	Encourages cooperation, minimizes risks, reduces anxiety.
b. Explain importance of coughing during procedure. Practice now, if able.	Facilitates secretion removal and may reduce frequency of future suctioning.
c. Assist client to assume position comfortable for nurse and client, usually semi-Fowler's or Fowler's. If unconscious, place in side-lying position.	Promotes client comfort; prevents muscle strain. Promotes maximum lung expansion and deep breathing. Also reduces risk of aspiration.
d. Place towel across client's chest.	Reduces transmission of microorganisms.
2. Wash hands and don goggles if appropriate.	Reduces transmission of microorganisms.
3. Turn suction device on and set vacuum regulator to appropriate negative pressure (see box on page 431).	Excessive negative pressure damages tracheal mucosa and can induce greater hypoxia.

Steps	Rationale
4. Connect one end of connecting tubing to suction machine and place other end in convenient location.	Prepares suction apparatus.
5. If using sterile suction kit: a. Open package. If sterile drape is available, place it across client's chest.	Prevents contamination of clothing.
b. Open suction catheter package. Do not allow suction catheter to touch any nonsterile surface.	Prepares catheter and prevents transmission of microorganisms.
c. Unwrap or open sterile basin and place on bedside table. Be careful not to touch inside basin. Fill with about 100 ml sterile normal saline.	Prepares catheter and prevents transmission of microorganisms.
6. If indicated, open lubricant. Squeeze onto sterile catheter package without touching package.	Prepares lubricant for use while maintaining sterility.
7. Apply one sterile glove to each hand or apply nonsterile glove to nondominant hand and sterile glove to dominant hand.	Reduces transmission of microorganisms and allows nurse to maintain sterility of suction catheter.
8. Pick up suction catheter with dominant hand without touching nonsterile surfaces. Pick up connecting tubing with nondominant hand. Secure catheter to tubing.	Maintains catheter sterility.
9. Check that equipment is functioning properly by suctioning small amount of saline from basin.	Ensures equipment function; lubricates catheter and tubing.

Steps	Rationale
10. Coat distal 6 to 8 cm of catheter with water-soluble lubricant. In some situations catheter is lubricated only with normal saline. Nursing assessment indicates need for lubrication.	Promotes easier catheter insertion. If lubricant is needed, it must be water soluble to prevent petroleum-based aspiration pneumonia. Excessive lubricant can adhere to artificial airway.
11. Remove oxygen or humidity delivery device with nondominant hand.	Exposes artificial airway.
12. Hyperinflate and/or oxygenate client before suctioning, using manual resuscitation (AMBU) bag or sigh mechanism on mechanical ventilator.	Hyperinflation decreases atelectasis caused by negative pressure. Preoxygenation converts large proportion of resident lung gas to 100% O_2 to offset amount used in metabolic consumption while ventilator or oxygenation is interrupted, as well as to offset volume lost out of suction catheter (Luce, 1993).
13. Without applying suction, gently but quickly insert catheter with dominant thumb and forefinger into artificial airway (best to time catheter insertion with inspiration).	Places catheter in tracheobronchial tree. Application of suction pressure while introducing catheter into trachea increases risk of damage to tracheal mucosa, as well as increased hypoxia caused by removal of inhaled oxygen present in airways.
14. Insert catheter until resistance is met, then pull back 1 cm.	Stimulates cough and removes catheter from mucosal wall.
15. Apply intermittent suction by placing and releasing nondominant thumb over vent of catheter and slowly withdraw catheter while rotating it back and forth between dominant thumb and forefinger. Encourage client to cough.	Intermittent suction and rotation of catheter prevents injury to tracheal mucosal lining. If catheter "grabs" mucosa, remove thumb to release suction.

Steps	Rationale
16. Replace oxygen delivery device. Encourage client to deep breathe.	Reoxygenates and reexpands alveoli. Suctioning can cause hypoxemia and atelectasis.
17. Rinse catheter and connecting tubing with normal saline until clear. Use continuous suction.	Removes catheter secretions. Secretions left in tubing decrease suction and provide environment for microorganism growth.
18. Repeat Steps 12 through 17 as needed to clear secretions. Allow adequate time (at least 1 full minute) between suction passes for ventilation and reoxygenation.	Repeated passes with suction catheter clear airway of excessive secretions and promote improved oxygenation.
19. Assess client's cardiopulmonary status between suction passes.	Suctioning can induce dysrhythmias, hypoxia, and bronchospasm.
20. When artificial airway and tracheobronchial tree are sufficiently cleared of secretions, perform nasal and oral pharyngeal suctioning to clear upper airway of secretions. After nasal and oral pharyngeal suctioning are performed, catheter is contaminated; do not reinsert into endotracheal (ET) or tracheostomy tube (TT).	Removes upper airway secretions. Upper airway is considered "clean" while lower airway is considered "sterile." Therefore, same catheter can be used to suction from sterile to clean areas, but not from clean to sterile areas.
21. Disconnect catheter from connecting tubing. Roll catheter around fingers of dominant hand. Pull glove off inside out so that catheter remains in glove. Pull off other glove in same way. Discard into appropriate receptacle. Turn off suction device.	Reduces transmission of microorganisms.

Steps	Rationale
22. Remove towel and place in laundry, or remove drape and discard in appropriate receptacle.	Reduces transmission of micro-organisms.
23. Reposition client.	Promotes comfort. Sims' position encourages drainage and reduces risk of aspiration.
24. Discard remainder of normal saline into appropriate receptacle. If basin is disposable, discard into appropriate receptacle. If basin is reusable, place it in soiled utility room.	Reduces transmission of micro-organisms.
25. Wash hands.	Reduces transmission of micro-organisms.
26. Place unopened suction kit on suction machine or at head of bed.	Provides immediate access to suction catheter.
27. Record respiratory assessment before and after suctioning, size of suction catheter used, duration of suction procedure, secretions, and client's tolerance to procedure.	Documents cardiopulmonary status, nursing care given, and provides baseline for further assessments.

Nurse Alert

When a client has a tracheostomy tube, there is a loss of upper airway function that includes warming, filtering, and humidifying. When thick, sticky secretions are present, assess hydration and monitor for the presence of infection.

Teaching Considerations

Clients in the home care environment need to be taught how to safely suction the tracheostomy tube. In addition, these clients must know when to use clean or sterile suction techniques and when to notify their physician.

Tracheostomy Care

Clients who have tracheostomy tubes require specialized nursing care to manage the tracheostomy tube itself and the stoma in the client's neck. The stoma provides the access for the tracheostomy tube in the client's tracheal airway.

Potential Nursing Diagnoses

Client data derived during the assessment reveal defining characteristics to support the following nursing diagnoses in clients requiring this skill:

Infection, high risk for
Skin integrity, impaired

Equipment (Fig. 157)

Bedside table
Towel
Tracheostomy suction supplies
Sterile tracheostomy care kit, if available (be sure all supplies listed that are not available in kit are assembled)
Sterile 4 × 4 gauze—3 pkg
Hydrogen peroxide
Normal saline
Sterile cotton-tipped swabs
Sterile tracheostomy dressing (precut and sewn surgical dressing)
Sterile basin
Small sterile brush
Roll of twill tape or tracheostomy ties
Scissors
2 sterile gloves
Face shield/goggles

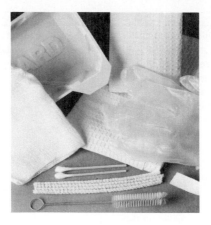

Fig. 157

Steps	Rationale
1. Have another nurse assist in this procedure (optional).	Prevents accidental extubation of tracheostomy tube.
2. Prepare client:	
a. Explain procedure and client's participation.	Encourages cooperation, minimizes risks, and reduces anxiety.
b. Assist client to position comfortable for both nurse and client (usually supine or semi-Fowler's).	Promotes client comfort, prevents nurse muscle strain.
c. Place towel across client's chest.	Reduces transmission of microorganisms.
3. Wash hands and apply gloves and face shield if applicable.	Reduces transmission of microorganisms.
4. Administer tracheostomy suctioning. Before removing gloves, remove soiled tracheostomy dressing and discard in glove with coiled catheter.	Removes secretions so as not to occlude outer cannula while inner cannula is removed.

Steps	Rationale
5. While client is replenishing oxygen stores, prepare equipment on bedside table. Open sterile tracheostomy kit. Open three 4 × 4 gauze packages aseptically and pour normal saline on one package and hydrogen peroxide on another. Leave third package dry. Open two cotton-tipped swab packages and pour normal saline on one package and hydrogen peroxide on the other. Open sterile tracheostomy dressing package. Unwrap sterile basin and pour about 1.8 ml (0.75 in) in hydrogen peroxide into it. Open small sterile brush package and place aseptically into sterile basin. If using large roll of twill tape, cut appropriate length of tape and lay aside in dry area. Do not recap hydrogen peroxide and normal saline.	Prepares equipment and allows for smooth organized completion of tracheostomy care.
6. Apply gloves. Keep dominant hand sterile throughout procedure. (For TT with inner cannula, complete Steps 7 through 19. For TT with no inner cannula or Kistner button, complete Steps 11 through 19).	Reduces transmission of microorganisms.
7. Remove oxygen source and then inner cannula with nondominant hand. Drop inner cannula into hydrogen peroxide basin.	Removes inner cannula for cleaning. Hydrogen peroxide loosens secretions from inner cannula.

Steps	Rationale
8. Place tracheostomy collar oxygen source over outer cannula. Place T-tube (Briggs) and ventilator oxygen sources over or near outer cannula. NOTE: T-tube and ventilator oxygen devices cannot be attached to all outer cannulas when the inner cannula is removed.	Maintains supply of oxygen to client.
9. To prevent oxygen desaturation in affected clients, quickly pick up inner cannula and use small brush to remove secretions inside and outside cannula.	Tracheostomy brush provides mechanical force to remove thick or dried secretions.
10. Hold inner cannula over basin and rinse with normal saline, using nondominant hand to pour normal saline.	Removes secretions and hydrogen peroxide from inner cannula.
11. Replace inner cannula and secure "locking" mechanism. Reapply T-tube (Briggs) and ventilator oxygen sources.	Secures inner cannula and reestablishes oxygen supply.
12. Using hydrogen peroxide-prepared cotton-tipped swabs and 4 × 4 gauze, clean exposed outer cannula surfaces and stoma under faceplate extending 4 to 8 cm (2 to 4 in) in all directions from stoma. Clean in circular motion from stoma site outward using dominant hand to handle sterile supplies.	Aseptically removes secretions from stoma site.

Steps	Rationale
13. Using normal saline-prepared cotton-tipped swabs and 4 × 4 gauze, rinse exposed outer cannula surfaces and stoma under faceplate extending 4 to 8 cm (2 to 4 in) in all directions from stoma. Rinse in circular motion from stoma site outward using dominant hand to handle sterile supplies.	Rinses hydrogen peroxide from surfaces.
14. Using dry 4 × 4 gauze, pat lightly at skin and exposed outer cannula surfaces.	Dry surfaces prohibit formation of moist environment for microorganism growth and skin excoriation.
15. Instruct assistant, if available, to securely hold TT in place. With assistant holding TT, cut ties. Assistant must *not* release hold on tracheostomy tube until new ties are firmly tied. If no assistant, do not cut old ties until new ties are in place and securely tied:	Promotes hygiene, reduces transmission of microorganisms. Secure TT.
a. Cut a length of twill tape long enough to go around client's neck twice; cut ends on diagonal.	Cutting ends of tie on diagonal aids in inserting tie through eyelet.
b. Insert one end of tie through faceplate eyelet and pull ends even.	
c. Slide both ends of tie behind head and around neck to other eyelet and insert one tie through second eyelet.	
d. Pull snugly.	

Steps	Rationale
e. Tie ends securely in double square knot allowing space for only one finger in tie.	One finger slack prevents ties from being too tight when tracheostomy dressing is in place.
16. Insert fresh tracheostomy dressing under clean ties and faceplate (Fig. 158).	Absorbs drainage.

 Fig. 158

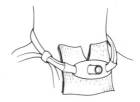

Steps	Rationale
17. Remove gloves and discard in appropriate receptacle with soiled tracheostomy ties.	Reduces transmission of microorganisms.
18. Replace cap on hydrogen peroxide and normal saline bottles. Store reusable liquids and unused supplies in appropriate place.	Once opened, normal saline can be considered free of bacteria for 24 hours, after which it should be discarded.
19. Position client comfortably and assess respiratory status.	Promotes comfort. Some clients may require posttracheostomy care suctioning.
20. Wash hands.	Reduces transmission of microorganisms.
21. Record assessment of client's respiratory status and status of skin around stoma, frequency of care, and tolerance to care.	Documents cardiopulmonary and tracheostomy site status, nursing care, and client's response to procedure.

Nurse Alert

There are alternate methods to apply tracheostomy ties. The one presented here is the safest and easiest to master. Commercial products that use Velcro and similar fastening devices are avail-

able in some institutions. Clients with new tracheostomy frequently have blood secretions for 2 to 3 days after procedure or
for 24 hours after each tracheostomy tube change.

Do not cut 4 × 4 gauze. Loose strings that enter stoma can
cause infection and irritation.

Some institutions use disposable (sterile) inner cannulas,
which are removed and discarded every 8 to 12 hours and new
ones inserted.

Teaching Considerations

Clients who are sent home with a tracheostomy tube must be
taught how to complete tracheostomy care safely and correctly.
Even when the client is able to complete the care, a family member or close friend should also learn the procedure in the event
that the client is unable to complete the procedure.

Care of
Chest Tubes

Trauma, disease, or surgery can result in air or fluid leaking into the intrapleural space. Small leaks are absorbed spontaneously. Closed chest drainage systems restore optimal lung expansion and promote the drainage of fluid and blood from the pleural space. There are two types of commercial systems: the water-seal and the waterless systems.

Potential Nursing Diagnoses

Client data derived during the assessment reveal defining characteristics to support the following nursing diagnoses in clients requiring this skill:

> Anxiety
> Gas exchange, impaired
> Pain

Equipment

Prescribed drainage system:
Water-seal system (Fig 159).
> Sterile water or N/S to cover lower one inch of water-seal U-tube.
> Sterile water or N/S to pour into the suction control chamber if suction is to be used.
Waterless system
> Vial of 30-ml injectable NaCl or water
> 20-ml syringe
> 21 gauge needle
> Antiseptic swab
Chest tube or trocar tray
> 1 knife handle
> Chest tube clamp

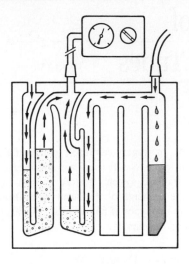

Fig. 159

Small sponge forceps
Needle holder
Knife blade #10
3-0 silk
Tray liner (sterile field)
2 curved 8-inch Kellys
10 4 × 4 sponges
Suture scissors
3 hand towels
Dressings
   Vaseline gauze
   Several 4 × 4 gauze dressings
   2 large dressings
   4-inch tape or elastoplast
Head cover
Face mask
Sterile gloves
Two shodded hemostats for each chest tube
1-inch adhesive tape for taping connections

Steps	Rationale
1. Assess client's cardiopulmonary status, observe for respiratory status, use of accessory muscles, color, pain, anxiety, and vital signs.	Provides continual data about client's status prior to, during, and after the chest tube procedure.
2. Review physician's role and responsibilities for chest tube placement (Table 5).	Helps differentiate doctor and nurse roles so that the nurse can function more effectively.

Table 5   Physician's role and responsibility in chest tube placement

1. Explain purpose, procedure, and possible complications to the client.	Provides informed consent.
2. Wash hands. Cleanse chest wall with antiseptic.	Reduces transmission of microorganisms.
3. Don mask and gloves.	Maintains surgical asepsis.
4. Drape area of chest tube insertion with sterile towels.	Maintains surgical asepsis.
5. Inject local anesthetic and allow time to take effect.	Decreases pain during procedure.
6. Use blunt or sharp dissection to create incision in the skin and chest wall.	Opens chest for insertion of chest tube. A trochar is outdated and increases risk of tissue damage.
7. Thread a clamped chest tube through the incision. Physician clamps chest tube until system is connected to water seal.	Inserts chest tube into the intrapleural space. Clamping prevents entry of atmospheric air into the chest and worsening of the pneumothorax.
8. Suture chest tube in place, if suturing is policy or physician preference.	Secures chest tube in place.

Continued.

Table 5   Physician's role and responsibility in chest tube placement—cont'd

9. Cover the chest insertion site with a large, sterile occlusive pressure dressing.	Holds chest tube in place and prevents air leakage around the tube to prevent additional atmospheric air from entering the intrapleural space.
10. Remove connector cover from client's end of chest drainage tubing, using sterile technique. Secure drainage tubing to the chest tube and drainage system.	Physician is responsible for making certain that the system is set up properly, the proper amount of water is in the water-seal, the dressing is secure, and the chest tube is securely connected to the drainage system.
11. Connect system to suction or supervise a nurse connecting it to suction, if suction is to be used.	The physician is responsible for determining and checking the amount of water that is to be added to the suction-control bottle/chamber and prescribing the suction setting.
12. Unclamp the chest tube.	Connects chest tube to the water-seal drainage and suction, thus promoting drainage of fluid or air from the intrapleural space and allowing the lung to reexpand.
13. Order and review chest x-ray.	Verifies correct chest tube placement.

Steps	Rationale
3. Explain procedure to client.	Reduces anxiety and promotes patient cooperation.
4. Wash hands.	Reduces transmission of microorganisms.
5. Set up the prescribed drainage system:	

Steps	Rationale
a. Water-seal system: ▪ Obtain a water-seal chest drainage system. Remove wrappers and prepare to set up the system. Can be set up as a two- or three-chamber system.	Maintains sterility of the system. The system is packaged in this manner so it can be used under sterile operating room conditions (Carroll, 1986). If a two-chamber system is prescribed, do not carry out steps to use the suction chamber or suction source.
▪ While maintaining sterility of the drainage tubing, stand the system upright and add sterile water or saline to the appropriate compartments.	Reduces possibility of contamination.
▪ For a two-chamber system (without suction), add sterile solution to the water-seal chamber (second chamber), bringing fluid to the required level as indicated.	Maintains water-seal.
▪ For a three-chamber system (with suction), add sterile solution to the water-seal chamber (second chamber). Add amount of sterile solution prescribed by physician to the suction control (third chamber), usually 20 cm (7.9 inches). Connect tubing from suction control chamber to suction source.	Depth of rold below fluid level dictates the highest amount of negative pressure that can be present within the system, (i.e., 20 cm of water is approximately -20 cm. of water pressure). Any additional negative pressure applied to the system will be vented into the atmosphere through the suction-control vent. This safety device prevents damage to pleural tissues from an unexpected surge of negative pressure from the suction source.

Steps	Rationale

b. Waterless system:
- Obtain a waterless system. Remove sterile wrappers and prepare to set up.

Maintains sterility of the system. The system is packaged in this manner so it can be used under sterile operating room conditions (Carroll, 1986).

- For a two-chamber system (without suction) nothing is added or needs to be done to the system.

The waterless two-chamber system is ready for connecting to the client's chest tube upon opening the wrappers.

- For a three-chamber waterless system with suction connect tubing from suction control chamber to the suction source.

The suction source provides additional negative pressure to the system.

- Instill 15 ml of sterile water or saline into the diagnostic indicator injection port located on top of the system.

Not necessary for mediastinal drainage because there will be no tidaling. Also, in an emergency this is not necessary because the system does not require water for set-up.

6. Tape all connection in a spiral fashion using 1-inch adhesive tape.
- Check both systems for patency by:
  Clamping the drainage tubing that will connect the client to the system. Connecting tubing from the float ball chamber to the suction source. Turning on the suction to the prescribed level.

Prevents atmospheric air from leaking into the system and the client's intrapleural space. Provides a chance to ensure an airtight system before connecting it to the client. Allows correction or replacement of system if it is defective before connecting it to the client. NOTE: Bubbling will be seen at first because there is air in the tubing and system initially. This should stop after a few minutes unless there are other sources of air entering the system. If bubbling continues, check connections and locate source of the air leak as described in Table 6.

Table 6   Problem-Solving with Chest Tubes

Problem	Solution
Air Leak in Water-Seal System	
Continuous bubbling in the water-seal chamber, indicated leak between client and the water seal.	Locate leak. Tighten loose connections between client and water seal. Loose connections cause air to enter the system. Leaks are corrected when constant bubbling stops.
Bubbling continues, indicating the air leak has not been corrected.	Cross-clamp chest tube close to client's chest. If bubbling stops, the air leak is inside the client's thorax (client-centered) or at the chest tube insertion site (Palau and Jones, 1986). *Unclamp tube and notify physician immediately.* Reinforce chest dressing. Leaving chest tube clamped with a client-centered leak can cause collapse of the lung, mediastinal shift, and eventual collapse of the other lung from the buildup of air pressure within the pleural cavity.
Bubbling continues, indicating leak is not client centered.	In an alternating fashion, gradually move clamps down the drainage tubing away from the client and toward the suction control chamber, moving one clamp at a time. When bubbling stops, leak is in the section of tubing or connection that is in between the two clamps. Replace tubing or secure connection and release clamps.
Bubbling continues, indicating leak is not in the tubing.	Leak is in the drainage system. Change drainage system (Palau and Jones, 1986).
Water-seal is disconnected.	Connect water seal and tape connection.

Continued.

Table 6   Problem-Solving with Chest Tubes—cont'd

Problem	Solution
Water-seal U-tube is not longer submerged in sterile fluid.	Add sterile solution to the water-seal bottle until the distal tip is 2 cm under surface level or set the water-seal bottle upright so that the tip is submerged.
Air Leak in the Waterless System	Locate leak.
Continuous left-to-right bubbling in the diagnostic air-leak indicator.	Tighten loose connections between client and water seal. Loose connections allow air to enter the system. Recheck for source of air leak if bubbling continues.
Negative pressure display ceases to display "yes" on inspiration (Davol Inc.).	
Bubbling and lack of display "yes" continues, indicating leak is not in connections.	Cross-clamp chest tube close to client's chest. If bubbling stops, the air leak is inside the client's thorax (client-centered) or at the chest tube insertion site (Palau and Jones, 1986). *Unclamp tube and notify physician immediately.* Reinforce chest dressing. Leaving chest tube clamped with a client-centered leak can cause collapse of the lung, mediastinal shift, and eventual collapse of the other lung from the buildup of air pressure within the pleural cavity.
Bubbling continues, indicating the leak is not client centered.	In an alternating fashion, gradually move clamps down the drainage tubing away from the client and toward the suction-control chamber, moving one clamp at a time. When bubbling stops, leak is in the section of tubing or connection that is in between the two clamps. Replace tubing or secure connection and release clamps.

Bubbling continues, indicating leak is not in the tubing.	Leak is in the drainage system. Change drainage system (Palau and Jones, 1986).
In Both Systems Air Leaks Can Lead To:	
Tension pneumothorax Severe respiratory distress Chest pain	Determine that chest tubes are not clamped, kinked, or occluded. Obstructed chest tubes trap air in the intrapleural space when there is a client-centered leak.
Absence of breath sounds on affected side	Notify physician immediately.
Hyperresonance on affected side	Prepare immediately for another chest tube insertion; obtain a one-way valve or large-gauge needle for short-term emergency release of air in the intrapleural space; have emergency equipment such as oxygen and code cart near the client.
Mediastinal shift to unaffected side Hypotension Tachycardia Supraclavicular bulging on affected side	
Trapping of fluid in dependent loops of drainage tubing	Drain tubing contents into drainage bottle. Coil excess tubing on mattress and secure in place.

Steps	Rationale
7. Turn off suction source and unclamp drainage tubing before connecting client to the system.	Having the client connected to suction when it is initiated could cause damage to pleural tissues from sudden increase in negative pressure. The suction source is turned on again after the client is connected to the three-chamber system.
8. Position the client:	
a. Semi-Fowler's to high-Fowler's position to evacuate air (pneumothorax).	Permits optimal drainage of fluid and/or air. Air rises to the highest point in the chest. Pneumothorax tubes are usually placed on the anterior aspect at the midclavicular line, second or third intercostal space (Carroll, 1986).
b. High-Fowler's position to drain fluid (hemothorax).	Permits optimal drainage of fluid. Posterior tubes are placed on the midaxillary line, eighth or ninth intercostal space.
9. Wash hands and don gloves.	Reduces transmission of microorganisms.
10. Administer parenteral premedications, such as sedatives, analgesics as ordered.	Reduces client anxiety and pain during procedure.
11. Assist physician in providing psychologic support to the client. (See physician's responsibilities in Table 5.) a. Reinforce preprocedure explanation. b. Instruct client throughout procedure.	Reduces client anxiety and assists in efficient completion of procedure.
12. Show anesthetic to physician.	Allows physician to read label of drug before administering it to client.

Steps	Rationale
13. Hold anesthetic solution bottle upside down with label facing physician. Physician will withdraw solution. a. Physician places chest tube. (A standard procedure is detailed in Table 5.)	Allows physician to withdraw solution properly while maintaining surgical asepsis.
14. Assist physician to attach drainage tube to chest tube.	Connects drainage system and suction (if ordered) to the chest tube.
15. Tape the tube connection between the chest and drainage tubes.	Secures chest tube to drainage system and reduces risk of air leaks causing breaks in the air-tight system.

16. Check patency of air vents in system:
   a. Water-seal vent must be without occlusion.
   b. Suction-control chamber vent must be without occlusion, when using suction.
   c. Waterless systems have relief valves without caps.
	Permits the displaced air to pass into the atmosphere.
	Provides safety factor of releasing excess negative pressure into the atmosphere.

17. Coil excess tubing on mattress next to the client. Secure with a rubber band and safety pin or the system's clamp.	Prevents excess tubing from hanging over the edge of the mattress in a dependent loop. Drainage could collect in the loop and occlude the drainage system.
18. Adjust tubing to hang in a straight line from top of the mattress to the drainage chamber.	Promotes drainage.

Steps	Rationale
19. If the chest tube is draining fluid indicate the date, time (e.g., 0900) that drainage was begun on the drainage chamber's write-on surface. Postoperative assessment is done every 15 minutes for the first 2 hours. This assessment interval then changes *based on client's status*. Mark the time and level of drainage on the calibrated write-on strip periodically.	Provides a baseline for continuous assessment of the type and quantity of drainage. Permits timely and efficient account of amount of drainage from the chest tube. Drainage is marked at specified periods of time and documented on the nurse's notes and I & O sheet. Ensures early detection of complications.
20. Strip or milk chest tube only if indicated: a. Postoperative mediastinal chest tubes are manipulated if nursing assessment indicates an obstruciton of drainage secondary to clots or debris in the tubing.	Stripping is controversial and should be performed only if hospital policy permits and there is a physician's order (Phipps et al, 1991; Johanson et al, 1988). Stripping creates a high degree of negative pressure and has potential of pulling lung tissue or pleura into drainage holes of the chest tube (Duncan, Erickson, and Weigel, 1987).
21. Provide two shodded hemostats for each chest tube. Shodded hemostats are usually attached to the top of the client's bed with adhesive tape or clamped to client's clothing during ambulation.	Chest tubes are double-clamped under specific circumstances a. To assess for an air leak (see Table 6). b. To empty or change the collection bottle or chamber (Farley, 1988). This procedure is performed only by physician or nurse who has received training in the procedure.

Steps	Rationale
	c. To change disposable systems have new system ready to be connected before clamping the tube, so that transfer can be rapid and the drainage system reestablished.
	d. To assess if client is ready to have chest tube removed. This is done by physician's order (Farley, 1988). In this situation, nurse must monitor client for the recreation of a pneumothorax (see Table 6).
22. Assist client to a comfortable position.	Reduces client anxiety and promotes cooperation.
23. Remove gloves and dispose of used, soiled equipment.	Prevents accidents involving contaminated equipment.
24. Wash hands.	Reduces spread of microorganisms.
25. Record procedure and client's cardiopulmonary assessment.	Documents procedure and client response.

Nurse Alert

Client with a hemothorax, who is also on anticoagulants, may need to have anticoagulant therapy reduced or discontinued until the hemothorax is resolved or controlled.

Teaching Considerations

Teach clients and families to:
- Inform the nurse of increased chest pain or difficult breathing.
- Never lift drainage system higher than the chest tube insertion site.

- Notify nurse immediately if a bottle breaks.
- Keep system upright at all times.
- Prevent pulling on the chest tube.
- Notify nurse immediately if there are changes in the way the system is functioning.

Applying a
Nasal Cannula

A nasal cannula is a simple device that can be inserted into the nares for delivery of oxygen and that allows the client to breathe through his mouth or nose. It is available for all age groups and is adequate for both short- and long-term use in the hospital or at home.

Potential Nursing Diagnoses

Client data derived during the assessment reveal defining characteristics to support the following nursing diagnoses in clients requiring this skill:

   Gas exchange, impaired

Equipment

Nasal cannula
Oxygen tubing
Humidifier
Oxygen source with flowmeter
"No smoking" signs

Steps	Rationale
1. Wash hands.	Reduces transmission of micro-organisms.
2. Attach cannula to oxygen tubing.	Establishes connection with oxygen source. Oxygen tubing has extension length so client has some mobility.

Steps	Rationale
3. Adjust oxygen flow to prescribed rate, usually between 1 and 6 L/min. Observe that water in humidifier is bubbling.	Administers oxygen at prescribed rate. Oxygen flow rates greater than 6 L/min do not increase oxygen concentration but do irritate nasal mucosa, causing swallowing of gas and abdominal distention.
4. Place prongs of cannula in client's nose and adjust band to client's comfort (Fig. 160).	Reduces chance that client will remove cannula because of discomfort.

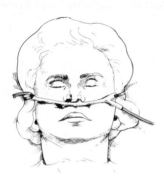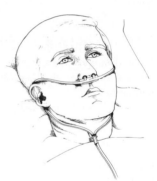

Fig. 160

5. Check cannula every 8 hours.	Patency of cannula and oxygen flow are ensured.
6. Keep humidification jar filled at all times.	Inhalation of dehumidified oxygen is prevented.
7. Assess client's nares, external nose, and ears for mucosal and/or skin breakdown every 6 to 8 hours.	Prolonged use of nasal oxygen can increase risk of mucosal breakdown in nares. Tape can irritate bridge of nose. Elastic band can excoriate ears.
8. Check oxygen flow rate and physician's orders every 8 hours.	Delivery of prescribed oxygen flow rate is ensured.

Steps	Rationale
9. Record in client's record time that therapy was initiated, oxygen flow rate, route of administration, and client's response.	Documents that procedure was performed.

Nurse Alert

In clients with underlying obstructive lung disease the flow rate of oxygen should not exceed 2 L/min. Higher rates can depress the stimulus to breathe.

Client Teaching

Clients may be placed on home oxygen via nasal cannula. They and their families must then be taught the hazards of oxygen therapy, the rationale for it, the correct flow rate, and the proper use and cleaning of oxygen equipment.

Pediatric Considerations

In general, oxygen is delivered via an oxygen tent to a child.

Geriatric Considerations

Frail elderly clients are at increased risk of skin breakdown resulting from the placement of an oxygen cannula. The sites for skin breakdown include the nares and ears. Skin breakdown can be minimized by frequent assessment of and care to these areas.

Measuring Peak Expiratory Flow Rates

The use of pulmonary function studies are essential for diagnosis of pulmonary disease. For patients with chronic airflow obstruction, such as asthma, measurement of the peak expiratory flow rate (PEFR) gives objective data about the severity of the airway obstruction. The PEFR is the maximum flow rate, in liters, that can be generated during a forced expiratory maneuver (NIH, 1991). The PEFR is measured using a peak flow meter. The peak flow meter is a simple device that records the PEFR in liters (Janson-Bjerklie and Shnell, 1988).

Potential Nursing Diagnoses

Client data derived during the assessment reveal defining characteristics to support the following nursing diagnoses in clients requiring this skill:

Gas exchange, impaired
Breathing pattern, ineffective
Knowledge deficit regarding use of PEFR

Equipment

Peak flow meter

Steps	Rationale
1. Observe for signs of airway obstruction: shortness of breath, wheezing, use of accessory muscles of respiratory, cyanosis, and nasal flaring.	Indicates client in distress. Airway obstruction can be life-threatening and needs immediate intervention.

Steps	Rationale
2. Observe for patient airway and remove secretions.	Secretions increase airway resistance.
3. Complete total respiratory assessment.	Provides objective baseline data.
4. Review client's medical record for order to measure PEFR and expected rate to be achieved by the client.	Requires physician order. Provides expected rate client is to achieve when at effective treatment levels.
5. Place indicator at base of the numbered scale (Fig. 161).	Starts all reading from zero.
6. Have client stand up.	Increases lung expansion.
7. Have client take a deep breath.	Maximal effort required for an accurate reading.
8. Have client place meter in the mouth and close lips around the mouth piece.	Increases accuracy of measurement.
9. Have client blow out as hard and as fast as he can (Fig. 162).	Maximal effort required for an accurate reading

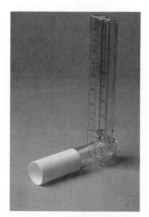

Fig. 161

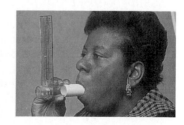

Fig. 162

Steps	Rationale
10. Have client repeat Steps 1 through 5 twice more, noting the highest number achieved (Janson-Bjerklie and Shnell, 1988; NIH, 1991).	Demonstrates the best effort.
11. Determine the client's PEFR and compare to the client's personal best.	Provides objective measure of client's symptoms. The personal best PEFR is obtained after the client is on effective therapy and has been determined to be maximally bronchodilated (NIH, 1991).
12. Reassess client for improvement in symptoms if bronchodilator therapy has been initiated.	PEFR is frequently measured following bronchodilator therapy to measure the client's response.

Nurse Alert

Be sure the client does not become light-headed while performing the PEFR measurement. If the client does, allow more time between measurements.

Teaching Considerations

Instruct client on care of peak flow meter. The client should be able to perform the measurement independently if it is required after discharge. The nurse needs to instruct the client on the technique itself, recognition of the best PEFR reading, recording of the measurement, and the care of the peak flow meter. A return demonstration by the client before discharge will determine his ability to perform the skill in the home. Review use of the peak flow meter with the client, the client's record of PEFR measurement, and the plan for notification of the physician when there are changes in the PEFR.

Cardiopulmonary

Resuscitation

(Two Nurses)

The purpose of cardiopulmonary resuscitation (CPR) is to restore an airway, breathing, and circulation to a client who has sustained catastrophic disruption of these functions.

Cardiopulmonary arrest is characterized by an absence of pulse and respirations and by dilated pupils. CPR is a basic emergency procedure for life support, consisting of artificial respiration and manual external cardiac massage.

Potential Nursing Diagnoses

Client data derived during the assessment reveal defining characteristics to support the following nursing diagnoses in clients requiring this skill:

Cardiac output, decreased
Gas exchange, impaired
Tissue perfusion, altered

Equipment

Oral airway if immediately available
Automatic manual breathing unit (AMBU) bag if immediately available
CPR pocket mask, if available
Chest compression board, if available
Resuscitation cart, if available
Face shield, if available

Steps	Rationale
1. Determine if person is unconscious by shaking him or shouting at him, "Are you OK?"	Confirms that person is unconscious as opposed to intoxicated, sleeping, or hearing impaired.
2. Determine presence of carotid pulse and respirations.	Presence of pulse *and* respiration contraindicates initiation of CPR.
3. Call for assistance, seek help from passerby, call for additional nurses. Goals of care: restore airway, breathing, circulation.	One person cannot maintain CPR indefinitely. Without relief, rescuer fatigues, chest compressions are ineffective, and volume of air ventilated into victim's lungs decreases.
4. Place victim on hard surface such as floor, ground, or backboard.	External compression of heart is facilitated. Heart is compressed between sternum and hard surface.
5. Place yourself in correct position, that is also somewhat comfortable:	You may be administering CPR for extended period, particularly in community setting. Correct, comfortable position decreases skeletal muscle fatigue.
a. *Two-person rescue:* One person faces victim, kneeling parallel to victim's head. Second person moves to opposite side and faces victim, kneeling parallel to victim's sternum.	Allows one rescuer to maintain breathing while other maintains circulation, without getting in each other's way.
6. Restore open airway:	
a. *Head tilt-chin lift* (Fig. 163): Elevate chin with one hand and apply downward pressure on forehead until teeth are almost together but mouth is still open.	Airway obstruction from tongue is relieved. If necessary, remove foreign body.

Steps   Rationale

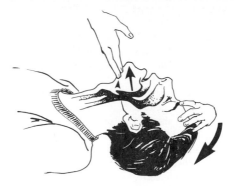

Fig. 163

b. *Jaw thrust maneuver*
   (Fig. 164) can be used
   by health professionals
   but is not taught to general public. Grasp an-
   gles of victim's lower
   jaw and lift with both
   hands, displacing the
   mandible forward while
   tilting the head back-
   ward.

Jaw thrust maneuver should be
used whenever cervical neck
injury is suspected. This permits
opening of airway without ma-
nipulating spinal column.

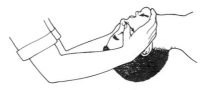

Fig. 164

7. If readily available, insert
   oral airway.

Maintains tongue on anterior
floor of mouth and prevents obstruction of posterior airway by
tongue.

Steps	Rationale

8. Administer artificial respiration:
   a. Mouth-to-mouth:
      - *Adult:* Pinch victim's nose and occlude mouth with yours. Blow 2 full breaths into victim's mouth (each breath should take 1.5 to 2.0 seconds); allow victim to exhale between breaths. Continue, giving 10 to 12 breaths per minute.

        Airtight seal is formed and air is prevented from escaping from nose. Hyperventilation is promoted and assists in maintaining adequate blood oxygen levels. In most adults this volume is 800 to 1200 ml and is sufficient to make the chest rise. An excess of air volume and fast inspiratory flow rates are likely to cause pharyngeal pressures that exceed esophageal opening pressures, allowing air to enter the stomach and result in gastric distention, thereby increasing the risk of vomiting.

      - *Child:* Place your mouth over child's nose and mouth (Fig. 165).

        For mouth-to-mouth resuscitation of child, administer two slow breaths lasting 1 to 1.5 seconds with a pause in between. Continue giving 20 breaths per minute.

        Airtight seal is formed and air is prevented from escaping from nose. Because an infant's air passages are smaller with resistance to flow quite high, it is difficult to make recommendations about the force or volume of the rescue breaths. However, three factors should be remembered: (1) rescue breaths are the single most important maneuver in assisting a nonbreathing child, (2) an appropriate volume is one that makes the chest rise and fall, and (3) slow breaths provide an adequate volume at the lowest possible pressure, thereby reducing the risk of gastric distention.

Steps	Rationale

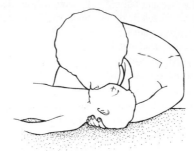

Fig. 165

b. AMBU:
   ■ *Adult and child:* For AMBU bag resuscitation use proper size face mask and apply it under chin, up and over victim's mouth and nose (Fig. 166).

Airtight seal is formed as bag is compressed and oxygen enters client.

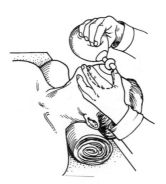

Fig. 166

Steps	Rationale
9. Observe for rise and fall of chest wall with each respiration. If lungs do not inflate, reposition head and neck and check for visible airway obstruction, such as vomitus.	Ensures that artificial respirations are entering lungs.
10. Suction secretions if necessary or turn victim's head to one side.	Suctioning prevents airway obstruction. Turning client's head to one side allows gravity to drain secretions.
11. Reassess for presence of carotid pulse (adults) or brachial pulse (infants) after restoring breathing.	Carotid artery pulse will persist when the more peripheral pulses are no longer palpable. Performing external cardiac compressions on a victim who has a pulse may result in serious medical complications.

12. If pulse is absent, initiate chest compressions:
  a. Assume correct hand position:
    ■ *Adult:* Place hands 1 to 2 cm above xiphoid process on sternum. Keep hands parallel to chest and fingers above chest. Interlocking fingers is helpful. Extend arms and lock elbows. Maintain arms straight and shoulders directly over victim's sternum (Fig. 167).
	Places hands and fingers over heart in proper position. Prevents xiphoid process and rib fracture, which can further compromise cardiopulmonary status.

Steps   Rationale

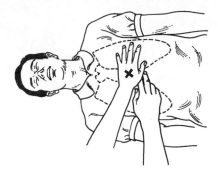

Fig. 167

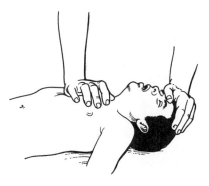

Fig. 168

- *Child:* Place heel of
  one hand 1 to 2 cm
  above xiphoid process
  (Fig. 168).

Steps	Rationale

- *Infant:* Place index and middle fingers of one hand on sternum above xiphoid process. Fingers should be 1 cm below nipple line (Fig. 169).

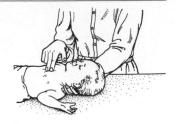

Fig. 169

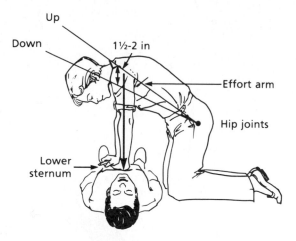

Fig. 170

b. Compress sternum to proper depth from shoulders. Do not rock, but transmit weight vertically and then release.

Compression occurs only on sternum. Pressure necessary for external compression is created by nurse's upper arm muscle strength. When the compression is released, the heart fills.

- Adult and adolescent: 4 to 5 cm (1.5 to 2 inches) (Fig. 170)
- Older child: 3 to 4 cm (1 to 1.5 inches)

Steps	Rationale

■ Toddler and pre-schooler: 2 to 4 cm (0.75 to 1.5 inches).

■ Infant: 1 to 2 cm (0.5 to 1 inches).

NOTE: Ratio of compressions to breaths for two rescuers is 5 to 1.

c. Maintain proper rate of compression:

Proper number of compressions/min should be delivered to ensure adequate cardiac output.

■ Adult and adolescent: 80/min (count one 1000; two 1000).

■ Older child: 100/min.

■ Infant and toddler: 100 to 200/min.

d. Continue mouth-to-mouth or AMBU ventilations.

Adequate ventilations promoted.

■ Adult and adolescent: every 5 seconds (12/min).

■ Older child: every 4 seconds (15/min).

■ Infant and toddler: every 3 seconds (20/min).

13. Palpate for carotid pulse with each external chest compression for first full minute. If carotid pulse is not palpable, compressions are not strong enough or hand position is incorrect.

Assessment of pulse validates that adequate stroke volume is achieved with each compression.

14. Continue CPR until relieved or until victim regains spontaneous pulse and respirations.

Artificial cardiopulmonary function is maintained.

Nurse Alert

If CPR must be interrupted, the interruption should not last longer than 5 to 30 seconds. CPR is interrupted when changing personnel, during defibrillation, or when transporting the victim. The nurse should remind rescue team members of the number of seconds elapsing.

Venipuncture

Venipuncture is a technique in which a vein is punctured transcutaneously by a sharp rigid stylet (such as with a butterfly needle, an angiocatheter, a needle attached to a syringe, or a Vacutainer). The general purposes of venipuncture are to collect blood, instill a medication, start an IV infusion, or inject a radiopaque substance for x-ray examination of a body part or system. The present skill deals with obtaining a blood specimen. Skill 13-2 discusses venipuncture for the purpose of initiating an IV infusion.

Nursing Diagnoses

Client data derived during the assessment reveal defining characteristics to support the following nursing diagnoses in clients requiring this skill:

Anxiety
Injury, high risk for
Skin integrity, impaired, high risk for
Pain

Equipment

Disposable gloves
Specimen tubes
Alcohol and Betadine (povidone-iodine) cleaning swabs
Rubber tourniquet
Towel to place under client's arm
Sterile gauze pads (2 × 2)
Band-Aid or adhesive tape

Syringe method
   Sterile needles (20- to 21-gauge for adult; 23- to 25-gauge for
      child)
   Sterile syringe of appropriate size
Vacutainer method
   Vacutainer tube with needle holder
   Sterile double-ended needles

Steps	Rationale
1. Wash hands and apply disposable gloves.	Reduces transmission of microorganisms. Gloves should be worn when handling items soiled by body fluids (CDC, 1987; OSHA, 1991).
2. Gather all equipment needed and bring to client.	Maintains organization and avoids your having to leave client while you get more equipment.
3. Close bedside curtain or room door.	Provides for client's privacy.
4. Organize equipment on clutter-free surface.	Reduces risk of contamination and accidents.
5. Assist client to supine or semi-Fowler position with his arm extended straight. Place small towel under upper arm.	Stabilizes client's arm and provides easy access to venipuncture site.
6. Open sterile packages using sterile technique.	Prevents contamination of sterile objects.
7. Select distal site in vein to be used. Veins frequently used for blood sampling include those in antecubital fossa and those in lower arm.	If sclerosing or other damage occurs to vein, proximal site in same vein is still usable.
8. If possible, place client's arm in dependent position.	Permits venous dilation, thereby improving visibility of vein.

Steps	Rationale
9. Place tourniquet 5 to 15 cm (2 to 6 inches) above venipuncture site. Encircle client's arm and pull one end of tourniquet tightly over other, looping one end under other. Do not use a knot.	Allows vein to distend with blood, for better visibility. Permits quick release of tourniquet with one hand.
10. Palpate distal pulse below tourniquet.	Pressure from tourniquet should not impede arterial flow.
11. Select well-dilated vein. It may help to have client make fist. Do not keep tourniquet on longer than 1 to 2 minutes.	Muscle contraction increases venous distention. Prolonged tourniquet time may cause venous stasis and thereby alter test results.
12. Clean venipuncture site with povidone-iodine (Betadine) solution and follow with alcohol. Move in circular motion out from site approximately 5 cm (2 inches).	Betadine is a topical anti-infective; alcohol, a topical antiseptic. Together these agents reduce skin surface bacteria.
13. Remove needle cover from syringe or Vacutainer and inform client that he is about to feel a stick.	Client has better control over his anxiety when he knows what to expect.
14. Place thumb or forefinger of your nondominant hand 2.5 cm (1 inch) below site and pull client's skin taut toward you.	Stabilizes vein and prevents rolling during needle insertion.
15. Hold syringe or Vacutainer and needle at 15- to 30-degree angle from client's arm with bevel of needle up.	Reduces chance of penetrating both sides of vein during insertion. Bevel up causes less trauma to vein.

Steps	Rationale
16. Slowly insert needle into vein.	Prevents puncture of entire vein.
17. With syringe, pull back gently on plunger while securing barrel. Hold Vacutainer securely and advance specimen tube into needle of holder.	Secure hold on syringe or Vacutainer prevents needle from advancing. Pulling on syringe plunger or inserting tube creates vacuum needed to draw blood into syringe or Vacutainer.
18. Note flow of blood into syringe or tube.	If blood fails to appear, indicates that needle is not in vein or vacuum has been lost in specimen tube.
19. Obtain desired amount of blood.	Test results are more accurate when specified amount is drawn.
20. Once specimen obtained, release tourniquet.	Reduces bleeding at site when needle is withdrawn.
21. Remove needle from vein: place gauze 2 × 2 or alcohol pad over venipuncture site without applying pressure. Using other hand, withdraw needle by pulling straight back from venipuncture site.	Pressure over needle can cause discomfort. Straight removal of needle from vein prevents injury to vein and other surrounding tissues.
22. Apply pressure to site.	Pressure controls bleeding. If client has been anticoagulated, pressure may be necessary for 3 to 5 minutes to prevent hematoma formation.
23. For blood obtained by syringe, transfer specimen to tube. Insert needle through stopper of blood tube and allow vacuum to fill tube. Do not force.	Vacuum present in specimen tube causes blood to enter. Forcing blood into tube can cause hemolysis.

Steps	Rationale
24. For blood tubes containing additives, gently rotate back and forth 8 to 10 times.	Additives mixed to prevent clotting.
25. Inspect puncture site for bleeding and apply Band-Aid.	Keeps puncture site clean and controls final oozing.
26. Attach properly completed identification label to each tube, affix requisition, and send to lab.	Tests should be performed properly. Incorrect labeling can cause diagnostic error.
27. Dispose of needles, syringes, and soiled equipment; remove gloves and wash hands.	Reduces transmission of microorganisms.

Nurse Alert

Pressure must be applied to the venipuncture site in clients with a bleeding disorder or low platelet count or in those receiving anticoagulant therapy. It will decrease the risk of hematoma formation.

Client Teaching

If a woman has impaired lymphatic drainage (as may occur following a mastectomy), she should be instructed to tell care givers to avoid blood sampling from that arm. Impaired lymphatic drainage results in edema, and venipuncture in that extremity is difficult. Lack of lymphatic flow also predisposes the client to infection from skin puncture.

Pediatric Considerations

The nurse should not make numerous punctures in a child's arm for blood sampling. This can be extremely upsetting. A young child who requires venous sampling may need restraining by a staff member or parent. This will help immobilize the limb and prevent sudden movement that could result in serious injury to the blood vessel.

Geriatric Considerations

A frail, elderly client's veins are fragile, and venipuncture becomes more difficult. The nurse should carefully assess such a client before venipuncture so he does not have to be repeatedly stuck with the needle. Because the elderly client's veins are fragile, bleeding may occur more easily in the tissues once the needle is withdrawn.

Initiating Intravenous Therapy

Venipuncture is a technique in which a vein is punctured transcutaneously by a sharp rigid stylet, such as an angiocatheter, or by a needle attached to a syringe. The major use of this technique is to initiate and maintain IV fluid therapy. In many settings the nurse has primary responsibility for initiating IV therapy with an angiocatheter.

Potential Nursing Diagnoses

Client data derived during the assessment reveal defining characteristics to support the following nursing diagnoses in clients requiring this skill:

Fluid volume deficit, actual or high risk for
Infection, high risk for

Equipment

Correct IV solution
Proper needle/catheter for venipuncture
For IV fluid infusion
    Administration set (choice depends on type of solution and rate of administration; infants and children require microdrop tubing, which provides 60 gtt/ml)
    0.22 μm filter (if required by agency policy or if particulate matter is likely)
    Extension tubing (used when a longer IV line is necessary)
For heparin lock
    IV plug
    IV loop or short piece of tubing (if necessary)
    1 to 3 ml of saline or heparinized saline (10 to 100 U/ml)
    Syringes
Tourniquet

Disposable gloves
Arm board
2 × 2 gauze and povidone-iodine ointment; or, for transparent
dressing, povidone-iodine solution
Tape that is cut and ready to use
Towel to place under client's hand
Intravenous pole
Special gown with snaps at shoulder seams (makes removal with
IV tubing easier)—if available

Steps	Rationale
1. Wash hands.	Reduces transmission of micro-organisms.
2. Organize equipment on clutter-free bedside stand or over-bed table.	Reduces risk of contamination and accidents.
3. Open sterile packages using aseptic technique.	Prevents contamination of sterile objects.
4. For IV fluid administration: a. Check solution, using "five rights" of drug administration. Make sure prescribed additives, such as potassium and vitamins, have been added. Check solution for color, clarity, and expiration date.	IV solutions are medications and should be carefully checked to reduce risk of error. Solutions that are discolored, contain particles, or are expired are not to be used.
b. When using bottled IV solution, remove metal cap and metal and rubber disks beneath cap. For plastic IV solution bags, remove plastic sheath over IV tubing port.	Permits entry of infusion tubing into solution.
c. Open infusion set, maintaining sterility of both ends.	Prevents bacteria from entering infusion equipment and bloodstream.

Steps	Rationale
d. Place roller clamp about 2 to 4 cm (1 to 2 inches) below drip chamber and move roller clamp to "off" position (Fig. 171).	Close proximity of roller clamp to drip chamber allows more accurate regulation of flow rate. Moving clamp to "off" prevents accidental spillage of fluid on client, nurse, bed, or floor.

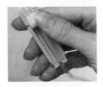

Fig. 171

e. Insert infusion set into fluid bag or bottle. ■ Remove protective cover from IV bag without touching opening (Fig. 172).	Maintains sterility of solution.

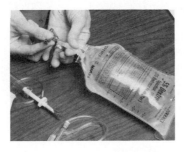

Fig. 172

Steps	Rationale
■ Remove protector cap from tubing insertion spike, not touching spike, and insert spike into opening of IV bag (Fig. 173). Or insert spike into black rubber stopper of IV bottle. Cleanse rubber stopper with antiseptic before insertion of spike.	Prevents contamination of solution from contaminated insertion spike.

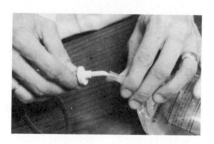

Fig. 173

f. Fill infusion tubing.

■ Compress drip chamber and release, allowing it to fill ⅓ to ½ full (Fig. 174).	Creates suction effect; fluid enters drip chamber to prevent air from entering tubing.
■ Remove needle protector and release roller clamp to allow fluid to travel from drip chamber through tubing to needle adapter. Return roller clamp to off position after tube is filled.	Removes air from tubing and permits tubing to fill with solution. Closing the clamp prevents accidental loss of fluid.

Steps   Rationale

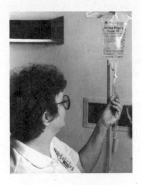

Fig. 174

■ Be certain tubing is clear   Large air bubbles can act as
  of air and air bubbles.   emboli. Remove air by allowing
                                     fluid to flow through tubing un-
                                     til tubing is free of air. Collect
                                     excess solution in basin and
                                     discard.

■ Replace needle protector.   Maintains system sterility.

5. For heparin lock:
   a. If a loop or short tubing   Removes air to prevent intro-
      is needed because of an   duction into the vein.
      awkward IV site place-
      ment, use sterile tech-
      nique to connect the IV
      plug to the loop or tub-
      ing. Inject 1 to 3 ml
      saline through the plug
      into the loop or tubing.

6. Select appropriate IV nee-   Necessary to puncture vein and
   dle or over-the-needle cath-   instill IV fluid.
   eter (ONC).

7. Select distal site of vein to   If sclerosing or damage to vein
   be used.   occurs, proximal site of same
                                     vein is still usable.

Steps	Rationale
8. If large amount of body hair is present at needle insertion site, clip it.	Reduces risk of contamination from bacteria on hair. Also assists in maintaining dressing intact and makes removal of tape less painful. Shaving may cause microabrasions and predispose to infection (Roth, 1992).
9. If possible, place extremity in dependent position.	Permits venous dilation and visibility.
10. Place tourniquet 10 to 12 cm (5 to 6 inches) above insertion site. Tourniquet should obstruct venous, not arterial, flow (Fig. 175). Check presence of distal pulse.	Diminished arterial flow prevents venous filling.

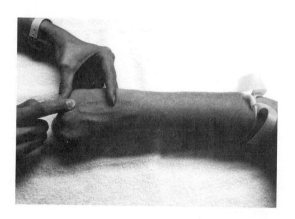

Fig. 175

11. Apply disposable gloves. Eye protection and mask can be worn to prevent spraying of blood on nurse's mucous membranes.	Decreases exposure to HIV, hepatitis, and other blood-borne organisms (CDC, 1987).

Steps	Rationale
12. Place needle adapter end of infusion set nearby on sterile gauze or towel.	Permits smooth, quick connection of infusion to IV needle once vein is punctured.
13. Select well-dilated vein. Methods to foster vein dilation include:	
■ Stroking the extremity from distal to proximal below the proposed venipuncture site.	Increases the volume of blood in the vein at the venipuncture site.
■ Opening and closing the fist.	Muscle contraction increases the amount of blood in the extremity.
■ Light tapping over the vein.	Fosters venous dilation.
■ Applying warmth to the extremity, for example, with a warm washcloth.	Increases blood supply and fosters venous dilation.
14. Cleanse insertion site with firm, circular motion with povidone-iodine solution; refrain from touching the cleansed site; allow the site to dry for at least 30 seconds. If the client is allergic to iodine, use 70% alcohol for 60 seconds (Fig. 176).	Povidone-iodine is a topical antiinfective that reduces skin surface bacteria; touching would introduce organisms from the nurse's hand to the site. Povidone-iodine must dry to be effective.
15. Perform venipuncture. Anchor vein by placing thumb over vein and by stretching the skin against the direction of insertion 2 to 3 inches distal to the site. *Butterfly needle:* Hold needle at 20- to 30-degree angle with bevel up slightly distal to actual site of venipuncture.	Places needle parallel to vein. When vein is punctured, risk of puncturing posterior vein wall is reduced.

Steps   Rationale

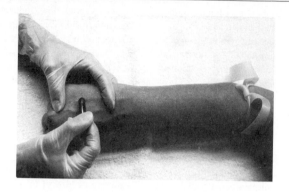

Fig. 176

ONC: Insert with bevel up
at 20- to 30-degree angle
slightly distal to actual site
of venipuncture in the direction of the vein (Fig.
177).

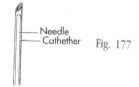

Needle
Cathether   Fig. 177

16. Look for blood return
    through tubing of butterfly
    needle or flashback cham-
    ber of ONC, indicating that
    needle has entered vein.
    Lower needle until almost
    flush with skin. Advance
    butterfly needle until hub
    rests at venipuncture site.
    Advance ONC catheter ¼
    inch into vein and then
    loosen stylet (Fig. 178).
    Advance catheter into vein
    until hub rests at venipunc-
    ture site. Do not reinsert
    the stylet once it is loos-
    ened.

Reinsertion of the stylet can
cause catheter breakage in the
vein.

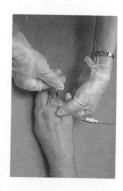

Fig. 178

Steps	Rationale
17. Stabilizing catheter with one hand, release tourniquet and remove stylet from ONC. Do not recap the stylet. quickly connect needle adapter of administration set or heparin lock to hub of ONC or butterfly tubing. Do not touch point of entry of needle adaptor.	Permits venous flow, reduces backflow of blood, and allows connection with administration set. Occupational transmission of HIV and hepatitis B is most commonly caused by needlestick injury (Gerberding, 1990). Prompt connection of infusion set maintains patency of vein. Maintains sterility.
18. Release roller clamp to begin infusion at a rate to maintain patency of IV line (not necessary with a heparin lock).	Permits venous flow and prevents clotting of vein and obstruction of flow of IV solution.
19. Secure IV catheter or needle. (Procedures can differ; check agency policy.) ■ Place narrow piece (½ inch) of tape under catheter with sticky side up and cross tape over catheter (Fig. 179).	Prevents accidental removal of catheter from vein. Prevents back-and-forth motion, which can irritate the vein and introduce bacteria on the skin into the vein.

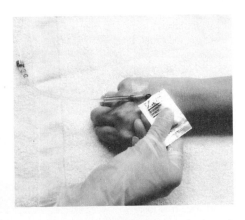

Fig. 179

Steps	Rationale
■ If gauze dressing is used, place povidone-iodine ointment at venipuncture site. If transparent dressing is used, place povidone-iodine solution at site; allow solution to dry.	Topical antiseptic germicide reduces bacteria on skin and decreases risk of local or systemic infection. Use of solution increases adherence of transparent dressing.
■ Place second piece of narrow tape directly across hub of catheter.	
■ Place 2 × 2 gauze pad over insertion site and catheter hub and secure with 1-inch piece of tape or place transparent dressing over IV site in direction of hair growth (Fig. 180). Do not cover connection between IV tubing and catheter hub.	Dressing protects site from bacterial contamination. Connection between administration set and hub needs to be uncovered to facilitate changing the tubing if necessary.

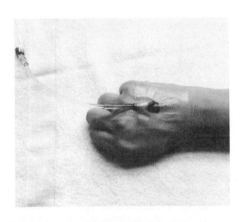

Fig. 180

Steps	Rationale
■ Secure a loop of infusion tubing to dressing with piece of 1-inch tape.	Stabilizes connection of administration set to catheter. Prevents weight of tubing from pulling catheter or needle out of venipuncture site.
20. For *IV fluid administration*, adjust flow rate to correct drops per minute (Skill 13-4).	Maintains correct rate of flow for IV solution.
■ For *heparin lock*, flush with 1 to 3 ml of sterile saline or heparinized saline (10 to 100 U/ml).	Maintains patency of IV catheter.
21. Write date and time of placement of IV line and gauge of catheter on dressing.	Provides immediate access to data as to when IV was inserted and when subsequent dressing changes are needed.
22. Remove gloves. Discard supplies and wash hands.	Reduces transmission of microorganisms.
23. Record in nurse's notes type of fluid, insertion site, flow rate, size and type catheter or needle, when infusion was begun, and how client tolerated procedure. A special parenteral therapy flowsheet may be used.	Documents initiation of therapy as ordered by physician. A special form provides a record of total intravenous therapy.

Nurse Alert

Venipuncture is contraindicated in a site that shows signs of infection, infiltration, or thrombosis. Infection is indicated by redness, tenderness, swelling, and warmth. Infiltration is identified by localized edema, blanching, and coolness of the surrounding tissues. Thrombosis is indicated by pain, swelling, and inflammation along the vein. To avoid displacement of the angiocatheter, an arm board is used.

Client Teaching

Clients and their families should be instructed not to move the extremity with the angiocatheter in place. Excessive motion can cause the angiocatheter to become displaced, resulting in an infiltration.

Pediatric Considerations

Most IV infusions in pediatric clients require a 22- to 24-gauge ONC (Whaley and Wong, 1993). When child is critically ill or long-term IV access is anticipated, surgical cutdown may be used to access a larger vein.

Geriatric Considerations

In older clients, use the smallest gauge possible. This is less traumatizing to the vein and allows better blood flow to provide increased hemodilution of the IV solution or medications (Coulter, 1992). Using an angle of 5 to 15 degrees on insertion is helpful because the elderly person's veins are more superficial (Coulter, 1992).

Initiating Peripherally
Inserted Central
Catheters

Peripherally inserted central catheters (PICCs) provide alternate access when the client requires intermediate-length (greater than 7 days to 3 months or longer) venous access. The PICC can be inserted by an RN. In comparison to centrally placed venous catheters, the PICC has less risk of pneumothorax, hemothorax, or air embolism, and costs less. Compared with peripheral IV catheters, the PICC can be kept in place longer (more than 48 to 72 hours), costs less, and is associated with less risk of infiltration and phlebitis because the IV fluids and medications are diluted in the greater volume of blood flow present in the larger veins (subclavian or superior vena cava) where the tip of the catheter is placed. For the catheter to be successfully placed, the client must have a palpable cephalic or basilic vein in the antecubital fossa. In addition to phlebitis, other complications associated with PICC use include clotting and leaking or breaking of the catheter.

Potential Nursing Diagnoses

Client data derived during the assessment reveal defining characteristics to support the following nursing diagnosis in clients requiring this skill:

> Fluid volume deficit, high risk for
> Infection, high risk for

Equipment

(Many manufacturers of peripherally inserted central catheters provide an insertion kit that provides all the required equipment; check how equipment is supplied in each agency.)

2 pairs of sterile gloves
2 drapes (1 fenestrated, 1 nonfenestrated)
Sterile forceps (nontoothed)
Sterile scissors
2 sterile 4 × 4 gauze pads
Tourniquet
3 Povidone-iodine swab sticks
3 alcohol swab sticks
2 sterile 2 × 2 gauze pads
Transparent dressing
Steri-strips
6 10-ml syringes with 1-inch, 21-gauge needles
4-inch extension tubing (one for each lumen)
Injection cap (one for each lumen)
2 10-ml vials of sterile normal saline for injection
10-ml vial of heparin 10 to 100 U/ml
Peripherally inserted central catheter (size depends on size of client's vein and type of infusion ordered)
2 tape measures (one sterile and one unsterile)
Face mask, gown, and goggles

Steps	Rationale
1. Review physician's order for client's name, type of catheter, type of infusion, desired placement of the catheter.	Ensures safe and correct initiation of the PICC. The catheter can be placed in either the subclavian vein or in the superior vena cava.
2. Know agency's policy concerning personnel who may start PICCs.	Most agencies require special training for persons who insert PICCs.
3. Explain the procedure to the client, including position that will be used and possible complications.	Providing information helps to minimize anxiety.

Steps	Rationale
4. Verify that a consent form has been signed.	Many agencies require a consent form.
5. Measure circumference of client's upper arm.	Provides a baseline for subsequent comparison to determine swelling, which can be associated with the advent of complications.
6. Wash hands.	Reduces transmission of microorganisms.
7. Organize equipment on clutter-free bedside stand or overbed table.	Reduces risk of contamination and accidents.
8. Identify an appropriate vein in the antecubital fossa by placing a tourniquet around the right upper arm close to the axilla and examining the veins in the antecubital fossa; release tourniquet, leaving it in place beneath the arm.	Either the basilic or the cephalic vein may be used; the basilic vein is preferred because it is less tortuous. Veins that are sclerosed (often from frequent blood drawing) should be avoided because the catheter will be difficult to advance. Releasing the tourniquet prevents venous engorgement.
9. Position the client flat in bed with the arm at a 90-degree angle (Fig. 181).	This provides a straighter course for advancing the catheter to the large veins in the chest.
10. Measure the distance from the insertion site to the proposed site for the catheter tip. For subclavian placement, measure from the proposed insertion site up the arm to the shoulder and across to the midclavicular line. For superior vena cava placement, continue to the sternal notch and down to the third intercostal space on the right of the sternum.	Desired position of the catheter may be indicated in the physician's order or by the type of therapy to be given (total parenteral nutrition and any irritating solution should be infused in the superior vena cava where the blood flow is highest). These landmarks correspond to the venous structures underneath.

Steps	Rationale

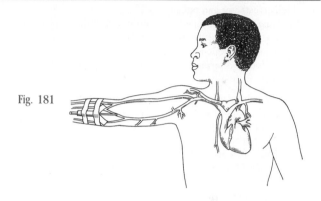

Fig. 181

11. Put on mask and gown. Client may also wear mask. — Reduces transmission of microorganisms.

12. Open the sterile supplies or kit. Using the kit's wrap as a sterile field, arrange supplies for efficient use; drop the 4 × 4 gauze, the extension tubings, and the injection cap(s) onto the field. Cleanse the top of the normal saline vial with alcohol and set aside. — Provides and sterile working surface. Facilitates efficient technique by having all supplies ready and accessible.

13. Clip hair if necessary. — Assists in maintaining adherence of dressing and tape. Makes removal of dressing less painful. Clipping prevents the microabrasions caused by shaving, thus decreasing the risk for infection.

14. Don sterile gloves. — Reduces transmission of microorganisms.

Steps	Rationale
15. Prepare catheter and tubing:	
■ Using the sterile tape measure to measure the catheter to the length previously determined plus 1 inch.	Ensures that distal tip of catheter will be properly positioned. The extra length will extend out from the venipuncture site.
■ Using the sterile scissors, cut the catheter at the appropriate length. Check agency policy about whether a straight cut or a 45-degree bevel cut should be used. Another method is to insert the uncut catheter the appropriate length and coil the excess catheter on the arm.	A straight cut may prevent the catheter end from lying on the intima and obstructing blood flow.
■ Attach the injection cap to the extension tubing (one set for each lumen). Using a 4 × 4 gauze to hold the vial, draw up 5 ml of normal saline into a syringe for each lumen of the catheter and flush each cap and tubing with 2 ml. Remove the needle from the syringe and flush the catheter, leaving the syringe in place. If the catheter is a triple-lumen catheter, two lumens must be flushed; all three lumens must be flushed if a guidewire is not used for insertion.	Removes air from tubing and catheter; ensures patency of catheter, detects any leaks.
■ Inspect the equipment for defects such as cracks or kinks. Verify patency of introducer.	Ensures proper function during and after insertion.

Steps	Rationale

Prepare the insertion site:

■ Place a sterile drape under the access arm.

Reduces transmission of microorganisms.

■ Vigorously scrub the insertion site using three alcohol swab sticks followed by three povidone-iodine swab sticks. A circular area from the middle of the forearm to the middle of the upper arm should be cleaned with each swab stick, starting at the venipuncture site and cleansing in a circular motion. Let the povidone-iodine dry completely.

Alcohol defats the skin; povidone-iodine is a topical antiinfective that reduces skin surface bacteria. The circular motion moves bacteria on the skin away from the insertion site. Use of separate swab sticks prevents bacteria from being reintroduced to the venipuncture site. Povidone-iodine must dry to be effective.

16. Remove gloves; reapply tourniquet if a single non-sterile tourniquet is used.

Tourniquet is not sterile; application of tourniquet impedes venous blood flow, resulting in an engorged vein to foster ease of venipuncture.

17. Don a new pair of sterile gloves; use talc-free gloves or rinse gloves with sterile water.
Place a sterile 4 × 4 over the tourniquet or apply a sterile tourniquet.

Reduces the transmission of microorganisms; rinsing gloves prevents talc adherence to the catheter.
Allows removal or tourniquet without contaminating glove.

Steps	Rationale
18. Place fenestrated drape over the insertion site, being careful to avoid contamination of the site.	Provides a sterile field around the venipuncture site.
Some agencies recommend administration of 0.1 to 0.2 ml of 1% lidocaine at the insertion site. Insert the introducer needle at a 20- to 30-degree angle, bevel up. Look for a brisk blood return through the introducer. Verify that blood return is venous, not arterial (arterial blood is pulsatile and bright red).	Local anesthetic reduces discomfort. Angle lessens risk of puncture of posterior wall of vein. The introducer is large bore. The brachial vein is close to the brachial artery and the artery may be inadvertently cannulated.
19. Lower the introducer parallel to the skin and advance ¼ to ½ inch further into the vein.	Ensures that vein is securely cannulated.
20. Insert the catheter through the introducer needle and advance it slowly approximately 2 to 3 inches using the nontoothed forceps. Agency policy differs concerning the use of a guidewire or stylet. If a guidewire is used ensure that it remains well within the lumen of the PICC during insertion. Take care that the catheter remains on the sterile field during insertion.	Allows the catheter to travel through the introducer into the vein. Slow advancement prevents trauma to the intima of the vein (Loughran, Edwards, and McClure, 1992). The guidewire provides more rigidity to the catheter to aid insertion. No significant difference was found between clients whose PICCs were begun with guidewires and those for whom guidewires were not used (Loughran, Edwards, and McClure, 1992). If the catheter leaves the sterile field, it is considered contaminated.
21. Release the tourniquet, using the sterile 4 × 4 gauze if a nonsterile tourniquet is used.	Allows further catheter advancement. Prevents contamination of glove.

Steps	Rationale
22. Advance the catheter an additional 6 inches (or more depending on client size) until tip of catheter is at the shoulder. The catheter is marked at 10-cm intervals to facilitate identification of location of tip.	The client's position needs to change to facilitate entry into the subclavian vein.
23. Instruct the client to turn the head toward the side of the venous access and drop the chin to the chest.	This position closes the internal jugular vein and prevents accidental cannulation.
24. Continue to slowly advance the catheter until the predetermined length is reached.	Ensures proper placement of the tip of the catheter in the superior vena cava.
25. Fully withdraw the introducer needle. Either use the forceps to maintain the position of the catheter or apply light pressure 2 inches above the insertion site while the introducer is withdrawn.	The introducer is removed to prevent accidental puncture of the vein. Ensures that the catheter will not be withdrawn with the introducer. Pressure any closer to the introducer may cause the introducer to nick the catheter.
NEVER WITHDRAW THE CATHETER THROUGH THE INTRODUCER NEEDLE.	May shear off the catheter, causing a catheter embolism.
26. When the introducer is out, press the wings together until they snap, then peel the needle from around the catheter.	Removes the needle so that the catheter cannot be inadvertently punctured.
■ Tell the client that a snapping sound will be heard.	Prevents anxiety.
27. Remove the guidewire using a gentle twisting motion.	Allow use of the lumen, prevents damage to the catheter and vein.

Steps	Rationale
28. Attach a syringe filled with 3 ml of normal saline to the lumen where the guidewire had been, aspirate for a blood return, and flush the catheter.	Verifies patency of distal lumen, prevents clotting.
29. Remove the syringe from each lumen and attach the extension tubing and cap to the lumen.	Prevents blood loss, maintains closed system.
30. Anchor the hub of the catheter to the skin with Steri-strips placed over the catheter's hub. Some agencies suggest that the PICC should be sutured in place.	Maintains the catheter's position for long-term use.
31. Place 2 × 2 gauze pads over the insertion site. Cover this with a transparent dressing.	Provides pressure on the insertion site for 24 hours to control oozing caused by large-gauge introducer.
32. Coil the extension tubings and tape securely to the client's arm. Do not pull or apply undue pressure to the catheter when manipulating it. Label dressing with date and time of insertion and gauge of catheter.	Prevents inadvertent dislodgement. Prevents catheter breakage.
33. Draw up 3 ml of heparin solution for each lumen of the catheter and flush each lumen:	Maintains patency of each lumen.
34. Dispose of equipment appropriately. Wash hands.	Reduces transmission of microorganisms.
35. Follow agency policy for x-ray verification of placement.	X-ray examination is usually done to verify placement in the superior vena cava before start of infusion therapy.

Steps	Rationale
36. Record PICC's gauge and length, insertion site, data and time of insertion, radiographic confirmation of location of catheter tip, presence or absence of signs and symptoms of complications.	Documents correct initiation of therapy, client's response.

Nurse Alert

When the PICC is to be placed in the superior vena cava, try to use the dominant arm because movement accelerates blood flow and reduces the risk of dependent edema. However, the placement of some catheters and their dressings may restrict flexion of the elbow on the side of insertion. Use an 18-gauge or larger catheter when infusion of blood or blood products is anticipated.

Teaching Considerations

Instruct client and caregiver about signs and symptoms of the most common complications of phlebitis, clotting, and catheter leaking or breaking and how to handle them. Because the dressing is the anchor for the PICC, the client and caregiver need to notify the nurse if the dressing becomes loose. The nurse does the dressing change. If the PICC becomes clotted, the client should promptly seek care so that declotting measures can be instituted.

Pediatric Considerations

An advantage of the use of PICCs for neonates is the longer duration of use as compared with traditional peripheral catheters (average duration was 24 days in a study by Oellrich et al, 1991); this decreases the frequency of noxious stimuli that can have adverse physiologic results such as lower oxygen saturation. In neonates the antecubital veins, long saphenous vein, superficial temporal vein, external jugular vein, popliteal vein, veins in the ankle, and axillary veins may be used.

SKILL 13-4

Regulating Intravenous Flow Rates

Once an IV infusion is in place and secured, the nurse has the responsibility of regulating its rate according to physician's orders. An infusion rate that is too slow can lead to further cardiovascular and circulatory collapse in a client who is dehydrated, in shock, or critically ill. A too-rapid infusion rate can result in fluid overload. The nurse calculates the infusion rate to prevent incorrect fluid administration.

Potential Nursing Diagnoses

Client data derived during the assessment reveal defining characteristics to support the following nursing diagnoses in clients requiring this skill:

Fluid volume deficit, high risk for
Fluid volume excess

Equipment

Paper and pencil
Watch with second hand

Steps	Rationale
1. Read physician's orders and follow "five rights" to be sure that you have correct solution and proper additives.	IV fluids are medications; following the "five rights" decreases chance of medication error.
2. Know calibration in drops per milliliter (gtt/ml) of infusion set: a. Microdrip 60 gtt/ml	Microdrip tubing, also called pediatric tubing, universally delivers 60 gtt/ml and is used when small or very precise volumes are required.

Steps	Rationale

    b. Macrodrip (Metheny, 1992)

Abbott Lab	15 gtt/ml
Travenol Lab	10 gtt/ml
McGraw Lab	15 gtt/ml

3. Select one of the following formulas to calculate flow rate after determining ml/hr (if necessary):

$$\text{ml/hr} = \frac{\text{total infusion (ml)}}{\text{hours of infusion}}$$

(1) $\dfrac{\text{ml/hr}}{60 \text{ minutes}} = $ ml/minute

(2) Drop factor × ml/minute = drops/minute

—OR—

$$\frac{\text{ml/hr} \times \text{drop factor}}{60 \text{ minutes}} = \text{drops/minute}$$

4. IV fluids are usually ordered for 24-hour period, indicating how long each liter of fluid should run. For example:

    Bottle 1— 1000 ml D5W c̄ 20 mEq KCl 8 AM - 4 PM

    Bottle 2— 1000 ml D5W c̄ 20 mEq KCl 4 PM - 12 MN

    Bottle 3— 1000 ml D5W c̄ 20 mEq KCl 12 MN - 8 AM

    Total 24-hour IV intake: 3000 ml.

Determines volume of fluid that should infuse hourly.

5. To determine hourly rate, divide volume by hours:

$$\frac{3000 \text{ ml}}{24} = 125 \text{ ml/hr.}$$

Provides even infusion over 24 hours.

6. IV fluid orders for 24-hour period may also be written as:

    Bottle 1— 1000 ml D5W c̄ 20 mEq KCl 8 AM - 4 PM

    Bottle 2— 1000 D5W c̄ 20 mEq KCl 4 PM - 12 MN

    Bottle 3— 500 D5W 12 MN - 8 AM.

Fluid needs vary. Rate must be as ordered.

Steps	Rationale

Hourly rate would be:

$$\frac{2000}{16} = 125 \text{ ml}$$
(8 AM - 12 MN)

$$\frac{500}{8} = 63 \text{ ml}$$
(12 MN - 8 AM).

7. Place adhesive tape on IV bag next to volume markings. This figure is based on 125 ml in 8-hour period (Fig. 182). | Time taping of IV bag gives you visual cue as to whether fluids are being administered at proper rate.

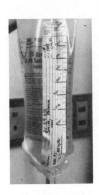

Fig. 182

8. Once hourly rate has been determined, minute rate is calculated based on drop factor of infusion set. | Allows you to calculate hourly flow rate based on this formula:
$$\frac{\text{Total volume} \times \text{Drop factor}}{\text{Infusion time in minutes}}$$

9. Using formula, calculate minute flow rates:
Bottle 1 (1000 ml c̄ 20 mEq KCl)
Microdrip | Volume is divided by time.

$$\frac{125 \text{ ml} \times 60 \text{ gtt/ml}}{60 \text{ minutes}} = \frac{7500 \text{ gtt}}{60 \text{ min}} = 125 \text{ gtt/min}$$

Steps	Rationale

Macrodrip

$$\frac{125 \text{ ml} \times 15 \text{ gtt/ml}}{60 \text{ minutes}} = 31 \text{ to } 32 \text{ gtt/min}$$

10. Time the flow rate by counting drops in drip chamber for 1 minute by watch, then adjust roller clamp to increase or decrease speed of infusion. Check this rate hourly (Fig. 183).	Determines if fluids are being administered too slowly or too fast.

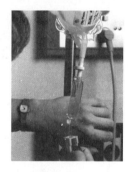

Fig. 183

11. Record in nurse's notes if IV is patent and infusing on time.	Documents IV status and client's response.

Nurse Alert

An IV that fails to infuse on time may be an early sign of infiltration. If an infusion pump is used, the nurse should still monitor the rate of flow of the IV solution at least hourly. If IV fluids are excessively slow or fast, the physician should be contacted for revision of the IV flow rate before the flow is increased or decreased.

Client Teaching

The client should be instructed to report any tenderness or swelling at the venipuncture site. If an infusion pump is used, the client should know its preset rate and the significance of alarms.

Pediatric Considerations

IV flows in children should always be maintained at the prescribed rate because fluid imbalances can occur rapidly. Pediatric settings usually require that infusion pumps or volume control devices be used with IV therapy.

Geriatric Considerations

Fluid imbalances occur rapidly in the older adult population. Careful monitoring of flow rates assists in preventing electrolyte imbalances and circulatory overload.

Changing Intravenous Solutions

The nurse changes IV solutions using sterile technique to discontinue a specific solution or to remove an empty solution container and reconnect the tubing to a new container.

Potential Nursing Diagnoses

Client data derived during assessment reveal defining characteristics to support the following nursing diagnosis in clients requiring this skill:

Infection, high risk for

Equipment

Correct IV solution (or D5W to maintain patency of IV line)
Roller clamps
IV pole and bag

Steps	Rationale
1. Wash hands.	Reduces transmission of microorganisms.
2. Have next IV solution prepared at least 1 hour before it is needed. If solution is prepared in pharmacy, be sure that it has been delivered to floor. Check that it is correct and properly labeled.	Prevents finding empty IV bag without having replacement bag. Also prevents medication error.
3. Prepare to change solution when it remains in neck of bag or bottle.	Prevents air from entering IV tubing and vein from clotting because of lack of IV flow.

Steps	Rationale
4. Be sure that drip chamber is half full.	Provides IV fluid while bag is being changed.
5. Prepare new solution for hanging: ■ Plastic bag—Remove protective cover from entry site. ■ Glass bottle—Remove metal cap, metal disk, and rubber disk.	Permits quick, smooth, and organized change from old solution to new.
6. Move roller clamp to reduce flow rate.	Prevents solution remaining in drip chamber from emptying.
7. Remove old solution bag or bottle from IV pole.	Brings work to eye level.
8. Quickly remove spike from old container and, without touching tip, insert it in new container.	Reduces risk that solution in drip chamber (Step 3) will run dry. Also maintains sterility.
9. Hang new bag.	Allows gravity to assist with delivery of fluid.
10. Check for air in tubing.	Reduces risk of embolus.
11. Make sure that drip chamber contains solution.	Reduces risk that air will enter tubing.
12. Regulate flow rate as prescribed.	Maintains measures to restore fluid balance.
13. Record in nurse's notes amount and type of fluid infused and amount and type of new fluid.	Documents that solution has infused and new infusion has been started.
14. Stabilize hub of IV catheter or needle. Gently pull out old tubing. Maintaining stability of hub, insert needle adapter of new tubing into hub.	Prevents accidental displacement of catheter or needle.
15. Open roller clamp.	Permits new intravenous solution to enter catheter or needle.

Steps	Rationale
16. Regulate IV drip according to physician's orders.	Maintains fluid and electrolyte balance.
17. Record in nurse's notes changing of tubing and solution.	Documents that measures to maintain sterility were carried out.
18. Wash your hands.	Reduces transmission of microorganisms.

Nurse Alert

An IV tubing change is easier if the nurse organizes it to occur when a new solution bag is being hung. There are times, however, when it is not possible to have the two procedures occur simultaneously, as when tubing is accidentally punctured with a needle.

Irrigating a
Heparin Lock

A heparin lock is an IV needle with a small "well" covered by a rubber diaphragm (Fig. 184). This device decreases costs by reducing the need for continuous IV therapy with clients who require only IV medications and not fluids. In addition, a heparin lock increases the client's mobility, safety, and comfort.

When clients have heparin locks, the lock must be flushed on a routine basis and after IV medications. Flushing of the heparin maintains patency of the cannulated vein. (Policies may differ from agency to agency as to the frequency of irrigation and the irrigant used.) This skill focuses on the irrigation of the heparin lock.

Fig. 184

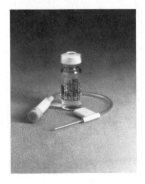

Potential Nursing Diagnoses

Client data derived during assessment reveal defining characteristics to support the following nursing diagnoses in clients requiring this skill:

Infection, high risk for

Pain

Equipment

Heparin flush solution: 1 ml/100 units or 1 ml/10 units
Sterile normal saline vial
Medication ticket, card, or form
Prepared medication
2 3-ml syringes used for heparin or saline flush
25-gauge needles to attach to syringes to irrigate heparin lock
Antiseptic swab
Watch with second hand—used for timing of IV bolus or IV pig-
    gyback medication

Steps	Rationale
1. Wash hands.	Reduces transmission of micro-organisms.
2. Verify physician's order and prepare medication.	Ensures that proper medication is given to the right client.
3. After preparing medication, apply small-gauge needle to syringe.	Used to insert through IV line or heparin lock.
4. Check client's identification by looking at armband and asking full name. Compare with medication ticket.	Ensures drug is administered to correct client.

5. Flush heparin lock.
a. Heparin only:
  ▪ Prepare a syringe with 1 ml of heparin flush solution.
  ▪ Prepare a syringe with 1 ml of normal saline. Attach 25-gauge needle to syringe.
b. Saline only:
  ▪ Prepare two syringes with 2 ml of normal saline each. Attach 25-gauge needle to each syringe.
	Flush solution keeps heparin lock patent after drug is administered.
	Used to assess for blood return in heparin lock.
	
	Normal saline has been found to be effective in keeping IV locks patent.

Steps	Rationale
c. Heparin and saline:	
■ Clean the lock's rubber diaphragm with the antiseptic swab.	Cleaning prevents introduction of microorganisms during needle insertion.
■ Insert needle of syringe containing normal saline through center of diaphragm. Pull back gently on syringe plunger and look for blood return.	Determines if IV needle or catheter is positioned in vein. (At times a heparin lock will not yield a blood return even though lock is patent.)
■ Flush reservoir with 1 cc saline by pushing slowly on the plunger.	Cleans needle and reservoir of blood.
■ Remove needle and saline-filled syringe.	
■ Clean the lock's diaphragm with the antiseptic swab.	Prevents transmission of infection.
■ Insert the needle of syringe containing prepared medication through center of diaphragm.	Using center of diaphragm prevents leakage.
■ Inject medication bolus slowly over several minutes. (Each medication has a recommended rate for bolus administration. Check package directions.) Use a watch to time the administration.	Rapid injection of an intravenous drug can kill a client.
■ After administering the bolus, withdraw the syringe.	
■ Clean the lock's diaphragm with an antiseptic swab.	Prevents transmission of infection.

Steps	Rationale
d. Heparin flush: ■ Insert needle of syringe containing the heparin through the diaphragm. Inject 1 ml heparin slowly, then remove syringe.	Maintains patency of needle by inhibiting clot formation. Diluted heparin avoids anticoagulation.
e. Saline flush: ■ If using only saline to flush the reservoir, inject 2 cc of saline after each use of the IV lock.	
6. Wash hands.	Reduces transmission of microorganisms.
7. Dispose of uncapped needles and syringes in proper container.	Prevents accidental needlesticks.
8. Record patency of heparin lock, drug, dosage, route, irrigation of heparin lock procedure, and assessment of venipuncture site.	Accurate documentation reduces risk of future medication errors. Provides data for ongoing assessment of heparin lock system.

Nurse Alert

Be sure to loosen tape or dressing over IV site to see it clearly before administering drug.

Administering a
Blood Transfusion

Blood products are ordered by the physician to restore circulatory blood volume, improve hemoglobin, or correct serum protein levels. Administration of blood or blood components is a nursing procedure.

Potential Nursing Diagnoses

Client data derived during assessment reveal defining characteristics to support the following nursing diagnoses in clients requiring this skill:

Fluid volume deficit, high risk for
Cardiac output, decreased

Equipment

In addition to that used to initiate an IV infusion
Normal saline IV solution, 0.9%
Infusion set with inline filter (Fig. 185).
Large catheter (18- or 19-gauge)
Correct blood product
Another nurse to double-check correct blood product with correct client
Disposable gloves

Steps	Rationale
1. Wash hands.	Reduces transmission of microorganisms.
2. Apply disposable gloves.	Reduces transmission of blood-borne pathogens. Gloves should be worn when handling items soiled by body fluids (CDC, 1987; OSHA, 1991).

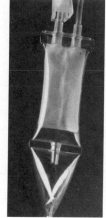

Fig. 185

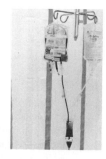

Fig. 186

Steps	Rationale
3. Explain procedure to client. Determine if there has been any previous transfusion and note reactions, if any.	Clients who have had blood transfusion in the past may have greater fear of transfusion.
4. Ask client to immediately report any of following symptoms: chills, headache, itching, rash.	These can be signs of a transfusion reaction. Prompt reporting and discontinuation of transfusion will help minimize reaction.
5. Be sure that client has signed any necessary consent forms.	Some agencies require clients to sign consent forms before receiving any blood component transfusions.
6. Establish IV line with large (18- or 19-gauge) catheter.	Permits infusion of whole blood and prevents hemolysis.
7. Use infusion tubing that has in-line filter. Tubing should also be Y-type administration set (Fig. 186).	Filter removes any debris and tiny clots from blood. Using Y-type set permits (a) administration of additional products or volume expanders easily and (b) immediate infusion of 0.9% sodium chloride solution after completion of initial infusion.

Steps	Rationale
8. Hang solution container of 0.9% normal saline to be administered after blood infusion.	Prevents hemolysis of red blood cells.
9. Follow agency protocol in obtaining blood products from blood bank. Request blood when you are ready to use it.	Whole blood or packed red blood cells must remain in a cold (1°-6° C) environment.
10. With another nurse, correctly identify blood product and client:	One nurse reads out loud while other nurse listens and double-checks information.
■ Check compatibility tag attached to blood bag and information on bag itself.	Verifies that ABO group, Rh type, and unit number match.
■ For whole blood, check ABO group and Rh type (on client's chart).	Verifies that they match those on compatibility tag and blood bag.
■ Double-check blood product with physician's order.	Verifies correct blood component.
■ Check expiration date on bag.	After 21 days, blood has only 70% to 80% of its original cells and 23 mEq/L of potassium.
■ Inspect blood for clots.	Anticoagulant, citrate-phosphate-dextrose (CPD), is added to blood and permits preserved blood to be stored for 21 days. Newer anticoagulant, citrate-phosphate-dextrose-adenine (CPD-A), allows storage for 35 days. If clots are present, return blood to blood bank.
11. Obtain baseline vital signs within 30 minutes before administering transfusion. Report any temperature elevation to the physician.	Verifies client's pretransfusion temperature, pulse, blood pressure, and respirations and allows detection of reaction by noting changes in vital signs.

Steps	Rationale
12. Have client void or empty urine drainage collection container.	If a transfusion reaction occurs, the urine specimen obtained needs to be urine produced after the initiation of the transfusion.
13. Open blood administration set.	Prepares blood administration tubing.
a. For Y-tubing administration, set all three roller clamps to "off" position.	Moving roller clamp(s) to "off" position prevents accidental spilling, and wasting of blood.
b. For single tubing administration, set roller clamp to "off" position.	
14. For Y-tubing:	Use of Y-tubing permits nurse to quickly switch from infusion of 0.9% normal saline to blood unit. Dextrose solutions are never used because they can cause coagulation of the donor blood. When unit is finished, nurse is able to maintain patency of vein by infusing normal saline. Y-tubing administration sets should be used when multiple blood transfusions are anticipated. Follow manufacturer's guidelines regarding number of units that can be given before tubing is changed.
a. Spike 0.9% normal saline IV bag.	
b. Prime tubing with 0.9% normal saline.	
■ Open roller clamp on Y-tubing connected to normal saline bag and release roller clamp on unused inlet tube until tubing from normal saline bag is filled.	Allows fluid to flow from normal saline bag to drip chamber.
■ Close clamp on unused tubing.	Prevents waste of IV solution.

Steps	Rationale
■ Squeeze sides of drip chamber. Allow filter to be partially covered.	Prevents air bubbles from entering system.
■ Open lower roller clamp and allow infusion tubing to fill with normal saline.	Removes all air from system.
■ Close lower roller clamp.	Prevents waste of IV fluid.
c. Gently invert blood bag 1 to 2 times to equally distribute cells. Spike blood or blood component container, open clamps on inlet tube and lower tubing, and fill tubing completely covering the filter with blood.	Prevents clumping of cells, which can block outlet of bag or lead to clotting. Fragile blood cells may be damaged if they hit an uncovered filter.
d. Close lower clamp.	
15. For single tubing administration: a. Spike blood unit. b. Squeeze drip chamber; allow filter to be filled with blood. c. Open roller clamp and allow infusion tubing to fill with blood.	Prepares administration filter and tubing with blood. Promotes quick connection of prepared infusion tubing to IV catheter.
d. When a single tubing administration set is used, another IV tubing with 0.9% normal saline infusing is piggybacked to the blood administration set. Use tape to secure all connections.	The blood product should not be piggybacked into the normal saline line to avoid forcing fragile blood cells through both a needle and an IV catheter, which could cause mechanical trauma to cells.

Steps	Rationale
16. Attach blood transfusion tubing to IV catheter maintaining sterility. Open lower clamp.	Initiates infusion of blood product into the client's vein.
17. Remain with client during first 15 to 30 minutes of transfusion. Initial flow rate during this time should be 2 to 5 ml/minute.	Most reactions occur during the first 15 to 30 minutes of a transfusion. Infusing a small amount initially minimizes the volume of blood to which the client is exposed, which limits the severity of the reaction. This also allows prompt treatment of a transfusion reaction.
18. Monitor client's vital signs: every 5 minutes for first 15 minutes; every 15 minutes for next hour; hourly until unit of blood is infused; for one hour after the infusion is completed.	Be alert for any change in vital signs that could be early warning of transfusion reaction.
19. Regulate infusion according to physician's orders. Packed cells usually run over 1½ to 2 hours while whole blood runs over 2 to 3 hours.	Client's condition dictates rate at which blood should infused. Drop factor for blood tubing is 10 gtt/ml. See Skill 13-4 for formula for regulating IV fluids.
20. After blood has infused, clear IV tubing with 0.9% normal saline and place blood bag in plastic bag to return to the lab.	Infuses remainder of blood in IV line; 0.9% normal saline prevents hemolysis of red cells.
21. Dispose of all supplies appropriately. Remove gloves and wash hands.	Reduces transmission of microorganisms.
22. Record type and amount of blood component administered and client's response to blood therapy. A separate transfusion record is usually used.	Documents administration of blood component and client's reaction.

Nurse Alert

Never inject any medication into an IV line with blood or a blood product infusing because of possible incompatibility and bacterial contamination of the blood product. When client requires rapid infusion of multiple units of blood, the infusion tubing itself should be warmed with a special blood warmer (LaRocca and Otto, 1989). A unit of blood and blood filter should not be allowed to hang longer than 4 hours because of danger of bacterial growth.

Teaching Considerations

Client is instructed to notify nurse of signs of itching, swelling, dizziness, dyspnea, or chest pain. Clients and caregivers are taught signs of long-term reactions, such as delayed hemolysis, so they can notify their doctor and receive treatment.

Pediatric Considerations

In the child, the first 50 ml of blood should be infused over 30 minutes. If no reaction occurs, flow rate is increased accordingly to infuse the remainder of 275 ml over 2-hour period (Whaley and Wong, 1991). Blood for the newborn is cross-matched with the mother's serum because it may have more antibodies than the newborn's and allows easier identification of an incompatibility.

Geriatric Considerations

Elderly clients may have decreased cardiac function or suffer from chronic anemia, thus they may require slower transfusion times.

NANDA-APPROVED
NURSING DIAGNOSES

Activity intolerance
Activity intolerance, high risk for
Adjustment, impaired
Airway clearance, ineffective
Anxiety
Aspiration, high risk for
Body image disturbance
Body temperature, altered, high risk for
Bowel incontinence
Breastfeeding, effective
Breastfeeding, ineffective
Breastfeeding, interrupted
Breathing pattern, ineffective
Cardiac output, decreased
Caregiver role strain
Caregiver role strain, high risk for
Communication, impaired verbal
Constipation
Constipation, colonic
Constipation, perceived
Coping, defensive
Coping, family: potential for growth
Coping, ineffective family: compromised
Coping, ineffective family: disabling
Coping, ineffective: individual
Decisional conflict (specify)
Denial, ineffective
Diarrhea
Disuse syndrome, high risk for
Diversional activity deficit

Dysreflexia
Family processes, altered
Fatigue
Fear
Fluid volume deficit (1)
Fluid volume deficit (2)
Fluid volume deficit, high risk for
Fluid volume excess
Gas exchange, impaired
Grieving, anticipatory
Grieving, dysfunctional
Growth and development, altered
Health maintenance, altered
Health-seeking behaviors (specify)
Home maintenance management, impaired
Hopelessness
Hyperthermia
Hypothermia
Incontinence, functional
Incontinence, reflex
Incontinence, stress
Incontinence, total
Incontinence, urge
Infant feeding pattern, ineffective
Infection, high risk for
Injury, high risk for
Knowledge deficit (specify)
Management of therapeutic regimen (individuals), ineffective
Mobility, impaired physical
Noncompliance (specify)
Nutrition, altered: less than body requirements
Nutrition, altered: more than body requirements
Nutrition, altered: high risk for more than body requirements
Oral mucous membrane, altered
Pain
Pain, chronic
Parental role conflict
Parenting, altered
Parenting, altered, high risk for
Peripheral neurovascular dysfunction, high risk for
Personal identity disturbance

Poisoning, high risk for
Post-trauma response
Powerlessness
Protection, altered
Rape-trauma syndrome
Rape-trauma syndrome: compound reaction
Rape-trauma syndrome: silent reaction
Relocation stress syndrome
Role performance, altered
Self-care deficit, bathing/hygiene
Self-care deficit, dressing/grooming
Self-care deficit, feeding
Self-care deficit, toileting
Self-esteem disturbance
Self-esteem, chronic low
Self-esteem, situational low
Self-mutilation, high risk for
Sensory/perceptual alterations (specify) (visual, auditory, kines-
    thetic, gustatory, tactile, olfactory)
Sexual dysfunction
Sexuality patterns, altered
Skin integrity, impaired
Skin integrity, impaired, high risk for
Sleep pattern disturbance
Social interaction, impaired
Social isolation
Spiritual distress (distress of the human spirit)
Suffocation, high risk for
Swallowing, impaired
Thermoregulation, ineffective
Thought processes, altered
Tissue integrity, impaired
Tissue perfusion, altered (specify type) (renal, cerebral, cardio-
    pulmonary, gastrointestinal, peripheral)
Trauma, high risk for
Unilateral neglect
Urinary elimination, altered
Urinary retention
Ventilation, inability to sustain spontaneous
Ventilatory weaning process, dysfunctional
Violence, high risk for: self-directed or directed at others

NORMAL REFERENCE
LABORATORY VALUES

Blood, plasma, or serum values

Determination	Reference Range	
	Conventional	SI
Acetoacetate plus acetone	0.3-2.0 mg/100 ml	3-20 mg/L
Aldolase	1.3-8.2 mU/ml	12-75 nmol · s^{-1}/L
Alpha amino nitrogen	3.0-5.5 mg/100 ml	2.1-3.9 mmol/L
Ammonia	80-110 μg/100 ml	47-65 μmol/L
Ascorbic acid	0.4-1.5 mg/100 ml	23-85 μmol/L
Barbiturate	0; coma level: phenobarbital, approximately 10 mg/100 ml; most other drugs, 1-3 mg/100 ml	0 μmol/L
Bilirubin (van den Bergh test)	1 minute: 0.4 mg/100 ml	Up to 7 μmol/L
	Direct: 0.4 mg/100 ml	Up to 17 μmol/L
	Total: 1.0 mg/100 ml	
	Indirect is total minus direct	
Blood volume	8.5%-9.0% of body weight in kg	80-85 ml/kg
Bromide	0; toxic level: 17 mEq/L	0 mmol/L
Bromsulfalein (BSP)	Less than 5% retention 45 min after 5 mg/kg IV	<0.051
Calcium	8.5-10.5 mg/100 ml (slightly higher in children)	2.1-2.6 mmol/L
Carbon dioxide content	24-30 mEq/L; 20-26 mEq/L in infants (as HCO$_3^-$)	24-30 mmol/L
Carbon monoxide	Symptoms with over 20% saturation	0(1)

Carotenoids	0.8-4.0 µg/ml	1.5-7.4 µmol/L
Ceruloplasmin	27-37 mg/100 ml	1.8-2.5 µmol/L
Chloride	100-106 mEq/L	100-106 mmol/L
Cholinesterase (pseudocholinesterase)	0.5 pH U or more/hr; 0.7 pH U or more/hr for packed cells	0.5 or more arb. unit
Copper	Total: 100-200 µg/100 ml	16-31 µmol/L
Creatine phosphokinase (CPK)	Female 5-35 mU/ml	0.08-0.58 µmol · s⁻¹/L
	Male 5-55 mU/ml	
Creatinine	0.6—1.5 mg/100 ml	60-130 µmol/L
Ethanol	0.3%-0.4%, marked intoxication; 0.4%-0.5%, alcoholic stupor; 0.5% or over, alcoholic coma	65-87 mmol/L
		87-109 mmol/L
		>109 mmol/L
Glucose	Fasting: 70-110 mg/100 ml	3.9-5.6 mmol/L
Iron	50-150 µg/100 ml (higher in males)	9.0-26.9 µmol/L
Iron-binding capacity	250-410 µg/100 ml	44.8-73.4 µmol/L
Lactic acid	0.6-1.8 mEq/l	0.6-1.8 mmol/L
Lactic dehydrogenase	60-120 U/ml	1.00-2.00 µmol · ⁻¹/L
Lead	50 µg/100 ml or less	Up to 2.4 µmol/L
Lipase	2 U/ml or less	Up to 2 arb. unit

Modified from Kaye DA and Rose LF: Fundamentals of internal medicine. St Louis, 1983, Mosby Year Book. Adapted from New Engl J Med 302:37, 1980.

Abbreviations used: *SI*, Système international d'Unités (The SI for the Health Professions. World Health Organization, Office of Publications, Geneva, Switzerland, 1977); *d*, 24 hours; *P*, plasma; *S*, serum; *B*, blood; *U*, urine; *L*, liter; *hr*, hour; and *sec*, second.

Blood, plasma, or serum values—cont'd

Determination	Reference Range	
	Conventional	SI
Lipids		
Cholesterol	120-220 mg/100 ml	3.10-5.69 mmol/L
Cholesterol esters	60-75% of cholesterol	
Phospholipids	9-16 mg/100 ml as lipid phosphorus	2.9-5.2 mmol/L
Total fatty acids	190-420 mg/100 ml	1.9-4.2 g/L
Total lipids	450-1000 mg/100 ml	4.5-10.0 g/L
Triglycerides	40-150 mg/100 ml	0.4-1.5 g/l
Lithium	Toxic level 2 mEq/L	2 mmol/L
Magnesium	1.5-2.0 mEq/L	0.8-1.3 mmol/L
5'Nucleotidase	0.3-3.2 Bodansky U	30-290 nmol · s^{-1}/L
Osmolality	285-295 mOsm/kg water	285-295 mmol/kg
Oxygen saturation (arterial)	96%-100%	0.96-1.00 L
P$_{CO_2}$	35-43 mm Hg	4.7-6.0 kPa
pH	7.35-7.45	Same
P$_{O_2}$	75-100 mm Hg (dependent on age) while breathing room air; above 500 mm Hg while on 100% O_2	
	10.0-13.3 kPa	
Phenylalanine	0-2 mg/100 ml	0-120 μmol/L

Phenytoin (Dilantin)	Therapeutic level: 5-20 µg/ml	19.8-79.5 µmol/L
Phosphorus (inorganic)	3.0-4.5 mg/100 ml (infants in 1st yr up to 6.0 mg/100 ml)	1.0-1.5 mmol/L
Potassium	3.5-5.0 mEq/L	3.5-5.0 mmol/L
Primidone (Mysoline)	Therapeutic level: 4-12 µg/ml	18-55 µmol/L
Protein: Total	6.0-8.4 g/100 ml	60-84 g/L
Albumin	3.5-5.0 g/100 ml	35-50 g/L
Globulin	2.3-3.5 g/100 ml	23-35 g/L
Electrophoresis	% of total protein	Of total protein
Albumin	52-68	0.52-0.68
Globulin:		
Alpha$_1$	4.2-7.2	0.042-0.072
Alpha$_2$	6.8-12	0.068-0.12
Beta	9.3-15	0.093-0.15
Gamma	13-23	0.13-0.23
Pyruvic acid	0-0.11 mEq/L	0-0.11 mmol/L
Quinidine	Therapeutic: 1.5-3 µg/ml	4.6-9.2 µmol/L
	Toxic: 5-6 µg/ml	15.4-18.5 µmol/L
Salicylate:	0	
Therapeutic	20-25 mg/100 ml; 25-30 mg/100 ml to age 10 yr 3 hr postdose	1.4-1.8 mmol/L
		1.8-2.2 mmol/L
Toxic	Over 30 mg/100 ml	>2.2 mmol/L
	Over 20 mg/100 ml after age 60	>1.4 mmol/L

Continued.

Blood, plasma, or serum values—cont'd

Determination	Reference Range	
	Conventional	SI
Sodium	135-145 mEq/l	135-145 mmol/L
Sulfate	0.5-1.5 mg/100 ml	0.05-1.2 mmol/L
Sulfonamide	0 mg/100 ml; therapeutic: 5-15 mg/100 ml	0 mmol/L
Transaminase (SGOT) (aspartate amino-transferase)	10-40 U/ml	0.08-0.32 μmol · s⁻¹/L
Urea nitrogen (BUN)	8-25 mg/100 ml	2.9-8.9 mmol/L
Uric acid	3.0-7.0 mg/100 ml	0.18-0.42 mmol/L
Vitamin A	0.15-0.6 μg/ml	0.5-2.1 μmol/L
Vitamin A tolerance test	Rise to twice fasting level in 3 to 5 hr	

Urine values

Determination	Reference Range	
	Conventional	SI
Acetone plus acetoacetate (quantitative)	0	0 mg/L
Alpha amino nitrogen	64-199 mg/d; not over 1.5% of total nitrogen	4.6-14.2 mmol/d
Amylase	24-76 U/ml	24-76 arb. unit

Calcium	150 mg/d or less	$3.8 \leq$ mmol/d
Catecholamines		
	Epinephrine: under 20 μg/d	<55 nmol/d
	Norepinephrine: under 100 μg/d	<590 nmol/d
Copper	0-100 μg/d	0-1.6 μmol/d
Coproporphyrin	50-250 μg/d	80-380 nmol/d
	Children under 80 lb 0-75 μg/d	0-115 nmol/d
Creatine	Under 100 mg/d or less than 6% of creatinine. In pregnancy: up to 12%. In children under 1yr: may equal creatinine. In older children: up to 30% of creatinine	<0.75 mmol/d
Cystine or cysteine	0	0
Follicle-stimulating hormone:		
Follicular phase	5-20 IU/d	Same
Midcycle	15-60 IU/d	
Luteal phase	5-15 IU/d	
Menopausal	50-100 IU/d	
Men	5-25 IU/d	
Hemoglobin and myoglobin	0	
5-Hydroxyindole acetic acid	2-9 mg/d (women lower than men)	10-45 μmol/d
Lead	0.08 μg/ml or 120 μg or less/d	$\leq$0.39 μmol/L
Phenolsulfonphthalein (PSP)	At least 25% excreted by 15 min; 40% by 30 min; 60% by 120 min	0.25 1
Phosphorus (inorganic)	Varies with intake; average 1 g/d	32 mmol/d

Continued.

Urine values—cont'd

Determination	Reference Range	
	Conventional	SI
Porphobilinogen	0	0
Protein:		
Quantitative	<150 mg/d	<0.15 g/d
Steroids		
17-Ketosteroids (per day)	*Male* *Female*	*Male* *Female*
	Age (mg) (mg)	(μmol/d) (μmol/d)
	10 1-4 1-4	3-14 3-14
	20 6-21 4-16	21-73 14-56
	30 8-26 4-14	28-90 14-49
	50 5-18 3-9	17-62 10-31
	70 2-10 1-7	7-35 3-24
17-Hydroxysteroids	3-8 mg/d (women lower than men)	8-22 μmol/d as hydrocortisone
Sugar		
Quantitative glucose	0	0 mmol/L
Identification of reducing substances		
Fructose	0	0 mmol/L
Pentose	0	0 mmol/L

	Conventional	SI
Titratable acidity	24-40 mEq/d	20-40 mmol/d
Urobilinogen	Up to 1.0 Ehrlich U	To 1.0 arb. unit
Uroporphyrin	0	0 nmol/d
Vanillylmandelic acid (VMA)	Up to 9 mg/d	Up to 45 μmol/d

Special endocrine tests

	Reference Range	
Determination	Conventional	SI
Steroid Hormones		
Aldosterone		
	Excretion: 5-19 μg/d	14-53 nmol/d
Fasting, at rest, 210 mEq sodium diet	Supine: 48 ± 29 pg/ml	180 ± 64 pmol/L
	Upright: (2 hr) 65 ± 23 pg/ml	
Fasting, at rest, 110 mEq sodium diet	Supine: 107 ± 45 pg/ml	279 ± 125 pmol/L
	Upright: (2 hr) 239 ± 123 pg/ml	663 ± 341 pmol/L
Fasting at rest, 10 mEq sodium diet	Supine: 175 ± 75 pg/ml	485 ± 208 pmol/L
	Upright: (2 hr) 532 ± 228 pg/ml	1476 ± 632 pmol/L
Cortisol		
Fasting	8 AM: 5-25 μg/100 ml	0.14-0.69 μmol/L
At rest	8 PM: Below 10 μg/100 ml	0-0.28 μmol/L
20 U ACTH	4 hr ACTH test: 30-45 μg/100 ml	0.83-1.24 μmol/L

Continued.

Special endocrine tests—cont'd

Determination	Reference Range		
	Conventional		SI
Dexamethasone at midnight	Overnight suppression test: Below 5 μg/100 ml		<0.14 nmol/L
			55-193 nmol/d
11-Deoxycortisol	Excretion: 20-70 μg/d		
	Responsive: over 7.5 μg/100 ml (after metyrapone)		>0.22 μmol/L
Testosterone	Adult male: 300-1100 ng/100 ml		10.4-38.1 nmol/L
	Adolescent male: over 100 ng/100 ml		>3.5 nmol/L
			0.87-3.12 nmol/L
	Female: 25-90 ng/100 ml		106-832 pmol/L
Unbound testosterone	Adult male: 3.06-24.0 ng/100 ml		3.1-44.4 pmol/L
	Adult female: 0.09-1.28 ng/100 ml		
Polypeptide Hormones			
Adrenocorticotropin (ACTH)	15-70 pg/ml		3.3-15.4 pmol/L
Calcitonin	Undetectable in normals		0
	>100 pg/ml in medullary carcinoma		>29.3 pmol/L
Growth hormone			
Fasting, at rest	Below 5 ng/ml		<233 pmol/L

After exercise	Child: Over 10 ng/ml	>465 pmol/L
	Male: Below 5 ng/ml	<233 pmol/L
After glucose	Female: Up to 30 ng/ml	0-1395 pmol/L
	Male: Below 5 ng/ml	<233 pmol/L
	Female: Below 10 ng/ml	0-465 pmol/L
Insulin		
Fasting	6-26 μU/ml	43-187 pmol/L
During hypoglycemia	Below 20 μU/ml	<144 pmol/L
After glucose	Up to 150 μU/ml	0-1078 pmol/L
Leuteinizing hormone	Male: 6-18 mU/ml	6-18 u/L
Pre- or postovulatory	Female: 5-22 mU/ml	5-22 u/L
Midcycle peak	30-250 mU/ml	30-250 u/L
Parathyroid hormone	<10 μl equiv/ml	<10 mEq/L
Prolactin	2-15 ng/ml	0.08-6.0 nmol/L
Renin activity		
Normal diet	Supine: 1.1 ± 0.8 ng/ml/hr	0.9 ± 0.6 (nmol/L)hr
	Upright: 1.9 ± 1.7 ng/ml/hr	1.5 ± 1.3 (nmol/L)hr
Low-sodium diet	Supine: 2.7 ± 1.8 ng/ml/hr	2.1 ± 1.4 (nmol/L)hr
	Upright: 6.6 ± 2.5 ng/ml/hr	5.1 ± 1.9 (nmol/L)hr

Continued.

Special endocrine tests—cont'd

Determination	Reference Range	
	Conventional	SI
Low-sodium diet	Diuretics: 10.0 ± 3.7 ng/ml/hr	7.7 ± 2.9 (nmol/L)hr
Thyroid Hormones		
Thyroid-stimulating hormone (TSH)	0.5-3.5 µU/ml	0.5-3.5 mU/L
Thyroxine-binding globulin capacity	15-25 µg T_4/100 ml	193-322 nmol/L
Total triiodothyronine by radioimmunoassay (T_3)	70-190 ng/100 ml	1.08-2.92 nmol/L
Total thyroxine by RIA (T_4)	4-12 µg/100 ml	52-154 nmol/L
T_3 resin uptake	25%-35%	0.25-0.35
Free thyroxine index (FT_4I)	1-4 ng/100 ml	12.8-51.2 pmol/L

Hematologic values

Determination	Reference Range	
	Conventional	SI
Coagulation factors		
Factor I (fibrinogen)	0.15-0.35 g/100 ml	4.0-10.0 µmol/L
Factor II (prothrombin)	60%-140%	0.60-1.40
Factor V (accelerator globulin)	60%-140%	0.60-1.40
Factor VII-X (proconvertin-Stuart)	70%-130%	0.70-1.30
Factor X (Stuart factor)	70%-130%	0.70-1.30
Factor VIII (antihemophilic globulin)	50%-200%	0.50-2.0
Factor IX (plasma thromboplastic cofactor)	60%-140%	0.60-1.40
Factor XI (plasma thromboplastic-antecedent)	60%-140%	0.60-1.40
Factor XII (Hageman factor)	60%-140%	0.60-1.40
Coagulation screening tests		
Bleeding time (Simplate)	3-9 min	180-540 sec
Prothrombin time	Less than 2-sec deviation from control	Less than 2-sec deviation from control
Partial thromboplastin time (activated)	25-37 sec	25-37 sec
Whole-blood clot lysis	No clot lysis in 24 hr	0/d

Continued.

Hematologic values—cont'd

Determination	Reference Range	
	Conventional	SI
Fibrinolytic studies		
Euglobulin lysis	No lysis in 2 hr	0 (in 2 hr)
Fibrinogen split products	Negative reaction at greater than 1:4 dilution	0 (at > 1:4 dilution)
Thrombin time	Control ± 5 sec	Control ± 5 sec
Complete blood count		
Hematocrit	Male: 45%-52%	Male: 0.42-0.52
	Female: 37%-48%	Female: 0.37-0.48
Hemoglobin	Male: 13-18 g/100 ml	Male: 8.1-11.2 mmol/L
	Female: 12-16 g/100 ml	Female: 7.4-9.9 mmol/L
Leukocyte count	4300-10,800/mm^3	4.3-10.8×10^9/L
Erythrocyte count	4.2-$5.9 \ 10^6$/mm^3	4.2-5.9×10^{12}/L
Mean corpuscular volume (MCV)	80-94 μm^3	80-94 fl
Mean corpuscular hemoglobin (MCH)	27-32 pg	1.7-2.0 fmol
Mean corpuscular hemoglobin concentration (MCHC)	32%-36%	19-22.8 mmol/L
Erythrocyte sedimentation rate (Westergren method)	Male: 1-13 mm/hr	Male: 1-13 mm/hr
	Female: 1-20 mm/hr	Female: 1-20 mm/hr

Erythrocyte enzymes		
Glucose-6-phosphate dehydrogenase	5-15 U/gHb	5-15 U/g
Pyruvate kinase	13-17 U/gHb	13-17 U/g
Ferritin (serum)		
Iron deficiency	0-20 ng/ml	0-20 μg/L
Iron excess	Greater than 400 ng/L	>400 μg/L
Folic acid		
Normal	Greater than 1.9 ng/ml	>4.3 mmol/L
Borderline	1.0-1.9 ng/ml	2.3-4.3 mmol/L
Haptoglobin	100-300 mg/100 ml	1.0-3.0 g/L
Hemoglobin studies		
Electrophoresis for A_2 hemoglobin	1.5%-3.5%	0.015-0.035
Hemoglobin F (fetal hemoglobin)	Less than 2%	<0.02
Hemoglobin, met- and sulf-	0	0
Serum hemoglobin	2-3 mg/100 ml	1.2-1.9 μmol/L
Thermolabile hemoglobin	0	0
LE (lupus erythematosus) preparation		
Heparin as anticoagulant	0	0
Defibrinated blood	0	0
Leukocyte alkaline phosphatase		
Quantitative method	15-40 mg of phosphorus liberated/hr 10^{10} cells	15-40 mg/hr
Qualitative method	Males: 33-188 U	33-188 U
	Females (off contraceptive pill): 30-160 U	30-160 U

Continued.

Hematologic values—cont'd

Determination	Reference Range	
	Conventional	SI
Muramidase	Serum, 3-7 µg/ml	3-7 mg/L
	Urine, 0-2 µg/ml	0-2 mg/L
Osmotic fragility of erythrocytes	Increased if hemolysis occurs in over 0.5% NaCl; decreased if hemolysis is incomplete in 0.3% of NaCl	
Peroxide hemolysis	Less than 10%	<0.10
Platelet count	150,000-350,000/mm^3	150-350 × 10^9/L
Clot retraction	50%-100%/2 hr	0.50-1.00/2 hr
Platelet aggregation	Full response to ADP, epinephrine, and collagen	1.0
Platelet factor 3	33-57 sec	33-57 sec
Reticulocyte count	0.5%-1.5% red cells	0.005-0.015
Vitamin B$_{12}$	90-280 pg/ml (borderline: 70-90)	66-207 pmol/L (borderline: 52-66)

Cerebrospinal fluid values

Determination	Reference Range	
	Conventional	SI
Bilirubin	0	0 μmol/L
Chloride	120-130 mEq/L (20 mEq/L higher than serum)	
Albumin	Mean: 29.5 mg/100 ml ± 2 SD: 11-48 mg/100 ml	0.295 g/L ± 2 SD: 0.11-0.48
IgG	Mean: 4.3 mg/100 ml ± 2 SD: 0-8.6 mg/100 ml	0.043 g/L ± 2 SD: 0-0.086
Glucose	50-75 mg/100 ml (30-50% less than blood)	2.8-4.2 mmol/L
Pressure (initial)	70-180 mm of water	70-80 arb. units
Protein		
Lumbar	15-45 mg/100 ml	0.15-0.45 g/L
Cisternal	15-25 mg/100 ml	0.15-0.25 g/L
Ventricular	5-15 mg/100 ml	0.05-0.15 g/L

Miscellaneous values

Determination	Reference Range	
	Conventional	SI
Autoantibodies in serum		
Thyroid colloid and microsomal antigens	Absent	
Stomach parietal cells	Absent	
Smooth muscle	Absent	
Kidney mitochondria	Absent	
Rabbit renal collecting ducts	Absent	
Cytoplasm of ova, theca cells, testicular interstitial cells	Absent	
Skeletal muscle	Absent	
Adrenal gland	Absent	
Carcinoembryonic antigen (CEA) in blood	0-2.5 ng/ml, 97% healthy nonsmokers	0-2.5 µg/L, 97% healthy non-smokers
Cryoprecipitable proteins in blood	0l	0 arb. unit
Digitoxin in serum	17 ± 6 ng/ml	22 ± 7.8 nmol/L
Digoxin in serum		
0.25 mg/d	1.2 ± 0.4 ng/ml	1.54 ± 0.5 nmol/L
0.5 mg/d	1.5 ± 0.4 ng/ml	1.92 ± 0.5 nmol/L

Duodenal drainage:

pH	5.5-7.5
Amylase	Over 1200 U/total sample
Trypsin	Values from 35%-160% "normal"
Viscosity	3 min or less
Gastric analysis	
	Basal
	Females 2.0 ± 1.8 mEq/hr
	Male 3.0 ± 2.0 mEq/hr
	Maximal (after histalog or gastrin)
	Females 16 ± 5 mEq/hr
	Males 23 ± 5 mEq/hr

pH	5.5-7.5
	>1.2 arb. unit
	0.35-1.60
	180 sec or less
	0.6 ± 0.5
	0.8 ± 0.6 µmol/sec
	4.4 ± 1.4 µmol/sec
	6.4 ± 1.4 µmol/sec

Gastrin-1 in blood	0-200 pg/ml	0-95 pmol/L
Immunological tests		
Alpha-feto-globulin	Abnormal if present	
Alpha 1-antitrypsin	200-400 mg/100 ml	2.0-4.0 g/L
Antinuclear antibodies	Positive if detected with serum diluted 1:10	
Anti-DNA antibodies	Less than 15 units/ml	
Complement, total hemolytic	150-250 U/ml	
C3	Range 55-120 mg/100 ml	0.55-1.2 g/L
C4	Range 20-50 mg/100 ml	0.2-0.5 g/L

Continued.

Miscellaneous values—cont'd

Determination	Reference Range	
	Conventional	SI
Immunoglobulins in blood:		
IgG	1140 mg/100 ml	11.4 g/L
	Range 540-1663	5.5-16.6 g/L
IgA	214 mg/100 ml	2.14 g/L
	Range 66-344	0.66-3.44 g/L
IgM	168 mg/100 ml	1.68 g/L
	Range 39-290	0.39-2.9 g/L
Viscosity	1.4-1.8 expressed as relative viscosity of serum compared to water	
Iontophoresis	Children: 0-40 mEq sodium/L	0-40 mmol/L
	Adults: 0-60 mEq sodium/L	0-60 mmol/L
Propranolol (includes bioactive 4-OH metabolite) in serum 4 hr after last dose	100-300 ng/ml	386-1158 nmol/L
Stool fat	Less than 5 g in 24 hr or less than 4% of measured fat intake in 3-day period	<5 g/day
Stool nitrogen	Less than 2 g/day or 10% of urinary nitrogen	<2 g/day

Synovial fluid		
Glucose	Not less than 20 mg/100 ml lower than simultaneously drawn blood sugar	See blood glucose mmol/L
Mucin	Type 1 or 2 Grades as: Type 1-tight clump Type 2-soft clump Type 3-soft clump that breaks up Type 4-cloudy, no clump	1-2 arb. unit
D-Xylose absorption	5-8 g/5 hr in urine 40 mg/100 ml in blood 2 hr after ingestion of 25 g of D-Xylose	33-53 mmol 2.7 mmol/L

Alspach JG, ed: *Core curriculum for critical care nurses,* ed 4, Philadelphia, 1991, WB Saunders.

American Heart Association: *Recommendations for human blood pressure determination by sphygmomanometers,* Pub. No. 701005 Dallas, 1987, The Association.

American Hospital Association: *Introduction to discharge planning for hospitals,* Chicago, 1983, American Hospital Publishing, Inc.

Arbiet JM, Way LW: Surgical metabolism and treatment. In LW Way (ed), *Current surgical diagnosis and treatment,* pp. 141-163, Norwalk, 1988, Appleton & Lange.

Baker NC et al: The effect of type of thermometer and length of time inserted on oral temperature measurements of afebrile subjects, *Nurs Res* 33:109, 1984.

Banasik J, Broderson M: The effect of lateral position on CVP, *Heart Lung* 23:296, 1991.

Bennett JV: Incidence and nature of endemic and epidemic nosocomial infections. In Bennett JF, Brachman PS, eds: *Hospital infection,* Boston, 1979, Little, Brown & Co.

Benner, P: *From novice to expert,* Menlo Park, 1984, Addison-Wesley.

Birdsall C: How do you manage peritoneal dialysis? *Am J Nurs* 88:592, 1988.

Blainey CG: Site selection in taking body temperatures, *Am J Nurs* 74:1859, 1974.

Breckenridge DM, Cupit MC, Raimondo JM: Systematic nursing assessment tool for the CAPD client, *Nephrol Nurse* 24, Jan/Feb, 1982.

Carden RG: The ins and outs of contact lenses, *RN* 48:48, Feb 1985.

Carlson JH et al: *Nursing diagnosis: a case study approach,* Philadelphia, 1991, Saunders.

Carnevali DL et al: *Diagnostic reasoning in nursing,* Philadelphia, 1984, Lippincott.

Carpenito LJ: *Nursing diagnosis: application to clinical practice,* ed. 5, Philadelphia, 1993, Lippincott.

Carroll PF: The ins and outs of chest drainage systems, *Nursing 86* 16(12):26, 1986.

Centers for Disease Control: Guidelines for intravascular infections, *Infect Control Hosp Epidemiol* 3:61, 1982.

Centers for Disease Control: Recommendations for prevention of HIV transmission in health care settings, *MMWR* (suppl) 36:SS, Aug 21, 1987.

Centers for Disease Control: Update: acquired immunodeficiency syndrome (AIDS) world wide, *MMWR* 37:286, 1988.

Clark JB et al: *Pharmacological basis of nursing practice,* ed 3, St Louis, 1990, The CV Mosby Co.

Connor PA: When and how do you use a Heimlich flutter valve? *Am J Nurs* 87:288, 1987.

Contact lens removal, *JEN* 6:15, 1980.

Corrado OJ: Hearing aids, *Br Med J* 296:33, 1988.

Coulter K: Intravenous therapy for the elder patients: implications for the intravenous nurse, *J Intraven Nurse* 15 (suppl):S18, 1992.

Davis M: Getting to the root of the problem: hair grooming techniques for black patients, *Nursing 77* 7:60, 1977.

Davis NM, Cohen MR: Learning from mistakes: 20 tips for avoiding medication errors, *Nursing 82* 12:65, 1982.

Dettenmeier PA: *Pulmonary nursing care,* St Louis, 1992, Mosby.

Duncan C, Erickson R: Pressures associated with chest tube stripping, *Heart Lung* 11(2):166, 1982.

Duncan C, Erickson R, Weigel RM: Effect of chest tube management on drainage after cardiac surgery, *Heart Lung* 16(1):1, 1987.

Ebersole P, Hess P: *Toward healthy aging: human needs and nursing response,* ed 3, St Louis, 1990, Mosby.

Egan D, Bennett E, Davis L: *Rigid lens care and handling,* Bethesda Eye Institute and St Louis University School of Medicine, Department of Opthalmology, St Louis, 1988 (unpublished).

Egan D, Bennett E, Davis L: *Soft lens care and handling,* Bethesda Eye Institute and St Louis University School of Medicine, Department of Opthalmology, St Louis, 1988 (unpublished).

Eoff MJ, Joyce B: Temperature measurements in children, *Am J Nurs* 81:1010, 1981.

Erickson R: Oral temperature differences in relation to thermometer and technique, *Nurs Res* 29:157, 1980.

Erickson R: Chest tubes: they're really not that complicated, *Nursing 81* 11(5):34, 1981a.

Erickson R: Solving chest tube problems, *Nursing 81* 11(6):62, 1981b.

Erickson RS et al: Comparison of tympanic and oral temperatures in surgical patients, *Nurs Res* 40:90, 1991.

Farley J: About chest tubes, *Nursing 88* 18(6):16, 1988.

Felton CL: Hypoxemia and oral temperatures, *Am J Nurs* 78:57, 1978.

Fowler EM: Equipment and products in management and treatment of pressure ulcers, *Nurs Clin North Am* 22(7):449, 1987.

Fowler E, Goupil DL: Comparison of wet-to-dry dressing and copolymer starch in the management of debrided pressure sores, *J Enterostomal Ther* 11:22, 1984.

Francis B: Hot and cold therapy, *J Nurs Care* 15:18, 1982.

Gannon EP, Kadezabek E: Giving your patients meticulous mouth care, *Nursing 80* 10:14, 1980.

Garner JS: *Guidelines for prevention of surgical wound infections,* 1985,

Hospital Infections Program, Centers for Disease Control, Public Health Service, and US Department of Health and Human Services.

Garner JS, Favero MS: *Guidelines for handwashing and hospital environmental control,* 1985, Hospital Infections Program, Centers for Disease Control, Public Health Service, and US Department of Health and Human Services.

Garner JS, Simmons BP: CDC guidelines for isolation precautions in hospitals, *Infect Control* 4(4):249, 1983.

Gerberding JL: Current epidemiologic evidence and case reports of occupationally acquired HIV and other bloodborne diseases, *Infect Control Hosp Epidemiol* 11(10):557, 1990.

Gordon M: *Nursing diagnosis: process and application,* ed 2, New York, 1987, McGraw-Hill Book Co.

Graves RD, Markarian MF: Three minute time interval when using an oral mercury-in-glass thermometer with or without J temp sheaths, *Nurs Res* 29:232, 1980.

Hanawalt A, Troutman K: If your patient has a hearing aid, *Am J Nurs* 84:900, 1984.

Holder L: Hearing aids, handle with care, *Nursing 82* 12:64, 1982.

Hollerbach AD et al: Accuracy of radial pulse assessment by length of counting interval, *Heart Lung* 19:258, 1990.

Hudson MP: Safeguard your elderly patient's health through accurate physical assessment, *Nursing 83* 13:58, 1983.

Iveson-Iveson J: The art of communication, *Nurs Mirror* p. 47, Feb 2, 1984.

Jacobsen G et al: Handwashing: ring-wearing and number of microorganisms, *Nurs Res* 34:186, 1985.

Janson-Bjerklie S, Shnell S: Effect of peak flow information on patterns of self-care in adult asthma. *Heart Lung* 17(5):543, 1988.

Johanson BC et al: *Standards for critical care,* ed 3, St Louis, 1988, Mosby.

Joint Commission on Accreditation of Healthcare Organizations: *Manual of accreditation,* Chicago, 1993, The Commission.

Kim MJ et al: *Pocket guide to nursing diagnoses,* ed 5, St Louis, 1993, Mosby.

Kirn TF: Contact lens need tender, loving care, ophthalmologists warn, or infection may result, *JAMA* 258:18, 1987.

Kosiak M: Etiology of decubitus ulcers, *Arch Phys Med Rehab* 42:19, 1961.

Krauss PJ: Chest tube stripping: is it necessary? *Foc Crit Care* 12(6):41, 1985.

Lane T, Stroshal V, Waldorf P: Standards of care for the CAPD Patient, *Nephrol Nurse* Sept/Oct:34, 1982.

LaRocca JC, Otto SE: *Pocket guide to intravenous therapy,* St Louis, 1989, Mosby.

Larsen EL: Quantity of soap as a variable in handwashing, *Infect Control* 8:371, 1987.

LaVelle BE, Snyder M: Differential conduction of cold through barriers: Ace bandages, padded Ace bandages, and compression dressings in the management of acute soft tissue trauma, *J Adv Nurs* 10(1):55, 1985.

Levine DL et al: *Care of the renal patient,* Philadelphia, 1983, WB Saunders.

Levin P: Safeguarding your patients against periodontal disease, *RN* 36:38, 1973.

Longworth JCD: Psychophysiological effects of slow stroke back massage in normotensive females. *ANS* 4:44, July 1982.

Loughran SC, Edwards S, McClure S: Peripherally inserted central catheters guidewire versus nonguidewire use: a comparative study. *J Intraven Nurs* 15(3):152, 1992.

Luce JM, Tyler ML, Pierson DL: *Intensive respiratory care,* ed 2, Philadelphia, 1993, Saunders.

McGinley KJ et al: Composition and density of micro flora in the sublingual space of the hand, *J Clin Microbiol* 26:950, 1988.

Metheny NM, ed: *Fluid and electrolyte balance: nursing considerations,* ed 2, Philadelphia, 1992, Lippincott.

Metheny N: Measures to test placement of nasogastric and nasointestinal feeding tubes: a review, *Nurs Res* 37:324, Nov/Dec 1988.

Millam DA: How to get into hard-to-stick veins, *RN* 48:34, April 1985.

Nash TB: What's new about new discharge planning standards? *Discharge Planning Update* 8(5):1, 1988.

National Heart, Lung, and Blood Institute: *Guidelines for the diagnosis and management of asthma,* National Asthma Education Program, Expert Panel Report, Pub No 91-3042, Bethesda, Md, 1991, The Institute.

National Institutes of Health: *Guidelines for the diagnosis and management of asthma,* Bethesda, Maryland, 1991, Pub No 91-3042, US Department of Health and Human Services.

Nichols GA, Kucha DW: Taking adult temperatures: oral measurement, *Am J Nurs* 72:1090, 1972.

Occupational Safety and Health Act: Bloodborne pathogens, *Fed Reg* 56(235):64, Dec 6, 1991.

Oellrich RG et al: The percutaneous central venous catheter for small or ill infants, *Am J Matern Child Nurs* 16(2):92, 1991.

Owen BD, Garg A: Reducing risk for back pain in nursing personnel, *AAOHN J* 39(1):24, 1991.

Palau D, Jones S: Test your skill at trouble-shooting chest tubes, *RN* Oct:43, 1986.

Perras ST et al: Primary nursing is the key to success in an outpatient CAPD teaching program, *Nephrol Nurse* 98, July/Aug 1983.

Phipps WJ et al: *Medical surgical nursing: concepts and clinical practices,* ed 4, St. Louis, 1991, Mosby.

Pollack S: Wound healing: a review. II. Environmental factors affecting wound healing, *J Enterostom Ther* 9:14, 1982.

Prescott PA, Dennis KE, Jacox AK: Clinical decision-making of staff nurses, *Image* 19:56, 1987.

Pugliese G, Lampinen T: Prevention of human immunodeficiency virus infection: our responsibilities as health care professionals, *Am J Infect Control* 17:1, 1989.

Quinn A: Thora-Drain III: closed chest drainage made simpler and safer, *Nursing 86,* 16(9):46, 1986.

Roth D: Intravenous therapy. In Metheny NM, *Fluid and electrolyte balance: nursing considerations,* ed 3, Philadelphia, 1992, Lippincott.

Schnapp LM, Cohen NH. Pulse oximetry: uses and abuses, *Chest* 98(5):1244, 1990.

Shinozaki T, Deane R, Perkins FM: Infrared tympanic thermometers: evaluation of a new clinical thermometer, *Crit Care Med* 16(2):148, 1988.

Shoemaker WC et al: *Textbook of critical care medicine,* ed 2, Philadelphia, 1989, Saunders.

Simmons BP: CDC guidelines for prevention of surgical wound infections, *Am J Infect Control* 11:133, 1983.

Spyr J, Prech MA: Pulse oximetry: understanding the concept, knowing limits, *RN* 53:38, 1990.

Stamps JL: "Back" to basics, *Emerg Med Services* 18(2):38, 1989.

Strangio, L: Believe it or not . . . peritoneal dialysis made easy, *Nurs 88* 18:43, 1988.

Strong R et al: Enteral feedings utilizing a pH sensor enteral feeding tube, *Nutr Support Serv* 8(8):11, 1988.

Tanner S: IV bolus leaves no room for error, *RN* 44:54, 1981.

Thomas DO: Fever in children, *RN* 48:18, 1985.

Thomason SS: Pressure ulcers: considerations of intervention strategies, *Ostomy/Wound Management* 19:48, 1988.

Thompson DR: Recording patients' blood pressure: a review, *J Adv Nurs* 6:283, 1981.

Trelease CC: Developing standards for wound care, *Ostomy/Wound Management* 20:46, 1988.

Ulrich BT: *Nephrology nursing: concepts and strategies,* Norwalk, Connecticut, 1989, Appleton & Lange.

Whaley LF, Wong DL: *Nursing care of infants and children,* ed 5, St. Louis, 1993, Mosby.

Williams WW: CDC guidelines for infection control in hospital personnel, *Infect Control* 4(4):325, 1983.

Williamson ML: Reducing post-catheterization bladder dysfunction in re-
   conditioning, *Nurs Res* 31:28, 1982.
Wilson D: Make mouth care a must for your patients, *RN* 49:39, 1986.
Young ME: Malnutrition and wound healing, *Heart Lung* 17(1):60,
   1988.

Index

t indicates a table

565